Study Guide for

Pharmacology for Canadian Health Care Practice

Third Canadian Edition

Study Guide for

Pharmacology for Canadian Health Care Practice

Third Canadian Edition

Linda Lane Lilley, RN, PhD
Shelly Rainforth Collins, PharmD
Julie S. Snyder, MSN, RN, BC
Beth Swart, BScN, MES

Study Guide prepared by

Julie S. Snyder, MSN, RN, BC
Adjunct Faculty
Old Dominion University
Norfolk, Virginia

Franklin F. Gorospe IV, RN, BScN, MN
Daphne Cockwell School of Nursing
Ryerson University
Toronto, Ontario

Student Study Tips prepared by

Diane Savoca
Coordinator of Student Transition
St. Louis Community College at Florissant Valley
St. Louis, Missouri

ELSEVIER

ELSEVIER

NOTICE

Knowledge and best practice in this field are constantly changing. As new research and experience broaden our understanding, changes in research methods, professional practices, or medical treatment may become necessary.

Practitioners and researchers must always rely on their own experience and knowledge in evaluating and using any information, methods, compounds, or experiments described herein. In using such information or methods, they should be mindful of their own safety and the safety of others, including parties for whom they have a professional responsibility.

With respect to any drug or pharmaceutical products identified, readers are advised to check the most current information provided (i) on procedures featured or (ii) by the manufacturer of each product to be administered, to verify the recommended dose or formula, the method and duration of administration, and contraindications. It is the responsibility of practitioners, relying on their own experience and knowledge of their patients, to make diagnoses, to determine dosages and the best treatment for each individual patient, and to take all appropriate safety precautions.

To the fullest extent of the law, neither the publisher nor the authors, contributors, or editors assume any liability for any injury and/or damage to persons or property as a matter of product liability, negligence, or otherwise, or from any use of any methods, products, instructions, or ideas contained in the material herein.

The Publisher

Library and Archives Canada Cataloguing in Publication

Lilley, Linda Lane, author
    Study guide for pharmacology for Canadian health care practice / Linda Lane Lilley, RN, PhD, Shelly Rainforth Collins, PharmD, Julie S. Snyder, MSN, RN-BC, Beth Swart, BScN, MES; study guide prepared by Julie S. Snyder, MSN, RN-BC (Adjunct Faculty, Old Dominion University, Norfolk, Virginia), Franklin F. Gorospe IV, RN, BScN, MN (Daphne Cockwell School of Nursing, Ryerson University, Toronto, Ontario); student study tips by Diane Savoca (Coordinator of Student Transition, St. Louis Community College at Florissant Valley, St. Louis, Missouri). Third Canadian edition.

Supplement to: Pharmacology for Canadian health care practice.
ISBN 978-1-77172-001-4 (paperback)

    1. Pharmacology—Canada—Problems, exercises, etc. 2. Nursing—Canada—Problems, exercises, etc.
I. Snyder, Julie S., author II. Swart, Beth, 1948-, author III. Savoca, Diane, author IV. Collins, Shelly Rainforth, author V. Gorospe, Franklin F., author VI. Title.

RM301.L54 2016 Suppl.   615.1076   C2016-901053-8

Vice President, Publishing: Ann Millar
Content Strategist (Acquisitions): Roberta A. Spinosa-Millman
Content Development Specialist: Sandy Matos
Publishing Services Manager: Hemamalini Rajendrababu
Senior Project Manager: Kamatchi Madhavan
Copyeditor: Michael Peebles
Proofreader: Wendy Thomas
Cover: Brett J. Miller, BJM Graphic Design and Communications
Cover Image: © Dmitry Yatsenko – Fotolia.com; © bitter – Fotolia.com
Typesetting and Assembly: GRAPHIC WORLD (INDIA)

Elsevier Canada
420 Main Street East, Suite 636, Milton, ON Canada L9T 5G3
Phone: 416-644-7053

Printed in Canada
2 3 4 5 20 19 18
Ebook ISBN: 978-1-927406-69-4

Student Study Tips

Time Management

TIME MANAGEMENT is a phrase used in a variety of contexts. Consider separating the two words TIME and MANAGEMENT. When these concepts are analyzed separately, we perceive MANAGEMENT as an organization of a particular focus—in this case, TIME. Now ask yourself, "Why consider MANAGEMENT in relation to TIME?"

For purposes of learning, consider the concept of money. Specifically, consider MONEY MANAGEMENT. Time and money have much in common. They can be spent, saved, invested, given away, stolen, and wasted. The big difference between these two commodities is that you can earn more money, but your time is limited. Learn to manage your time now, and the quality of your life will increase because you will have more time to do what you enjoy.

You may not enjoy studying. What you want is to be a nurse, but studying is one choice that will get you what you want. Being a nurse will bring you the satisfaction that you need. I, for one, am very thankful that you have made this decision. The world needs dedicated skilled nurses. To meet this need, you must make the decision to manage your time effectively.

General Guidelines
Establish Goals and Create Action Plans

One key to time management is having clear goals and an action plan to accomplish these goals. This is more than saying, "I want to be a nurse" or "I want to ace my pharmacology midterm." It is a decision to spend time now to get clarity and direction so that you will have more time later to relax. The following guidelines can help you get what you want.

Guidelines for Setting Goals

There are some basic guidelines to follow when setting goals:

- **Be realistic.** The goal must be something that you can reasonably expect to accomplish. A goal of scoring 100% on each and every unit test is not realistic, but a goal of scoring 85% or better is.
- **Be specific.** Goals must set out exactly what needs to be done. Do not simply state, "I will study for the exam." Specify how many hours, what days, and what times you will study. The more specific the goal statement, the easier it is to establish a plan, complete that plan, and thus achieve the goal set.
- **Establish a time limit.** Specify a time limit for completing each step in the plan and an overall deadline for accomplishing the goal.
- **Make the goal and actions measurable.** State the goal and each step in the plan for achieving it in a way that will enable you to measure your progress toward completion.
- **Commit to a list.** Write down your goals. Often we say we are going to do something in the moment, yet when the moment passes, we forget, watch other priorities set in, and say, "I'll get to it after." Make a list of your goals and prioritize them. Perceive this as a contract to yourself, a commitment you have to facilitate the accomplishment of your goals.

The following is an example of how this goal and action process works: You have a chapter test a week from today. The test will cover approximately 45 pages of text material, and there are 40 specific pharmacological terms you must know. In addition, you have been given about 20 pages of supplementary handouts in class. What will you do in the next 7 days to prepare for this test?

Goal statement:
I will study to do well on this exam.

This is a poor goal statement because it is not specific, sets no time limits, and offers no real way to measure progress. The intent is good, but the implementation of such a vague goal is usually poor and difficult.

Revision 1:
I will spend 2 hours a day studying for the next chapter test in order to get at least an 80% score.

This is a better goal statement. If one assumes that 2 hours per day is realistic, then the goal is more specific, the grade goal is measurable, and there is a time limit of sorts. This goal statement might be good enough, but it could still be improved.

Final version:
I will spend 2 hours per day, from 2:30 to 4:30 P.M., for the next 7 days studying for the chapter test in order to score at least 80%.

This is what is needed. This version states how much time, when, how many days, and for what purpose. Setting clear goals helps you get started and serves as a motivator to keep you working.

Guidelines for Action Statements

A goal, no matter how well stated, is not enough. There must be action statements to help you make day-to-day progress toward meeting the goal. The guidelines that apply to defining your goal also apply to establishing the action statements—they should be realistic, specific, measurable, and time limited. They spell out what is going to be done day to day. Here are three examples of good action statements for the sample goal:

- I will master six pharmacology terms each day.
- I will spend from 2:30 to 3:00 P.M. each day reviewing class handouts.
- I will review 10 pages of text material from 3:00 to 4:00 P.M. each day.

These examples should give you a good idea of how to go about developing a clear goal and a set of actions to carry out to achieve that goal.

Organize Tasks and Create Schedules

It takes time to make time. It is your choice. Either you set your schedule or others will do it for you. It is 2:30 P.M. The phone rings and friends want you to go out or your boss wants you to work overtime or your sister wants you to watch the kids. When you have an action plan and a schedule, your choices are clear. This is the time you scheduled to review class handouts. Can you reschedule this review, or do you want to keep this promise you have made to yourself to accomplish your goal? No matter what you decide, you have maintained control over your time.

Your goals and action plans are the foundation for your time management. The next key is to organize tasks and create schedules.

Guidelines for Organizing Tasks

1. Divide tasks into three categories:
   a. Jobs that **have to be done,** such as going to class, going to work, eating, and getting adequate rest. These jobs are the easiest to accomplish because the consequences of not doing them are serious. If you do not go to class, failure is almost a sure thing. If you do not go to work, soon there will be no paycheck. The consequences of not eating or sleeping are obvious.
   b. Jobs that **should be done,** such as studying, cleaning, and all of those other necessary but unpleasant tasks that are part of life. The "should-be-done" jobs are the most difficult to

accomplish because they are the jobs that are all too easy to put off doing. These are also the jobs for which time management skills are most essential.
   c. Things that you **want to do.** These include all of the fun things that provide pleasure and escape from the routines of class, study, and work. Most of us are successful at finding time to do what we want to do, even when there is a sizable backlog of "should-be-done" chores waiting. This choice can lead to procrastination and stress. The important things are maintaining balance and staying focused on your goals.
2. Prioritize items in your **"have-to-be-done" category** on the basis of your physical and mental health needs. Examine the consequences of not doing these activities. If you can live without doing an activity, then it is not a need.
3. Prioritize your **"should-be-done" category** on the basis your physical and mental health needs. Examine the consequences of not doing these activities. Can you accomplish your established goals without doing a given activity? If so, then it is not a need.
4. Prioritize your **"want-to-do" category**. Some recreational time is absolutely essential in any effective time management system. "Want-to-do" activities can often be used as incentives for completing what should be done.
5. Use incentives to accomplish what you should do. For each person the rewards will be different. Spend a little time determining what will work for you. It might be watching your favourite reality show, prime-time drama, or comedy show; going to the movie theatre to see a new release; reading a book for pleasure; or just spending some time with family or friends.

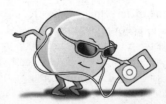

Guidelines for Creating Workable Schedules

You will need three types of schedules: **master, weekly,** and **daily.**

Start by developing a **master schedule** table on your computer that has 7 columns and 15 to 17 rows. The columns are the days in the week and the rows are the hours in the day. The left-hand column will represent Sunday and the far right will be Saturday. Start at the top of each column with the time you usually get up in the morning, and end each column with the time you usually go to bed. A typical master schedule might begin at 6 A.M. and end at 11 P.M.

Once the blank schedule sheet is prepared, the next step is to fill in those hours that correspond to the activities you have to do. These are the hours others control, and the activities are those that occur at the same hour, on the same day or days, and for several weeks or longer. For example, the semester's schedule of classes is the first set of activities to enter into the master schedule. Other activities such as work, travel, worship services, and any other regular activities also belong in the master schedule.

The master schedule should contain only those recurring activities that cannot be done at any other time. Activities such as doing the laundry, watching television, and shopping should not be included, because the time when you do them is more flexible. The idea behind compiling the master schedule is to establish those times of the day that are "spent" and therefore cannot be used for any other activities. The empty blocks that remain represent the time you have to do everything else. Figure 1-1 shows a sample master schedule.

Creating a master schedule takes no more than a half-hour, and it will generally serve you for an entire semester. The only reason to compile a new master schedule is that a significant schedule change has occurred. You may get a new work assignment or your nursing practicum site may change and require an additional 15 or 20 minutes of travel time. Then a new master schedule should be drawn up to accommodate the increase in time that is now necessary. Once the master schedule is completed, make four or five copies of it

These copies will be used to prepare the detailed weekly schedule.

Next, move on to developing your **weekly schedule.** The master schedule helps you identify the time you have available to complete the **"should-be-done"** and **"want-to-do"** task lists. The weekly schedule is more complex. It is intended to help you plan for study, recreation, family time, and all those other activities that you want to fit into a typical week. To prepare the detailed weekly schedule, take one of the copies you made of the master schedule and begin to fill in activities in the open blocks of time. The first blocks of time you should assign are the most important ones for any student: study time. This is what time management is all about—scheduling the needed hours of study (Figure 1-2 on the next page).

When filling in study hours, consider these important factors:

- **Amount of planned study time.** There is an old rule pertaining to study time, and even though it is an old rule, it is still a good guideline. The rule is to plan 2 hours of study time for each 1 hour spent in class. For example, a three-credit-hour course meets 3 hours per week, so you need to plan 6 hours of study time per week for this course. Remember, this is a general rule. Some courses will not actually require as much time as you allot whereas others will require more. The reason for beginning a semester with this approach is simple. It is easy to find things to do with time you do not need for study, but once a semester is under way it can be very difficult to

	SUN	MON	TUES	WED	THUR	FRI	SAT
7:00		GET UP		GET UP		GET UP	
8:00		TRAVEL		TRAVEL		TRAVEL	
9:00	GET UP	CLASS		CLASS		CLASS	
10:00	CHURCH	CLASS	TRAVEL	CLASS	TRAVEL	CLASS	
11:00	CHURCH		PRACTICUM		PRACTICUM		
12:00		CLASS	PRACTICUM	CLASS	PRACTICUM		
1:00			PRACTICUM		PRACTICUM		
2:00		PERSONAL	PRACTICUM		PRACTICUM		
3:00		PERSONAL					
4:00		AEROBICS		AEROBICS		AEROBICS	
5:00							
6:00		DINNER	DINNER	DINNER	DINNER	DINNER	
7:00							FUN
8:00							FUN
9:00							FUN
10:00							FUN
11:00	BEDTIME	BEDTIME	BEDTIME	BEDTIME	BEDTIME	BEDTIME	FUN

FIGURE 1-1 The master schedule. This is an essential first step in managing time effectively.

find additional study time. If you do not plan enough study time at the beginning, you will soon find yourself in a constant battle to keep up. The result is frustration, anxiety, and a sense of impending doom—feelings you do not need when you want to perform at your best.

- **Personal prime time.** Do you wake up early, ready to charge forward, but find it difficult to be productive after 10 P.M.? Do you do your best work in the afternoon and early evening and prefer to sleep until 10 A.M.? Are you a night owl? Answers to these questions will reveal your prime time, those times of the day when your ability to concentrate is at its best and you can accomplish the most. These are the times you want to use for study. It is not always possible, because of class and work schedules, to schedule all study time in your prime hours, but it is essential that those hours be used for study as much as possible. It would be foolish to plan to study your toughest material between 9 p.m. and 11 p.m. when you know that is a time when just reading the daily paper is a challenge.

- **Study hours for specific courses and general study hours.** The reason for scheduling both general and specific study times is that the study demands of different courses vary from day to day and week to week. For instance, you will need some hours of study every week to master new material, terms, and concepts in pharmacology, but the study time demands will increase in the days just before exams, midterms, and project due dates. The hours set aside for specific courses are for accomplishing the day-to-day study demands; the unassigned study hours are for meeting the changing demands posed by these special circumstances. These unassigned study hours also let you meet unexpected demands. No matter how carefully you plan your time, something will happen to prevent you from using the time block you had set aside for learning.

Be patient and evaluate what works for you. It usually takes two or three attempts over a period of 3 weeks to arrive at a detailed schedule that works well for you. There is a tendency on the first attempt to try to schedule some important activity for every waking hour. Ultimately such a schedule will make you feel as though there is no time for fun. Determine what is not working for you and make appropriate adjustments. Each week your schedule will come closer to being realistic and effective. The need to evaluate and revise is the reason for making several copies of the master schedule. Or you may want to use an electronic calendar. It saves time in the revision process, and saving time is, after all, what time management is all about.

Your last scheduling activity is to create **daily schedules and lists.** No matter how carefully and thoughtfully you prepare the detailed weekly schedule, it cannot include all the tasks you will face. You will have small tasks, infrequent tasks, and unexpected tasks that will need to be added to your schedule. Each day as you think of things you want or need to do the next day, it is easy to either write them down (carry a small notebook

	SUN	MON	TUES	WED	THUR	FRI	SAT
7:00		GET UP		GET UP		GET UP	
8:00		TRAVEL		TRAVEL		TRAVEL	
9:00	GET UP	CLASS	*STUDY*	CLASS	*STUDY*	CLASS	
10:00	CHURCH	CLASS	TRAVEL	CLASS	TRAVEL	CLASS	*STUDY*
11:00	CHURCH	*LUNCH*	PRACTICUM	*LUNCH*	PRACTICUM	*LUNCH*	*STUDY*
12:00		CLASS	PRACTICUM	CLASS	PRACTICUM		*PERSONAL*
1:00		*STUDY*	PRACTICUM	*STUDY*	PRACTICUM	*STUDY*	*PERSONAL*
2:00	*FREE*	*STUDY*	PRACTICUM	*STUDY*	PRACTICUM	*STUDY*	*PERSONAL*
3:00			*TRAVEL*		*TRAVEL*		
4:00		AEROBICS		AEROBICS		AEROBICS	
5:00							
6:00		DINNER	DINNER	DINNER	DINNER	DINNER	
7:00	*STUDY*	*STUDY*	*STUDY*	*STUDY*	*STUDY*	*STUDY*	FUN
8:00	*STUDY*		*STUDY*		*STUDY*		FUN
9:00	*STUDY*	*REVIEW*	*REVIEW*	*REVIEW*	*REVIEW*		FUN
10:00							FUN
11:00	BEDTIME	BEDTIME	BEDTIME	BEDTIME	BEDTIME	BEDTIME	FUN

FIGURE 1-2 The detailed weekly master schedule. Fill in the study times first.

that will fit into a pocket or purse) or make use of scheduling technology and input tasks into a handheld electronic device such as an iPhone, Blackberry, Palm Pilot, or personal digital assistant (PDA). Many devices offer calendar, memo, or task reminder features and allow users to organize a daily schedule that can also be synchronized to a desktop or laptop. The schedule can be reviewed regularly and revised as priorities change.

Consider the following when setting priorities:

- **There are only 24 hours in each day.** Be realistic about what you are able to accomplish. Do not plan to review three chapters of text material on a day when you know there will not be enough time to cover more than half of one chapter.
- **Everything is not important.** Rank your tasks as A, B, or C, with A being the most important and C being the least important. Then go about completing your As. Procrastinating about your B and C lists is not a sin. For example, going to the dry cleaners is critical if the outfit you must wear tomorrow is there, but if you do not absolutely have to have that outfit tomorrow, then the trip to the cleaners is a low priority and can be postponed to another day. Then it will be on your A list.
- **Rewriting to-do lists can steal your time.** You may want to make one weekly list and mark the tasks as A, B, or C. Put only A tasks on your daily to-do list. If you have extra time you can look at your weekly list. Or you can keep your tasks on note cards and then each day stack them in priority order.
- **Planning your route can save you time.** Look at the small tasks listed, such as picking up milk and dog food, dropping off dry cleaning, and going to the bank. Not only plan to do those errands but also think about the order in which they should be done. Planning your route so that it completes a circle from home to the cleaners to the grocery store to home will be much more time efficient than going from home to the grocery store, back home, then to the cleaners, and finally back home again.
- **As you complete a job on the daily list, cross it off.** Crossing it off tells you that you are making progress and motivates you to move to the next item on the list. If not every item is crossed off, remember that tomorrow is another day. Celebrate what you did get done, and create a plan for tomorrow that will help you accomplish your goals.
- **Remember your goals and planned action steps.** When unexpected daily tasks push them onto the B list, be sure to revise your plan to get back onto your time line. Put planning on your A list.
- **Waiting time can be a gift.** Small blocks of time are often lost or wasted because it does not seem as though anything significant could be accomplished during them. If you learn to use these small blocks effectively, you can free up larger blocks for more time-consuming or fun tasks. If a class ends 10 minutes early or if you are waiting for your ride, use the time for study. Take advantage of such "found" time to review five vocabulary terms, rework a set of class notes, or preview the next five pages of assigned reading. Using the odd minutes in the day to your advantage can really help you achieve your goals as a student.

Your time is a valuable resource for you to manage or to waste. The choice is yours. Stop for a few minutes and think over the previous strategies on how to manage your time: establishing goals and creating action plans, organizing tasks, and creating schedules. Which of these strategies will you choose to apply?

Choose to Use Your Resources

This Study Guide is one of the resources that will help you be successful in this course. When you choose to apply these study tips, they will help you to be successful in all of your course work. Three other resources are your textbook, your instructor, and your classmates.

Your Textbook

The authors of your textbook have taken great care in organizing the information provided in a manner that will assist your learning. Each part starts with study skills tips that build on the tips that are presented in the Study Guide. At the beginning of each chapter, you will find specific objectives describing what you are expected to know and be able to do as a result of studying each chapter. Each chapter also contains learning activities and a glossary of terms. Take 10 minutes right now to perform a survey of your textbook so that you know what to expect over the term of this course. Look for chapter titles and Points to Remember. Later in this Study Guide you will find tips for mastering your textbook.

Your Professor or Instructor

Your professor or instructor wants to hear your questions because this demonstrates that you are interested in learning and are actively engaged with the material in your textbook and lectures. The instructor is an expert on the content and the type of tests that will be given in the class. Ask questions about what will be covered on a test and the type of questions you can expect. Office hours are designed to make your instructor available to you. Choose to get your money's worth and use them!

Your Colleagues

We all have different learning styles, strengths, and perspectives on the course material. Participating in a study group can be a valuable addition to your nursing school experience. These groups can be a fun way to learn. Teaching others helps us to learn and aids in organizing the course material. A study group is made up of students who are in the same class and who want to learn by discussing the course material. There are guidelines for organizing successful study groups.

1. Carefully **select members** for your group.
   - Choose students who have **abilities and motivation** similar to your own. Socializing and gossiping can eat up valuable study time. Noncommitted and underprepared classmates can be a drain.
   - Look for students who have a **common time to meet.**
   - Select colleagues who have **different learning styles** from yours. They might understand the reading material or lecture material better than you. They may be able to draw a diagram that will help your learning.
   - Find students who have good communication skills—people who know how to listen, ask good questions, and explain concepts.
2. Clarify the **group's purpose and expectations.**
   - Where and when will you meet?
   - How often will you meet? How long will the meetings be?
   - How much individual preparation between meetings is expected?
3. **Exchange names, phone numbers, addresses, and email addresses.** Have a plan in case of emergencies.
4. **Plan an agenda** for each meeting.
   - Put the date and goal for the session on the top.
   - List the activities that will help you accomplish the goal.
   - At the end of the study session, list the results of your efforts and set the date and time for your next session.
   - Make assignments for the next session.

There are also some useful strategies to follow:
1. Exchange lecture notes and discuss content for clarity and completeness.
2. Divide up difficult reading material and develop a lesson to teach the information to each other.
3. Quiz each other by turning objectives at the beginning of each chapter into questions.
4. Use the Critical Thinking and Application and Case Study sections in this Study Guide as a basis for discussions.

5. Create and take your own practice tests. Discuss the results.
6. Develop flash cards that review key vocabulary terms.

This list could go on and on. Work with your group to design the strategy that works for you. Each study group you work with will be different.

Often in career programs like those in nursing, medical, and law schools, the course study group will turn into a learning group. **Learning groups may meet over several semesters even when the members are not taking the same classes.** Learning groups help you to prepare for licensing examinations, laboratory work, clinics, or practicum experiences. They focus on understanding and application in the field.

Choose to Develop Your Vocabulary

Participating in study groups and learning groups is an asset when you are working to develop a new vocabulary. Every specialty or discipline has its own language that must be learned for full mastery to occur. When you learn vocabulary with a group, you can hear others using the terms, and they start to become real to you. Courses such as this one on pharmacology contain extremely complex material, and terminology is a major component of that complexity. As you learn to integrate this vocabulary into your discussions of the discipline, it will seem less like a foreign language. In technological, scientific, and medical areas, mastering the vocabulary can make the difference between being successful and struggling constantly to understand the ideas and concepts being presented. It is therefore helpful to adopt some strategies that can make the process of vocabulary development easier and more effective. Working with a study group is one strategy, but there are several more.

Use Dictionaries

You must have a good current reference dictionary. A desk reference dictionary is a hard-bound dictionary and not a condensed or paperback version. *Current* means the most recent edition of whatever dictionary you choose. A dictionary published 10 or 15 years ago may contain most of what you need, but unless there have been periodic revisions, as shown on the copyright page, it is almost certain to lack some information, and this may cause you problems. Alternately, electronic dictionary subscriptions or credible online medical resources and dictionaries such as MedlinePlus provide quick access to current and relevant information as well as definitions.

Reference the Text Glossary

As soon as you look at any of the chapters in this text, you will discover the glossary. A glossary is nothing more than a text-specific dictionary. It contains the terms and definitions the authors consider essential for a full understanding of the material. The glossary will not necessarily contain every term that is unfamiliar to you. (This is why you need a good dictionary.) You can begin the process of mastering vocabulary by paying particular attention to the glossary and key terms.

Create Flash Cards

Obtain a supply of note cards. Pick the size that best accommodates your handwriting style and size. If 5 × 7 inch cards do not fit into your notebook, pocketbook, or book bag and this discourages you from carrying them around with you, then use 3 × 5 inch cards. Remember, the flash cards these become are among the best things you can study on the run.

Hypercholesterolemia, a condition in which greater-than-normal amounts of cholesterol..

Use What You Know

When you encounter an unfamiliar word, do not automatically assume that you have no idea what it means. Use the knowledge you have already acquired in other nursing courses and throughout your life.

For instance, *psychotherapeutic* appears in the chapter title for Chapter 17. Your first reaction may be that you do not know what this term means. By using what you know, however, you may be able to make an educated guess as to the meaning of the word without consulting either the text glossary or a dictionary.

This is how you make that educated guess: Consider that the first part of the word is *psycho*. By this point in your career as a student, you know that *psycho* refers to the mind. This is a good start. Now consider the next part of the word. The meaning of *therapeutic* may or may not be evident to you, but it should remind you of a simpler word, *therapy*, which is the treatment used to cure or alleviate an illness or condition. Put *mind* and *treatment* together, and it would seem that *psychotherapeutic* must refer to the treatment of mental problems.

Note that this is an educated guess. It may not be a perfect definition, but it will give you a basis for acquiring a fuller understanding when the term is defined in the glossary or introduced and defined in the text of the chapter. The first sentence in Chapter 17 confirms that this educated guess is very close to the actual meaning: "The treatment of emotional and mental disorders is called *psychotherapeutics*." Using this approach to analyzing the meaning of a word not only confirms that you have a basic understanding of the word but also cultivates a mental link between what you know and the more specific definition provided in the text. Words and their meanings learned in this way are usually easier to grasp and easier to retain. Unfortunately, this technique will not work with some of the terms used in pharmacology, because they are so specialized and specific to the field. This calls for the use of other techniques.

Learn the Standard Abbreviations

Make sure as you read that you pay attention to the "shorthand" used. For example, in Chapter 13, the abbreviation *CNS* is used repeatedly. The first time it is presented, the authors identify it as standing for *central nervous system* by putting the abbreviation in parentheses after the term. Thereafter, the abbreviation is used in lieu of the long term. The same thing is done for *REM* in this chapter. It is essential that you learn these abbreviations and recall each, not as a set of meaningless letters but as a key term that must be mastered.

Establish Relationships

REM is an abbreviation for *rapid eye movements*, and this term refers to a particular stage of sleep. Chapter 13 deals with CNS depressants. Relating REM to the focus of this chapter will help you remember that CNS depressants are used to influence sleep. The idea is to establish a clear relationship between the terms used and the ideas presented. Words should not be learned in isolation from the material; otherwise, you may know a lot of words and their meanings but not be able to relate them to ideas and content. On tests, you are not likely to be asked just to repeat memorized definitions. Instead, you will be asked to integrate these meanings into your answers to questions about nursing practices and applications.

Another important way of relating words to meanings is to link the meanings of closely related terms. The words *hypnotic* and *sedative* are good examples of this. In looking at the meanings in the glossary, you will find that each refers to a certain class of drugs. Both classes of drugs influence the CNS, but the drugs in each class have a somewhat different effect. It is useful to start with the understanding that both affect the CNS but then to appreciate how the terms relate to each other. Sedatives inhibit the CNS but do not cause sleep; hypnotics at low dosages have the same effect, but at higher dosages they may induce sleep. In this learning method, you learn meanings by looking at the general similarities and then at the specific differences between terms. In doing this, you have learned both words and should never have any problems relating the words to their meanings.

Choose to Take Effective Lecture Notes
Why Take Notes?

The primary reason for taking notes is to help your memory. It is impossible to remember everything that is said during a 1- to 2-hour lecture. The act of writing something down helps strengthen learning and memory. In addition, note taking helps to focus attention on the lecture. It is easy to take mental vacations during a lecture; note taking helps keep you involved.

Note-Taking Problems

1. **Selectivity** is the biggest challenge. How do you know what is really important?
2. **Unfamiliar vocabulary** causes confusion. This is particularly true in a course heavy in technical, medical, and pharmaceutical terminology such as this one.
3. Hard-to-read or even **illegible handwriting** is frustrating.
4. It is **difficult to listen and write at the same time**. It splits one's focus and often gets in the way of understanding.

Note-Taking Solutions

1. Realize that note takers are made, not born. You can learn to be more effective as both a note taker and note user, but **this requires some practice** and a willingness to adopt new techniques.
2. **Use the vocabulary development** strategies previously discussed so that you will have a better understanding of the lecture material.
3. **Note taking is a five-stage process** that is spread out over the days and weeks between lectures and the time when you are reviewing your notes in preparation for a test.

Stage 1: Be Prepared

Note taking begins before the lecture. Read assigned material before class. This provides you with the background needed to listen intelligently to the lecture and to be selective when taking notes. You will have less unfamiliar vocabulary. The lecture will bring the textbook content to life for you.

Go to class a few minutes early and review your notes from the previous lecture. This will help warm up your brain so it will be ready to receive new information.

Stage 2: Active Listening

Taking quality class notes requires active listening. This is one of the most challenging aspects of being a good note taker. It requires an awareness of both the lecturer's language and nonverbal style. You have to pay attention not only to what is said—the verbal aspect—but also to the visual, nonverbal aspect of the presentation.

Active listening requires selectivity. If you spend the lecture time trying to write down every word, you will not be able to listen to and thereby grasp the ideas. Focus on the most important ideas, terms, and facts to be recorded for later review. Writing less and listening more is a good rule to follow for note taking.

Learn to listen for key words and phrases. These vary with the subject content and with the individual lecturer, so there is no way to provide a single, definitive list of them. However, there are some verbal signals (words) that will give you clues that the lecturer is about to give important information:

- Sequence words—*first, second, next, then, last, finally*
- Contrast words—*but, however, on the other hand*
- Importance words—*significant, key, main, main point, most important*

The use of words and phrases such as these is the lecturer's way of signaling the relative importance and progression of certain facts and ideas. As important as these words are, however, it is also necessary to be aware of the volume, tone, and pace of delivery. Some instructors will slow down or repeat ideas that are important. Other instructors may speak louder and point into the air to emphasize a point. Get to know your instructor's style, and you will be able to anticipate what will be on the test. Of course, if the instructor says, "One of the most important drugs in the treatment of . . . ," then you should immediately know that what follows is an important point for your notes; the instructor has even told you it is important. As you practice active listening and observing in the lecture environment, you will find that your ability to discern the important ideas will improve.

Stages 1 and 2 are preparation for the real work that goes on in the last three stages.

Stage 3: In-Class Note Taking

The split-page note format requires a change in the way you set up your note paper. In this method, each sheet is divided into two parts by drawing a line down the full length of the page to create a left-hand column that is 6 to 8 cm in width and a right-hand column that is 14 to 15 cm in width. The right-hand column should be used for taking class notes. (The function of the left-hand column will be explained in the description of Stages 4 and 5.)

There is no magic formula for note taking. Simply take the best notes you can. Remember, notes are personal. Do not judge your notes against those of other classmates. Some will take a lot of notes, and others with a different background and expectations will take far fewer notes. The key point is to do what works for you. When what you are doing stops working, then try another strategy.

Here are some tips for taking effective lecture notes that may make the process easier and more effective for you:

- **Write in your own words** most of the time. Writing ideas in your own style will make them easier to learn and remember.
- **Leave space** between main points. When you sense that the lecturer has moved to a new idea, leave a couple of lines blank on your note paper. That way, if the lecturer returns to this point later, you will have room to add further notes. Even if there is no need for additional notes, the blank lines will help you see the organization of the ideas and the relationship between them. This space can also be used to add information that is from the textbook.
- Indicate **direct cues** from the lecturer, such as "This will be on the test," "This is a difficult concept," or even "Know this." Put a star or a check in your notes so you will remember to study this information when preparing for the test.
- Be especially aware of the **visual presentation**. This consists of information written on the chalkboard or presented using an overhead projector, slide projector, PowerPoint display, or other electronic display. Many lecturers outline key points on the chalkboard as a means of staying focused on the points they want to cover. Use this information to help you stay equally focused. Electronic displays are often chosen because the ideas can best be understood when they are presented visually.
- The **repetition** of certain points is the single most useful tip that they are really important. When an idea, term, or fact is important, the lecturer will almost certainly repeat it. For instance, the lecturer will introduce a new term, define it, give a couple of examples to clarify the definition, and finally redefine the term. This repetition is a signal that it is very important for you to learn the information.
- Be alert for **questions directed to the class**. These questions are another way the speaker stresses important information and are also a way for him or her to find out how well the students have understood

what has been said. Such questions are thus also cues that certain information is important.

- Be **actively involved** in what is going on in class. This means being willing to respond to a question directed to the class. It also means asking questions when things are not clear. Do not feel that because no one else is asking questions you are the only person who does not understand something. It is highly probable that there are others who are just as confused. Your objective in class is to understand the lecture and record key ideas in your notes so that you can study effectively. Questions are not dumb if they relate to the material being presented.

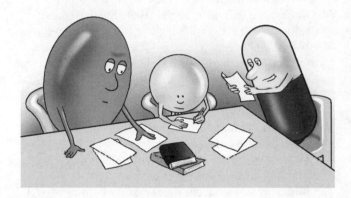

Stage 4: Out-of-Class Reworking

The notes you take in class are only one part of the effective study of lecture material. Out-of-class reworking of these notes is critical, and this is where the left-hand column of your note paper comes into use. Ideally, this reworking should be done immediately after the class ends, but this is not always possible. It must be done within 24 hours, however, to get full benefit from this strategy. Reworking class notes will not take more than 10 to 15 minutes to complete, but it will save you hours of study time later on.

The following is the recommended method for reworking your class notes:

- **Read over the class notes**. Look for major topics, key ideas, terms, and the organization pattern. At this point, you are not trying to remember everything you got from the lecture; you are looking for places where your notes are incomplete or confusing. If you read your notes soon after the lecture, you will be able to clarify points or add missing material, because most of what was said will still be fresh in your mind. If you wait until the next day (or worse, the next week), what is now only confusing will by then be a complete mystery. Taking the time to read your notes over soon after you take them will save much time and frustration later on.

■ **Write topic heads for lecture segments** in the empty left-hand column of your notes. As you read your notes, identify the major topics that were discussed. For example, look at Chapter 12 in the text. The chapter title tells you that it is about general and local anaesthetics, but the information does not stop there. Further topics are discussed and divided into subgroups. Headings are necessary to break down very complex material into understandable blocks. You should be doing the same thing with your notes. Limit your labels to three to five words. You are not trying to rewrite class notes but to make the organization of the ideas crystal clear. Sometimes the notes on the chalkboard or Power-Point slide will provide the labels for you. Sometimes the labels will be included in a lesson outline furnished by the instructor. Often, however, you will have to compose your own labels. With practice you will develop this skill. Keep at it. These labels are an essential aspect of the final stage of this note-taking method.

■ **List vocabulary.** The left-hand column is also a great place to put content-specific vocabulary. Look again at Chapter 12. Notice that there is a glossary of terms for that chapter. This is provided so that you can immediately begin to focus on the content-specific vocabulary you will have to master for that chapter. You can create your own personal glossary of the terms used in the lecture. As you read over your notes, each time you encounter terms from the text or new terms introduced in the lecture, note the word in the left-hand column. Doing this will help you learn the needed vocabulary.

■ **Expand.** Often during a lecture, you will only have time to write fragments of information. These may be meaningful at the time you write them but can be confusing later. Therefore, as you read your notes, fill in those places where there may be such gaps; otherwise, what was a small problem will become a big one later on. It will not take long, and it will pay off. You may use the left-hand column or the lines that you left blank for adding such information.

Remember: The reworking must be done the same day as the lecture for it to be efficient and productive. The longer the interval between the lecture and this reworking, the greater the likelihood of forgetting. When you read notes the same day as the lecture, you will be able to recall almost everything said. The reworking process will only take 10 minutes or so to complete, but it will pay off in a significantly improved set of class notes. Of equal importance is the fact that the reworking process is preparation for the final, critical stage in the note-taking process.

Stage 5: Frequent, Active Review

Notes, no matter how good, need to be **studied early and often.** Learning and memory depend on rehearsal or review, and this must be an active process. Rereading notes will improve your understanding and memory somewhat, but there is a technique you can use that will accomplish much more. This technique will help you to be an active learner and encourage frequent rehearsal. It is also efficient because it will only take you 10 to 15 minutes to completely review 2 or 3 days' worth of class notes.

When to Review. The first review of your notes should be performed within 2 days of the lecture. If the lecture has taken place on Monday, your review should occur on Tuesday or Wednesday. Do not wait more than 2 days. Studies have repeatedly shown that we forget nearly 50% of what we learn in the first 24 hours after we learn it. The reworking process will slow the forgetting process, but it will not stop it. The longer you wait to review your notes, the more time it will take and the more difficult it will be when you finally do it.

When to do a second, third, or any additional reviews depends on the success of the previous review. Review each day until you find that you remember and understand 80% or more of the material (you have to be the judge). When this is accomplished, the next review can wait for 3 or 4 days. If you find that after the first review you recall or understand only 70% of the material (an average amount), then the next review should occur within 2 or 3 days. If the amount you remember is less than 70%, you should review the material the next day. You must assess your own performance on each review to determine how soon to schedule another review. There are no hard and fast rules for this. A good review does not mean you have mastered the material forever, and what you remember clearly at one review may be the very thing you forget the next time around. **The only rule is to review frequently.** By doing this you will be well prepared for quizzes, tests, or any other measure of your learning.

How to Review. To review your notes, **cover the right-hand column** (class notes) with a blank sheet of paper. Look at the topics, vocabulary, and further notes that you added to the left-hand column during the reworking process; these will serve as your study guide for review. Look at the first topic heading you have written. It might be something like "Hypnotics." Turn that heading into one or more questions. What are hypnotics? When are they used? What are the adverse effects? Are there persons for whom hypnotics are inappropriate? Ask these questions aloud; do not just think them. **Framing questions orally is what makes this review active.** Now that you have asked a question, the next step is obvious: Answer it without looking at the covered notes. Say the answer aloud. This oral question-and-answer process forces you to state the information in your own words and style. In addition, you are relying on more faculties in your learning than just the visual one of rereading. You are speaking and listening, which is more active than just looking at the words. **Recall is strongly enhanced when you express the information in your own words.**

Another benefit of this review process is that it **helps identify what you do not know.** If you ask a question and find yourself struggling to respond, then it will be clear that this is something you have not yet mastered. When this happens, uncover the class notes pertaining to that topic and read what is needed. Sometimes only three or four words will be needed to trigger recall. When this happens, immediately cover the notes and resume your oral response. Sometimes you will have to read a large portion of the notes to trigger your memory. The reading is now focused on material that you have clearly identified as unknown. This means that your review time will be much more productive. Instead of reading everything known and unknown, you will now be concentrating on re-inforcing the known material and studying the unknown. **The best way to prepare for a test is to take a test.** By using the question-and-answer model, you are creating and taking your own test. You may discover that many of the questions you asked yourself also appear in some form on the classroom test covering that same material. If you have already answered the question several times for yourself, it will be easy to answer it on the test.

Two-Page Split-Note Variation. There is a variation of the split-page note paper format that some students find works better for them. If you find that the 15 cm–wide right-hand column is too narrow for taking class notes, simply take your class notes on the right-hand page in your notebook and use the left-hand page for the reworking process. This allows more room for the charts, diagrams, or complex formulas that are often part of the lecture material in courses such as pharmacology. This two-page method will also allow you to incorporate text notes. To do this, divide the left-hand page into two columns of equal width. Use the right-hand column for the reworking of class notes and the left-hand column for text notes on the same topic.

On-the-Run Action. Record the information you find to be most difficult to remember on 3 × 5 inch cards and carry them with you in your pocket or purse. When you are waiting in traffic or for an appointment, just pull out the cards and review again. This "found" time may add points lost in the past to your test scores.

Choose to Master Your Textbooks

Many students find themselves falling asleep while reading their textbooks. Text material can be long, complex,

sometimes confusing, and often highly technical. It can seem as though the more you read, the more there is to learn and the less you understand. Close the book and everything you have just read evaporates from your memory. If you feel like this, just remember that you are not alone. Every student feels this way. However, there are effective ways to maximize your learning and maybe even reduce the time it takes to do this.

Many different study systems have been devised to aid in the mastery of textbook material, and each has worked for some students. The model presented here is a combination of the best elements of this multitude of systems and is the best one for dealing with the subject matter in this pharmacology text.

Getting the most from a lecture requires active listening. The same active process applies to the reading of a textbook. Several techniques promote active reading. A good study system such as the PURR method presented in this textbook is one part of the process, but a good study system can be enhanced by reading with a pencil. Making text notations will help you concentrate and also make future review of the material more productive.

There are three notation systems:

- Highlighting and underlining
- Marginal notation
- Written text notes

Each of these notation systems has certain advantages and disadvantages. No single method will work perfectly all the time. Just as you must use different techniques to meet the different needs of your patients, you also need to use different techniques of text notation to meet the different needs you have as a learner. First, though, let's discuss two general guidelines that apply to the different systems of text notation.

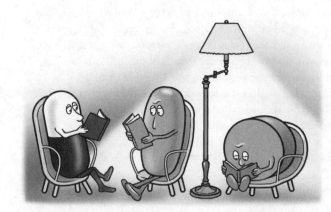

General Guidelines

1. **Read first.** Before you begin to make any text notations, you must first read the material. The objective of text notations is to identify the important ideas,

facts, and terms, just as this is the objective of listening during a lecture. If you attempt to mark text while reading it for the first time, everything will seem important, and you will find yourself making far too many notations or highlighting far too much material.

2. **Be selective.** The objective of text notation is much like that of taking notes during a lecture: to pick out the important ideas for immediate learning and for future review. If you have ever looked at a used textbook, you are sure to have seen that the previous owner has highlighted nearly every line on some pages. Excessive marking means the reader was not discerning the important ideas as he or she was reading. If you are taking separate handwritten notes, you should **limit what you write down** to the major headings and subheadings, important and unfamiliar vocabulary, and no more than two sentences of personal notes for each paragraph. The object is not to rewrite the chapter but to distill the important information. If you are highlighting, limit the material marked to no more than 20 to 25% of the total material. This is not to say that you must impose this limit on every paragraph, but it should be an overall goal.

Text Notation Systems
Text Conventions

As you read and prepare for making text notations, be aware of certain conventions used throughout the text. These help the reader focus on what the authors consider important. By now you have noticed the use of headings in this study tips chapter. Look back at some of them, and you will also notice that they are styled differently. Some are all capitals, others have only the first letter of each word capitalized. These represent main topics and subtopics. Now look at a chapter in your text. Examine the way headings and bold facing draw your eyes to certain words, phrases, and portions of the page. These are text conventions provided by the authors to help you understand the organization of the material and the relationships within the text content. Other text conventions that you should note are numbered lists, bulleted lists, special display material, and the like.

Language Conventions

Another important aspect of text notation is to become language sensitive. In a class lecture, when you hear a professor say, for instance, "One of the most important first-generation anaesthetics was . . . ," the words "most important" are a direct clue that this is a significant point for your notes. The same type of clues often occur in the text. The authors want to make certain that their important ideas are communicated to you, the reader. Because the authors cannot speak to you face to face, however, they must rely on a certain written style to get important points across. This means that you must become aware of that style so that you can identify these important ideas. For example, in a sentence saying, "Opioids can be classified into four main categories," the phrase "four main categories" is the author's way of telling you not only what is coming but also what you should be taking note of.

Pay attention if a paragraph begins with the phrase "The most significant effects. . . . " Whenever an author uses words or phrases such as these, it tells you that something important is being discussed. When you highlight text, phrases such as "most important," "four main categories," and "most significant" are the clues you should look for to help identify the most important information. The combination of text conventions and language conventions helps make the reading and marking of text more successful.

How to Highlight and Underline

Text marking is done to help in future review. This means that text marking is a personal process and should be used to point out only the most important information. The previous two sections on conventions gave you some concrete ideas on what to mark in your textbook. The main point is **read before you mark.**

It is essential that you read meaningful blocks of text before you do any marking. A meaningful block may be as little as a single paragraph but never less. It may be as much as an entire chapter. In a text such as *Pharmacology for Canadian Health Care Practice*, in which the material is highly technical and challenging, it is unlikely that you will want to read more than a section of the chapter at a time before going back to highlight.

Look at Chapter 13. The first paragraph mentions the boldfaced terms "**sedatives**" and "**hypnotics**." As you read this paragraph the first time, do not mark anything. Instead, **read for a general understanding of the content**. After this, go back to the beginning of the section, and note the following language conventions: two basic elements; different stages; summarized; is known as; and four distinct stages. These are all words and phrases that point out important information that should be highlighted. You may not actually need to highlight all the information flagged by these words and phrases. Some of it is probably already familiar to you because of earlier courses you have taken or earlier chapters you have read in this text. Avoid highlighting information you have already mastered.

Review
When

How soon after you have done some form of text notation should you review what you have highlighted?

Ideally, review should begin within 24 to 48 hours after the initial learning has occurred. Psychologists have studied learning, memory, and forgetting and have found that after the first day or two, we forget approximately 50% of what we learn. Therefore, the sooner you begin to review, the easier it is to move learning from short-term memory (quickly learned and quickly forgotten) to long-term memory.

How

The process for reviewing any text notations follows the same general principles that apply to lecture notes. The intent is to make your review an active process in which real learning takes place. For example, if you have written questions in the text's margins, try to answer these questions without rereading the text. If you are able to answer the question to your satisfaction, then move on to the next question. If you have highlighted terms and definitions, cover the definition and try to define the term without looking at the text. If you are able to do this, you have effectively moved material into long-term memory. If you cannot define the term, then read the text definition. As you read, think about the meaning and think about strategies you might use to help you remember the term and definition the next time. You will find additional memory strategies in the later section on studying for exams. The key is always to focus on being an active learner.

How Often

How often you review is a personal matter. The best way to judge is to be aware of your success, or lack of it, in the current review session. If you do very well at recalling information, then you can probably wait 3 to 4 days for the next review. If the review goes okay, then the next session should take place within 2 days. If you find yourself reviewing your own notations with little understanding and limited memory, the next review should take place the following day. Each time you review, it will get easier and faster, and as you practice this approach to reviewing your text notations, you will gradually acquire a good sense of how often you need to review to maintain mastery of the material.

Choose to be Successful in Exams

You can be successful in your exams by **applying the recommendations and strategies** offered in this section. Start by following the dozen basic rules of exam success.

Rules for Success on Exams

1. Accept your anxiety as normal. Tests are important, both in the short term, from the standpoint of grades and successful completion of this course, and also in the long term, from the standpoint of completing the program and getting your degree and eventually the job you want. This fact can cause stress.
2. Reduce your stress by **studying often, not long**. The most important rule in preparing for exams is simple—spend at least 15 minutes every day (Saturdays, Sundays, and holidays included) in reviewing the "old" material. The more time you can find for this each day, the better, but spend at least 15 minutes. This one action will do more to reduce test anxiety than anything else you do. The more time you devote to reviewing past material learned, the more confident you will feel about your knowledge of the topic. This confidence will accompany you into the classroom on the exam day, and it will help you get the test score that you want and are capable of. Just remember: **start the review process on the first day of the semester,** and do some review every single day until the final exam.
3. Balance your review time between your lecture notes, textbook notes or highlighting, and any handouts you may have been given.
4. Ask your instructor about the exam. If he or she says the test is mostly on the lecture, then you may want to spend more time reviewing your class notes. Ask about the type of questions that will be on the exam. Will the test consist entirely of multiple-choice questions? Will it have true-or-false items? Will there be matching, short-answer, or essay questions? You should not study any differently for a multiple-choice exam than you should for a short-answer or essay exam. However, knowing the type or types of questions that will be on the test will help you develop a strategy for quizzing yourself.
5. Work with your study group to create practice tests. For example, if you know the test will consist of multiple-choice questions, then as you do your review, think of the kinds of questions you would ask if you were composing the test. Consider what would be a good question, what would be the right answer, and what would be other answers that would appear right but would in fact be incorrect.
6. Take the practice tests in each chapter and on the Evolve website (http://evolve.elsevier.com/Canada/Lilley/pharmacology/). Practice writing out the answers of short-answer or essay questions. **The best way to prepare for a test is to take one.**
7. **Study wisely, not hard.** Use the study strategies offered in this guide so you can save time and be able to get a good night's sleep the night before your exam. Cramming is not smart, and it is hard work that increases stress while reducing learning. When you cram, your mind is more likely to go blank during a test. When you cram, the information is in your short-term memory so you will need to relearn

it before a comprehensive exam. Relearning takes more time. The stress caused by cramming may interfere with your sleep. Your brain needs sleep to function at its best.

8. Prepare for exams when and where you are most alert and able to concentrate. Use your personal prime time, which was discussed earlier in the time management section. If you are most alert at night, study at night. If you are most alert at 2 A.M., study in the early morning hours. Study where you can focus your attention and avoid distractions. This may be in the library or in a quiet corner of your home. The key point is to keep on doing what is working for you. If you are distracted or falling asleep, you may want to change when and where you are studying.

9. **Relax the last hour before an exam.** Your brain needs some recovery time to function effectively.

10. Survey the test before you start answering the questions. Plan how to complete the exam in the time allowed. Read the directions carefully, and answer the questions you know for sure first.

11. Before turning in the exam, make sure that you have answered all of the questions. If you are to fill in the boxes on an answer sheet that will be read electronically, be sure you have put only one answer per line and that you have answered each question. If you must make a correction, be sure to erase carefully and thoroughly.

12. Celebrate your success. Congratulate yourself for choosing to pass your exam by applying the exam preparation and exam-taking skills that have been proven to work.

Strategies for Reviewing Class Notes

Look at your class notes. If you have been using the split-page model described earlier, you have made your own topic headings in the left-hand column beside the class notes. Cover the class notes and turn each heading into one or more questions. Think carefully about the answers and then answer aloud. By answering questions aloud, you are forcing yourself to think about what you know and organizing that knowledge in the way that is most meaningful to you. If you can answer your questions, then you have demonstrated that you know the material, and there is no immediate need to reread that section of notes. If you cannot answer one of your questions, then you know you need to review that material more intensively. Uncover the notes and read the pertinent ones. You are now using your review time effectively, because instead of just rereading everything, which invites boredom—or worse yet, daydreaming— the rereading is directed at the material of which you are unsure. The result is more efficient use of your time and more effective learning.

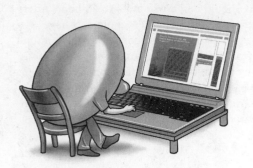

Strategies for Reviewing the Textbook

The technique you used for studying your class notes will also work for studying text material. As mentioned, in this book the authors have provided you with a variety of features that can help enormously. First, look at the objectives at the beginning of each chapter to be studied. Even if you have been assigned only small portions of the chapter, it is important to consider the objectives for the chapter as a whole. Ask yourself whether you have met these objectives. This is a quick way of assessing how much review may be necessary. If you feel confident that you have accomplished most of the objectives, then the review should go quickly. If you feel uncertain about many of them, then the review is going to take more time.

The next task is to consider the topic headings and language conventions. Use them in the same way as you have used the labels in your notes. Turn them into questions and answer these questions aloud. If you can answer them, then there is no need to reread. If you cannot, then you will need to reread the pertinent text.

Again, this way of reviewing is focusing your time and energy mostly where it is needed: on the material you have not yet mastered. Each time you review the text (or class notes), the sections of material you reread may differ. This is to be expected. You cannot remember everything forever, but if you spend time each day doing this type of review, you will remember more and for longer periods of time.

Strategies for Reviewing Terminology

One aspect of nursing that can seem overwhelming is the terminology. It is highly technical and specialized. Learning it poses the same kind of challenge as learning a foreign language. In fact, it almost is a foreign language. However, for the concepts and ideas to be mastered, the terms must be mastered. One of the best ways to go about doing this is to use a technique you probably learned in grade school: flash cards. Put each term on one side of a 3×5 inch note card and the definition or other essential information about the term on the back. Group together cards containing terms that have common word elements (e.g., terms beginning with "cardio") or that concern common concepts (e.g., terms to do with renal function). The more relationships you can establish between words, the easier it will be to learn and remember them.

On-the-Run Action

Get in the habit of carrying a deck of 10 to 15 of these cards with you. When you have a few minutes, review as many cards as time allows. Sometimes start with the term side of the card and try to recall what is written on the back. Other times look at the definition on the back of the card and try to recall the term. Do not focus exclusively on term-to-definition learning, because you may be given definitions or some variation on the exam and be asked to provide the terms.

Exam Time

This is it. The culmination of all your work—lectures, notes, flash cards, textbook readings, and handouts. **It is time to relax.** Test anxiety interferes with test performance. If you have put to use the learning techniques described in this chapter, you are ready for the exam. You have mastered the material, and you can do well on the exam. If you continue to experience test anxiety in spite of preparing thoroughly for the exam, it might be a good idea to visit a professional counselor on your campus.

Avoid cramming and remain confident in the learning techniques you have chosen to apply. This can usually control normal nervousness. Besides these learning techniques, however, techniques are also available for dealing with the various types of exam questions, and these are discussed in this section. None of these strategies can guarantee a 10-point jump in your test score. Only the degree to which you have mastered the material can make that sort of difference. However, each of the strategies described in this section may help you answer one or two questions correctly that you might otherwise have missed. **These test-taking strategies are not intended to replace regular study** and mastery; however, they are intended to enhance your test performance. If you use these strategies, you will see a positive gain in your test performance.

When the instructor passes out the exam, all your work and preparation are about to pay off, but do not just leap into the test. Take a couple of minutes to put yourself in a frame of mind for doing well on the test. At this point, you have a perfect test score; you have not answered any questions incorrectly yet. It is likely that you will get some answers wrong, but do not start out by making mistakes that cost you points that you should not have lost.

First, look over the entire test. Do not read it, but turn the pages and look at a question here and a question there. How many items are there on the test? Are all the questions of one type, or is there a mixture of types? Knowing in advance the length of the test and the types of questions helps you plan your strategy for taking the test.

Second, read the directions. This is the first opportunity you have to make a mistake that could cost points. Some directions for true-or-false questions may ask you to correct the statement and make it true. Others may ask you to justify your answer. When you respond with just a T or an F, you have lost important points because you did not read the directions.

Third, create a plan to complete the test in the time allowed. For example, if the test has 50 multiple-choice questions and the time limit is 40 minutes, then you know you will have to average a little better than one item per minute. Obviously you will need to allocate more time to essay questions if they are on the exam. Plan to glance at your watch or the classroom clock occasionally during the exam to make sure you are not losing time or going too quickly. Pace yourself. If you are answering questions quickly and are confident that the answers are right, do not worry about being ahead of schedule. If you spend too much time on individual questions, you may try to decide the answers to the last questions quickly, and this increases your chances of making errors. Planning a strategy for finishing the test within the time allowed helps you maintain a sharp focus on the task and enables you to do the best job possible.

Fourth, start answering the questions. If the test consists of only one type of question, then start with the first question. However, if the test has multiple-choice, true-or-false, and short essay questions, for example, you must decide where it is best for you to start. If you find essay questions easy to do, then perhaps you should start with these. There is no reason you have to begin with the multiple-choice questions. On the other hand, if you find essay questions a challenge, then do not start with them. Begin the test in a way that will give you confidence.

Tips for Answering the Questions

■ Start with the first question or with those types of questions you feel most confident answering. Wherever you choose to start, there is a strategy you can use that can improve your test performance.

■ Read the question carefully, and if you know the answer, indicate it and move on to the next question. If you cannot immediately think of the answer, give it a few seconds of thought. If the answer comes, indicate it and move on. If the answer still does not come or if the question is confusing, then skip to the next question.

■ In the first pass through the exam, answer what you know and skip what you do not know. Answering the questions you are sure of increases your confidence and saves time. This is buying you time to devote to the questions with which you have more difficulty.

- Notice that the subjects of the questions on a particular exam are related, that the answers to questions you have skipped may be provided by other questions on the test, or that a later question may trigger recall of the correct answer. Skipping questions you are unsure of offers one more opportunity to get the correct answer.

- After you have gone through the entire test completing the questions that you are confident you can correctly answer, go back to the items you skipped. First check the time, however, so you know how much time you have left to answer these questions. On this second pass through the exam, you will often be surprised at how many questions you now can answer that drew a complete blank before.

- Answer every question. A question without an answer is the same as a wrong answer. Go ahead and guess. You have studied for the test and you know the material well. You are not making a random guess based on no information. You are guessing based on what you have learned and your best assessment of the question.

- When you have answered all the questions on a page, put a check mark in the upper right corner of this page. Avoid going back and second-guessing yourself. There is nothing worse than changing right answers to wrong ones. Have confidence in your own knowledge and let go of the test. If you are the first person to complete a test and are sure of what you did, then turn it in. At the same time, do not let what others in the class are doing affect your test strategy. If you are the last person to turn the test in, it does not mean you know less than those who were faster. It simply means that you are a careful, thoughtful test taker.

Strategies for Specific Types of Questions

For each type of question there are particular strategies you can use that can help prevent incorrect responses. Many times students miss questions not because of a lack of information but because of a poor strategy. Sometimes the error stems from misreading a question—for instance, overlooking a key word such as "not" or choosing an answer that does not quite fit the question asked. Errors like these can be costly. Expect to find some questions on a test to which you do not remember the answer or that are worded in a confusing way. A perfect test score is a great goal, but be realistic and accept the fact that perfect scores may be few and far between. At the same time, do not lose points because of careless and preventable errors.

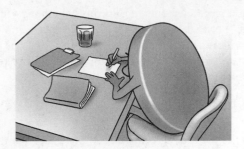

Strategy for Multiple-Choice Questions

Multiple-choice questions can be challenging because students think that they will recognize the right answer when they see it or that the right answer will somehow stand out from the other choices. This is a dangerous misconception. The more carefully the question is constructed, the more each of the choices will seem like the correct response. The successful student can do several things to improve performance on multiple-choice questions.

Before the strategies for analyzing multiple-choice questions are discussed, it is important to understand each part of a question and its purpose. There are three parts to a multiple-choice question: stem, distractors, and the correct choice.

First, there is the **question stem**. This is the complete question that one or more of the response choices will answer.

EXAMPLE:

If excessive amounts of water-soluble vitamins are ingested, what usually happens?

Notice that this could just as easily be a short-answer question. In this case, the stem is a complete sentence that should be answered by one of the response choices. The stem can also be an incomplete statement that one or more of the response choices completes correctly.

EXAMPLE:

The likelihood that a drug will have therapeutic effects increases dramatically when . . .

This statement is incomplete, and you must pick out the response choice that best completes it.

The second part of multiple-choice questions is the **distractors**. These are the response choices that do not best answer or complete the stem. They are known as distractors because their purpose is to distract you from the best choice. Good distractors are usually very similar to the best choice. If you have not studied enough, a good distractor will be a very tempting choice, but you must reduce the allure of distractors.

The third and final part of all multiple-choice questions is the **best choice**. This is the choice you want to pick. Notice that it is the "best" choice; in many multiple-choice questions there may be more than one response choice that appears to answer the stem, and the differences between the responses may be slight. Your task is therefore to identify the option that best answers the stem, not necessarily the only right choice.

Recall. The most reliable way to ensure that you select the correct response to a multiple-choice question is to recall it. Depend on your learning and memory to furnish the answer to the question. To do this, read the stem, and then *stop!* Do not look at the response options yet. Try to recall what you know and, based on this, what you would give as the answer. After you have taken a few seconds to do this, look at all of the choices and select the one that most nearly matches the answer you recalled. It is important that you consider all the choices and not just choose the first option that seems to fit the answer you recall. Remember the distractors. Choice B may look okay, but choice D may be worded in a way that makes D a slightly better choice. If you do not weigh all the choices, you are not maximizing your chances of correctly answering each question.

Once you have decided on an answer, there is one more important step before you mark it. Look at the stem again. Does your choice answer the question that was asked? If the question stem asks "why," be sure the response you have chosen is a reason. If the question stem is singular, then be sure the option is singular, and the same for plural stems and plural responses. Many times, checking to make sure that the choice makes sense in relation to the stem will reveal the correct answer.

This is the most reliable technique to use for answering multiple-choice questions. If you do this for every multiple-choice question on the test, your accuracy rate will be very high, and you will not need any further strategy. Unfortunately, however, recall does not always work, and when it does not, there are some additional strategies you can apply to improve your chances of picking the correct answer.

Recognition and Elimination. Read each of the answer options carefully. Usually at least one of them will be clearly wrong; eliminate this one from consideration. Now you have reduced the number of response choices by one and improved the odds. Continue to analyze the options. If you can eliminate one more choice in a four-option question, you have reduced the odds to 50/50, the same as the odds of correct random guessing for true-or-false questions. There are still some strategies that will help you pick the best choice. In addition, while you are eliminating the wrong choices, recall often occurs. One of the options may serve as a trigger that causes you to remember what a few seconds ago had seemed completely forgotten.

LOOK-ALIKE ANSWERS. After you have eliminated one or more choices, you may discover that two of the options are very similar. This can be very helpful, because it may mean that one of these look-alike answers is the best choice and the other is a very good distractor. Test both of these options against the stem. Ask yourself which one completes the incomplete statement grammatically and which one answers the question more fully and completely. The option that best completes or answers the stem is the one you should choose. Here, too, pause for a few seconds, give your brain time to reflect, and recall may occur.

ABSOLUTES. The presence of absolute words and phrases can also help you determine the correct answer to a multiple-choice item. If an answer choice contains an absolute (e.g., *none, never, must, cannot*), be very cautious. Remember that there are not many things in this world that are absolute, and in an area as complex as pharmacology, an absolute in an option may be reason to eliminate it from consideration as the best choice. This is only a guideline and should not be taken to be true 100% of the time; however, it can help you reduce the number of choices.

NEGATIVES AND EXCEPTIONS. In the stem "A drug reaction could include all but which of these symptoms?" the phrase all but tells you to choose the response that is an exception. All but one of the choice options is a symptom. In this case, the option that is not a symptom is the best choice. If you look at the options and see several that seem correct, look at the stem again; it may be that you have overlooked an exception phrase such as "all but" or "all but one." A similar stem wording that can throw you off is a negative or negative prefix. The stem "It is generally not a good idea to administer adult dosages to . . . " is asking you to select the answer that names the inappropriate, not appropriate, recipient of a medication. The word "not" helps identify the answer.

All these strategies can help you analyze the response choices so that you have the best possible chance of selecting the correct choice. When you are ready to mark the answer, keep in mind that the final step is always to test your response against the stem.

If after you have tried all of these strategies, you find yourself still unable to choose a response, there is one final strategy. Ask the instructor for clarification of the question. There is nothing to lose by asking and everything to gain. The worst that can happen is that the instructor will tell you that he or she cannot answer your question. The best that can happen is that the instructor will rephrase the question in a way that resolves the problem for you.

When asking for such clarification, try to phrase your question in a way that encourages a response. Do not simply state that you do not understand the question.

This is generally not the approach that invites an answer. If you are having trouble with a term in the stem or response choices, ask for a definition. If there is a phrase that is unclear or a response choice that is confusing, ask for clarification. Anything you do to make your question more specific increases the likelihood that the instructor will answer it.

After all other avenues have been exhausted, remember the final rule: **Never leave a question unanswered.** Even if answering is no more than an educated guess on your part, go ahead and mark an answer. You might be right, but if you leave it blank, you will certainly be wrong and lose precious points.

Strategy for Short-Answer and Essay Questions

Notice that this strategy applies to both short-answer and essay questions. Both types of questions require careful thought and planning before you write an answer. It is helpful to get into the habit of regarding short-answer questions as short-essay questions. Too often students lose points on short-answer questions by being too brief. A short answer should usually consist of three or four sentences, but frequently students interpret "short answer" to mean four or five words.

Start answering these questions by analyzing the question carefully and then framing a response that will fully answer it. Assume that the reader—in this case, the course instructor—does not know anything and that you have to explain it all. Short-answer and essay questions require you to show what you know. Do not assume that the instructor can read your mind or read between the lines of your response to discern what you knew but did not include. It is better to have a little more than was needed in your answer than not enough. Extra information will not hurt, but missing information will always cost points. Once again, remember that the idea is to gain a point here and there throughout the test, which will result in a higher score and a better grade for the course.

Two Key Issues

1. In writing answers to short-answer and essay questions, it is essential to answer exactly the question that is asked. This means that you must understand the question before you do any writing. Unlike with true-or-false and multiple-choice questions, which you should try to answer using every possible strategy before seeking help, you should ask for help with short-answer and essay questions before doing anything. The first opportunity you have to lose points in an essay question occurs with the first reading of the question. If you misread the question, you may write an excellent answer but not the right one. Such a mistake can be costly.

2. A good answer must be organized so that it is clear and logical to the reader. Do not read a question and start writing down whatever ideas spring to mind. Spend a minute or two thinking and planning the structure of the answer so that your ideas are clearly stated and the supporting details relate directly to each idea. Your instructor, the reader, will have a difficult time grading your essay if he or she has to read it two or three times to figure out what you are trying to say. Organization and clarity of expression really pay off in essay exams.

Five Steps to Good Essay Answers

1. **Read the questions carefully.** As was discussed earlier, misreading the question can result in a high-quality answer that does not address the question asked. Read and think about the question's major focus. Do not jump on the first familiar phrase or term and start writing without further thought.

2. **Decide on an approach.** Telling you to read the question carefully is good advice, but without some strategy to apply to the reading, it might be difficult advice to carry out. Here is a strategy to help you read carefully and begin to plan your answer. Look at the question as you read, and identify the words and phrases that tell you what to do. Some standard "what-to-do" words and phrases, such as *discuss, compare, contrast, explain, tell why,* and *analyze,* are used consistently in essay questions,. Circle each of these words or phrases as you read the question. The second part of the decision step is to underline what you are to write about. This circling and underlining will force a careful reading of the question and help you begin the process of organizing the answer. The sample question that follows is marked to show the circle and underline strategy.

   SAMPLE QUESTION:

   (Discuss) the <u>ways</u> in which <u>pediatric and elderly patients</u> are <u>alike</u> in <u>determining</u> appropriate dosage. (Explain) <u>why adult dosage</u> may be <u>inappropriate and</u> the <u>dangers</u> in <u>using adult dosage</u> in these special populations.

3. **Compile a brief written outline.** Before you start writing your answer, take a few minutes to organize the points you want to cover. This should not be an elaborate outline with roman numerals, capital letters, and Arabic numerals, but rather a quick sketch of the question and the points you want to make in the answer. The circle-and-underline step described earlier will help make this easy to do.

SAMPLE OUTLINE*
Discuss
- Child and older adult similarity with regard to drug dosage
  - Body weight factor
  - Organ function

Explain
- Reasons adult dosage inappropriate
  - Drugs not tested on pediatric and older-adult population
- Dangers of adult dosage
  - Possible organ damage
  - Increased absorption and possible adverse effects

Sketching out an outline like this will organize your ideas, speed your writing, and ensure that you are answering the question asked.

4. **Write an answer.** With the question analyzed and a quick outline in place, it is time to put your answer on paper. The basic structure of an exam essay or answer to a short-answer question is the same as that for an in-class composition on an assigned topic. Every rule on which composition teachers insist for writing assignments should be followed in writing essay answers.

Any answer of more than four or five sentences should follow the basic three-part essay structure of introduction, body, and conclusion.

The **introduction** should be only one or two sentences long. It tells the reader what you are going to present in your answer. There is a relatively simple way to write an essay introduction: State the question positively, adding a few words that show the main points you intend to make in your answer.

SAMPLE INTRODUCTION
Child and older-adult patients have a number of similarities that must be considered in determining drug dosage. Two of the most important are body weight and organ function, and these factors can make adult dosages inappropriate for these two populations.

These two sentences tell the reader exactly what you plan to discuss. From this point on, it becomes your task to explain why those two are important and how they affect drug dosage. You have told the reader what to expect, and you have begun to organize your answer.

The **body** is the most important part of any essay answer. In it you want to state the ideas, concepts, and points that you believe answer the question. These should be stated clearly and positively. Do not ramble on, trying to cover all the possible variations that might

fit into an answer. Decide on the most important, most significant points you have to make, then state them and support and explain with relevant details that show how and why your points answer the question. For short-answer questions in which three to five sentences are expected, drop the introduction and conclusion, and put all of your energy into a clear, concise body.

For the **conclusion**, there should be a concluding sentence or two to let the reader know that you have finished. Like the introduction, it should be brief and direct. Restate the question, and summarize the key points made in your answer.

SAMPLE CONCLUSION
It is evident that older-adult and child patients are very similar in their responses to drug dosages. Clearly, the factors of body weight and organ function will play a major role in determining the appropriate dosages for these two groups.

5. **Read the answer.** The writing has been completed. Before you turn in the paper, take another minute or two and read over what you have written. Look for errors that would make the reader pause, question what you have said, or be unable to read a word or phrase. Sometimes the mind works much faster than the pen, and a word or phrase is left out in writing. Use a caret (^) and insert the word or phrase where it belongs. If your writing got a little sloppy and a word is hard to read, cross it out and print it clearly right above. Proofreading and correcting small errors like these will make the answer easier to read and understand. Anything that contributes to the overall quality of an answer will influence the grade in a positive manner. You will not have time to rewrite an answer, but you should correct obvious errors.

Strategy for True-or-False Questions

True-or-false items outwardly appear to be fairly simple; after all, the statement is either true or false. The odds of answering correctly are 50/50, and if all else fails, a coin toss can decide the issue. Appearances are deceiving, however, and true-or-false questions can be challenging to answer. A good test strategy should be applied to answer all types of questions because the object is to get the best score you can, and this represents the total points for all correct answers.

Read the Question. Reading the question may seem like such an obvious part of all test-taking strategies that it may appear absurd even to be told to do this. If you do not pay careful attention to the wording of true-or-false statements, however, you are increasing the odds of making an otherwise avoidable error. Take the time to read and understand the statement. Read it all the way

*This is a model of the process of the Decision and Outline steps. It is not to be viewed as an accurate outline of pharmacological content.

through to the end. Do not jump to conclusions based on half the statement.

Assume That the Statement Is True. As you read each true-or-false statement, begin with the assumption that the statement is true. The idea behind this strategy is that it will cause you to read the statement carefully, which will result in your choosing the correct answer. This approach to reading the statement makes the reading an active process, because you are then reading to confirm the truth in the statement. You will be analyzing the statement as you read, looking for any information that would contradict or change the statement from true to false. You will also be choosing your answer as you read rather than waiting to the end to decide whether the statement was true or false. Obviously not every statement will be true, but this step makes you a much more thoughtful reader, and that encourages better test performance.

Remember one other important rule when analyzing true-or-false statements: If any part of the statement is false, then the entire statement is false. There may be only one altered word or prefix (such as un- or anti-) that changes a statement from true to false, but that is all that is required.

Strategies for Analysis. Sometimes, no matter how carefully you have read the question, the answer is not immediately obvious. When that happens, there are a number of strategies you can use to analyze the question. Using these strategies will not guarantee that you will get the correct answer, but they will often help you see something about the statement you might have overlooked and assist you in identifying the correct answer.

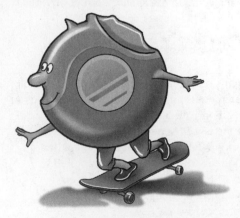

ABSOLUTES AND QUALIFIERS. Absolutes are words such as "none," "never," "all," and "always." These words mean that there are absolutely no exceptions to the statement. For instance, the statement "All birds fly" means just that. Every bird, past, present, and future, has flown or does fly. If there is or has been just one bird that has not flown or does not fly, then the statement is false. All in this statement is an absolute. True-or-false statements that contain such absolutes are usually false. In an area as complex as pharmacology, it is unlikely that there are many absolutes. If you are struggling with a question that has you stumped, look for absolute words; they may help you determine the answer.

On the other hand, there are words that suggest the possibility of exceptions. Such words or phrases are called qualifiers; examples of these are "some," "possibly," "in most cases," and "will generally." "Most birds can fly" is an example of a qualified statement. The word "most" tells you that some not precisely specified number of all birds can fly. This makes it more probable that the statement is true.

STATED IN THE NEGATIVE. A true-or-false statement that is rendered in the negative can be difficult to answer. To draw on the earlier example, "It is not true that all birds can fly" is such a statement. The word "not" in this statement can make it much more complex to read and answer. There is a relatively simple way to deal with this type of statement: Read it as though the negative were not included, so that it becomes "It is true that all birds can fly." This statement is clearly false. Because the word "not" reverses the meaning of the statement, this makes the statement "It is not true that all birds can fly" true. Simply put, if the statement is true without the negative, then it becomes false with the negative. Similarly, if it is false without the negative, then it is true with the negative.

STRINGS. A string is a true-or-false statement that requires careful attention. It is a statement that contains a list of several words or phrases, but often one or more of the words or phrases is false. It is easy to read the statement and see that the first two or three words or phrases are true but then overlook the one that is incorrect, with the consequence that you mark the answer as true when it is actually false. An example of a string is "First-generation cephalosporins, such as cefadroxil, cloxacillin, cefazolin, and cephalexin, are antibiotics specifically active against gram-negative bacteria." As you read this statement, it is easy to be lured by the words "such as" into thinking that the statement is true without noting the fact that cloxacillin is in fact a penicillinase-resistant penicillin, not a cephalosporin. The statement is false, but the string can trick you into thinking the statement is true.

These strategies for analyzing true-or-false items can help you increase the number of correct answers, but they are not intended to replace study and learning. The best way to perform well on any test is to know the answers based on your own learning. When the answer does not immediately come to mind, however, apply these strategies. Although they will not necessarily lead to a 10-point difference in your score, they may help you add 2 points to your score. Better scores mean better course grades, and of course, this results in improved self-confidence and improved chances of success.

Conclusion

Remember: It is up to you how many of these strategies you decide to implement. These study tips are only as valuable as you make them!

CHAPTER 1

Nursing Practice in Canada and Drug Therapy

Chapter Review and Examination Preparation

Choose the best answer for each of the following:

a 1. Which phase of the nursing process requires the nurse to establish a comprehensive baseline of data concerning a particular patient?
   a. Assessment
   b. Planning
   c. Implementation
   d. Evaluation

d 2. The nurse may revise or eliminate unrealistic goals during which phase of the nursing process?
   a. Assessment
   b. Planning
   c. Implementation
   d. Evaluation

c 3. The nurse prepares, then administers a prescribed medication. To what phase of the nursing process does this refer?
   a. Assessment
   b. Planning
   c. Implementation
   d. Evaluation

b 4. Which of the following must occur for a goal statement to be patient centred?
   a. The family must be involved in decision making.
   b. The patient must be involved in establishing the goal(s).
   c. The nurse must develop the goal(s).
   d. The physician must be involved in establishing the goal(s).

a,e,f 5. A nurse is completing a patient's medication history. The nurse should include information about which of the following? *(Select all that apply.)*
   a. Use of "street" drugs
   b. Current laboratory work
   c. Past history of surgeries
   d. Family history
   e. Recreational alcohol use
   f. Use of herbal products

b 6. The nurse prioritizes the nursing diagnoses during which phase of the nursing process?
   a. Assessment
   b. Planning
   c. Implementation
   d. Evaluation

d 7. The nurse is preparing to administer a medication order that reads "ibuprofen, 1 tablet PO, every four hours prn." What information is missing in this medication order?
   a. Frequency
   b. Time
   c. Route
   d. Dosage

8. Place the phases of the nursing process in a progressive numerical order (1 = first; 5 = last).
   _5_ a. Evaluation
   _2_ b. Formulation of nursing diagnosis
   _1_ c. Assessment
   _3_ d. Planning
   _4_ e. Implementation

Critical Thinking and Application

Label each of the following data gathered from an assessment of Ms. Biehl, a young woman visiting an outpatient clinic with what she describes as "maybe an ulcer," as either objective data (O) or subjective data (S):

9.

_____S_____ Ms. Biehl says that she smokes a pack of cigarettes a day.

_____O_____ She is 165 cm tall and weighs 61.2 kg.

_____O_____ The nurse finds that Ms. Biehl's pulse rate is 68 beats per minute and that her blood pressure is 128/72 mm Hg.

_____O_____ Her stool was tested for occult blood by a laboratory technician; the results were negative.

_____S_____ Ms. Biehl says that she does not experience nausea, but she reports pain and heartburn, especially after she eats popcorn (which she and her husband always do while watching television before bedtime).

_____S_____ She experiences occasional increases in stomach pain, "a feeling of heat" in her abdomen and chest at night when she lies down, and increased incidents of heartburn.

Answer the following questions on a separate document:

10. Identify the "10 Rights" of drug administration, and specify ways to ensure that each of these rights is addressed.
medication, dose, route, time, reason, documentation, right to refuse, right to be informed

11. The following items will help you review the nursing process. *& patient   right pt education, right evaluation*

Data are collected during the (a) _assessment_ phase of the nursing process.

Data can be classified as (b) _objective_ or (c) _subjective_.

To formulate the nursing diagnosis, the nurse must first (d) _cluster_ *analyze* the information collected.

The planning phase includes identification of (e) _outcomes_ *criteria* and (f) _timeframe_ *X goals*.

The (g) _implementation_ phase consists of the initiation and completion of the nursing care plan.

The (h) _evaluation_ phase is ongoing and includes monitoring the patient's response to medication and determining the status of goals.

12. During a busy shift, the nurse is preparing to administer a medication order listed as "amoxicillin 500 mg PO tid." What is the priority action the nurse must consider before administering this medication to the patient?
5 rights, allergy   clarify the order with the prescriber

Case Study

Read the scenario and answer the following questions on a separate document.

A 72-year-old woman has been admitted to the hospital because of uncontrolled nausea and vomiting. She has a concurrent diagnosis of hepatitis C. She says she stopped drinking 3 years ago but has had increasing problems with peripheral edema, shortness of breath, and getting out of bed and chairs independently. Laboratory results show elevated liver enzyme and decreased sodium and potassium levels. Her blood pressure is 160/98 mm Hg, her pulse rate is 98 beats/min regular, and her respiratory rate is 24 breaths/min. She is afebrile and states that she is having slight abdominal pain.

1. From the brief facts given, what information will be important to consider when obtaining a drug history?

2. The physician wrote the following drug order:

    October 27, 2017
    Give furosemide now.
                    Charles Simmons, MD

Patient's Name: Jane Doe	F	Age: 72
Medical Record No: 1234567		DOB: 16/1/44

    What elements, if any, are missing from the above medication order? What should the nurse do next?

3. After the order is clarified, the pharmacy sends up furosemide (Lasix) 80 mg tablets, but the patient is unable to swallow them because of her nausea. A colleague suggests giving the furosemide to her as an intravenous injection. What should the nurse do next?

4. After the patient has received the dose of furosemide, what priority actions should the nurse do?

CHAPTER 2

Pharmacological Principles

Chapter Review and Examination Preparation

Provide the best answer for each of the following:

1. Number the following forms of drug in order of speed of dissolution and absorption, with 1 being the fastest and 5 being the slowest:

   _4_ a. Capsules

   _5_ b. Enteric-coated tablets

   _1×2_ c. Elixirs

   _2×3_ d. Powders

   _3×1_ e. Orally disintegrating tablets ~sublingual~

_C_ 2. When considering the various routes of elimination of a drug, what priority body systems should the nurse monitor to ensure excretion is occurring?
   a. Kidney tubules and skin
   b. Skin and lungs
   c. Bowel and kidney tubules
   d. Lungs and gastrointestinal tract

_b_ 3. The nurse is aware that excessive dosages, poor circulation, faulty metabolism, or inadequate excretion may result in which drug effect?
   a. Tolerance
   b. Cumulative effect
   c. Incompatibility
   d. Antagonistic effect

_d_ 4. Which of the following defines a drug's half-life?
   a. The amount of time required for 50% of a drug to be absorbed by the body
   b. The amount of time a drug needs to reach a therapeutic level
   c. The strength of a drug required to exert a therapeutic response
   d. The amount of time required for 50% of the drug to be eliminated by the body

_a_ 5. Which route of drug administration should the nurse know will be altered by the first-pass effect?
   a. Oral
   b. Sublingual
   c. Subcutaneous
   d. Intravenous

_C_ 6. If a drug binds with an enzyme and thereby prevents the enzyme from binding to its normal target cell, it will produce an effect known as which of the following?
   a. Receptor interaction
   b. Enzyme stimulation
   c. Enzyme interaction
   d. Nonspecific interaction

_b_ 7. The nurse reviewing a list of a patient's medications notes that one of the drug is known to have a low therapeutic index. Which of the following statements accurately explains this concept?
   a. The difference between a therapeutic dose and a toxic dose is large.
   b. The difference between a therapeutic dose and a toxic dose is small.
   c. The dose needed to reach a therapeutic level is small.
   d. The drug has only a slight chance of being effective.

_C_ 8. A patient started a new medication that has a low therapeutic index. What is the most appropriate course of action for the nurse to follow to monitor trough level?
   a. Obtain the patient's blood sample immediately after the next medication dose.
   b. Draw blood samples from the patient's arterial blood flow.
   c. Obtain the patient's blood sample just before the next medication dose.
   d. Draw blood samples from the patient's venous blood flow.

d 9. Consider a medication that has a half-life of 2.5 hours.
At 0800 hours, the medication is measured as 100 mg/L.
What will the medication level be at 1300 hours?
   a. 100 mg/L
   b. 75 mg/L
   c. 50 mg/L
   d. 25 mg/L

Match each field of study with the corresponding job description of a person working in that field.

10. ___ c × b ___ Pharmaceutics

11. ___ h ___ Pharmacokinetics

12. ___ i ___ Pharmacodynamics

13. ___ f ___ Pharmacogenetics

14. ___ b × g ___ Pharmacotherapeutics

15. ___ a ___ Pharmacognosy

16. ___ d ___ Toxicology

17. ___ e ___ Teratogenesis

18. ___ g × c? ___ Prophylactic therapy

a. Pedro is researching botanical and zoological sources of drugs to treat multiple sclerosis. He is part of a university research team that is currently experimenting with varying the biochemical composition and therapeutic effects of several new drugs.

b. Norman works for a pharmaceutical corporation. One of its new drugs looks promising, and Norman's company is experimenting with dose forms for this investigational drug. He is responsible for measuring the relationship between the physiochemical properties of the dosage form and the clinical therapeutic response.

c. Liz examines case studies of patients with similar conditions and drug therapies to determine similarities based on clinical observations.

d. Hamische studies various poisons and is particularly concerned with the detection and treatment of the effects of drugs and chemicals in adolescents.

e. Dana represents a research firm that subcontracts with Health Canada to observe and report on drug-induced congenital anomalies and the toxic effects drugs can have on the developing fetus.

f. Nirmala and Phil have spent the last 3 years gathering family histories, legal case reports, and current clinical data to identify genetic factors that possibly influence individuals' responses to meperidine (Demerol) and related drugs.

g. Carmen is a manager for a company that is focused on studying the effects of a particular drug on several infectious conditions.

h. Rohit's laboratory monitors drug distribution rates between various body components, from absorption to excretion. Recently, her laboratory suggested a positive change in the dosage regimen of an injectable drug, earning her firm a prestigious award.

i. Malcolm's research unit recently recommended two new contraindications to a newly marketed drug after discovering its biochemical and physiological interactions with an unrelated drug.

Critical Thinking and Application

Answer the following questions on a separate document.

19. A patient is to receive a medication that is available in both intramuscular and subcutaneous forms. If this patient's condition requires fast absorption of this medication, which route of administration should the nurse use? What actions can the nurse take to promote faster absorption?

20. Patricia was diagnosed with hypertension a month ago. She has since been taking the antihypertensive medication amlodipine (Norvasc). What type of drug therapy is this known as (acute, maintenance, supplemental, or palliative)? Explain your answer.

21. Riley has a prescription for an extended-release enteric-coated tablet. The next day, his partner calls to ask about crushing the tablet, explaining that Mr. Bole "cannot swallow that big pill." What is the nurse's best response?

Case Study

Read the scenario and answer the following questions on a separate document.

A 65-year-old man with liver cirrhosis is admitted to the medical-surgical unit with nausea and vomiting. He also has a diagnosis of heart failure. The nurse notes that his serum albumin level is low. The physician has written admission orders, and the nurse is trying to make the patient comfortable. He is to take nothing by mouth except for clear liquids. An intravenous infusion of dextrose 5% in water at 50 mL/hr has been ordered, and the unit nurses have had difficulty inserting his intravenous line.

1. One of the drugs ordered is known to reach a maximum level in the body of 200 mg/L and has a half-life of 2 hours. If this maximum level of 200 mg/L is reached at 1600 hours, what will the drug's level in the body be at 2200 hours?

2. Explain what factors from this patient's history would affect the following:

   a. Absorption

   b. Distribution

   c. Metabolism

   d. Excretion

3. Placement of a peripherally inserted central catheter (PICC) has been ordered. The physician writes an order for a dose of an intravenous antibiotic to be given before this procedure is carried out. What is the reason for this order?

4. This patient is also receiving digoxin (Lanoxin) for heart failure. This drug is known to have a low therapeutic index. Explain the term "therapeutic index."

CHAPTER 3

Legal and Ethical Considerations

Chapter Review and Examination Preparation

Choose the best answer for each of the following:

1. What is the primary purpose of Health Canada's Therapeutic Products Directorate?
   a. To allow pharmaceutical companies a time frame of noncompetitiveness with generic drugs
   b. To ensure the safety, efficacy, and quality of drugs sold on the market
   c. To direct and monitor the clinical trials of therapeutic drugs
   d. To monitor the import and export of foods and drugs

2. Which of the following Health Canada regulations applies to the sale of probiotics, amino acids, and essential fatty acids?
   a. Natural Health Products Regulations
   b. Precursor Control Regulations
   c. Supplements and Dietary Products Regulations
   d. Benzodiazepines and Other Targeted Substances Regulations

3. Nurses are expected to enact the ethical principle of nonmaleficence with patients. What statement best exemplifies this principle?
   a. Promote independence.
   b. Do good.
   c. Keep health information private.
   d. Do no harm.

4. Which phase of the four clinical phases of investigational drug studies is focused on determining the drug's ability for therapeutic effect, the identification of adverse effects, and the refinement of therapeutic dosage ranges?
   a. Phase I: drug safety study
   b. Phase II: drug effectiveness study
   c. Phase IV: branded versus generic drugs comparison study
   d. Phase III: drug duration and long-term effects study

5. Which of the following is the correct definition of *placebo*?
   a. An investigational drug used in a new drug study
   b. An inert substance that is not a drug
   c. A legend drug that requires a prescription
   d. A substance that is not approved as a drug but is used as a natural health product

6. When a patient's health history is being taken, what cultural information important for medication administration is important for the nurse to consider? *(Select all that apply.)*
   a. The patient uses acetylsalicylic acid as needed for pain.
   b. The patient has a history of hypertension.
   c. The patient will eat only at nighttime for the next 4 weeks.
   d. The patient is allergic to shellfish.
   e. The patient does not eat pork products (for religious reasons).

Match each investigational drug study phase with its corresponding description.

7. ___d___ Phase I

8. ___a___ Phase II

9. ___c___ Phase III

10. ___b___ Phase IV

a. A study using small numbers of volunteers who have the disease or disorder that the drug is meant to diagnose or treat. Subjects are monitored for drug efficacy and adverse effects.

b. Postmarketing studies conducted by drug companies to obtain further proof of the drug's therapeutic effects.

c. A study that involves a large number of patients at research centres and is designed to monitor for infrequent adverse effects and identify any associated risks. Double-blind, placebo-controlled studies eliminate patient and researcher bias.

d. A study that uses small numbers of healthy volunteers, as opposed to volunteers afflicted with the target ailment, to determine dosage range and pharmacokinetics.

Match each cultural group with its corresponding cultural practice.

11. ___a x c___ Asian

12. ___c x a___ Hispanic

13. ___d___ Indigenous

14. ___b___ Caribbean — folk, spiritual

a. Some may seek a balance between the body and mind through the use of cold remedies or foods for "hot" illnesses, and vice versa.

b. Some may use folk medicine and be influenced by strong spiritual beliefs.

c. Some believe that opposing forces lead to illness or health, depending on which force is dominant in the individual and whether the forces are balanced, producing healthy states.

d. Some believe in the balance between body, mind, and environment to maintain health and harmony with nature.

Critical Thinking and Application

Answer the following questions on a separate document.

15. Identify a cultural group in your area, and explore the health belief practices of that group.

   a. Are there any barriers to adequate health care?

   b. What is the attitude toward Western medicines and health treatments?

   c. What questions should you ask in your ethnocultural assessment?

Case Study

Read the scenario and answer the following questions on a separate document.

The nurse works in an outpatient treatment clinic for patients with human immunodeficiency virus (HIV) infection. During a recent staff meeting, the medical director discussed a new drug that has shown good results in clinical trials in another country. This drug has not yet been tested in Canada. She stated that she hopes to start clinical trials of that drug in the HIV clinic.

The following week, the nurse is asked to give a new drug regimen for four patients with HIV. One of the drugs is unfamiliar to her, and when she asks about it, the medical director states, "Oh, that's the new drug I mentioned last week! One of my colleagues in that country sent me some samples, so we are going to try it here. Health Canada has already started trials in Canada. We will be comparing how these four patients do compared with four other patients who are in the same stages of HIV. The patients will not even know about this change."

1. Should the nurse administer the drugs as requested? If not, what should be done to correct the situation?

2. What ethical principle or principles guide the nurse's decision?

3. One of the potential study patients, brought in by his brother, seems reluctant to answer questions and says he "does not need any drugs." Upon further questioning, the nurse finds out that he would prefer to take some home remedies that his mother has made for him. How should the nurse handle this situation?

4. When the nurse meets with potential study patients, several mention that they fear others will find out about their illness if they participate in the study. What should the nurse tell these patients?

CHAPTER 4

Patient Focused Considerations

Chapter Review and Examination Preparation

Choose the best answer for each of the following:

_c_ 1. What physiological factor is most responsible for the differences in the pharmacokinetic and pharmacodynamic behaviour of drugs in neonates and adults?
   a. Infants' stature
   b. Infants' smaller weight
   c. Immaturity of neonatal organs
   d. Adults' longer exposure to toxins

_a,c,e_ 2. A public health nurse works in a health promotion program focused on reducing the rate of unhealthy pregnancies. What should the nurse do for a patient during the first trimester to decrease the risk of drug-induced developmental defects? _(Select all that apply.)_
   a. Reduce the patient's exposure to prescription drugs.
   b. Increase the patient's exposure to prescriptive drugs.
   c. Reduce the patient's exposure to illicit drugs.
   d. Increase the patient's exposure to illicit drugs.
   e. Reduce the patient's exposure's to non-prescription drugs.
   f. Increase the patient's exposure to non-prescription drugs.

_d_ 3. Most drug references recommend that dosages for children be based on which of the following?
   a. Total body water content
   b. Fat-to-lean mass ratio
   c. Height in centimetres
   d. Milligrams per kilogram of body weight

_a_ 4. Dosages in older adults are based
   a. more on age than on height or weight.
   b. more on weight than on age.
   c. on total body water content.
   d. on the glomerular filtration rate.

_a,b + d_ 5. When administering medications to the older adult, what age-related conditions can the nurse expect to note? _(Select all that apply.)_
   a. Decreased total body water content as body composition changes
   b. Less acidic gastric pH due to reduced hydrochloric acid production
   c. Increased protein albumin binding sites because of decreased protein
   d. Increased fat content, resulting from changes in lean body mass and total body water
   e. Increased absorptive surface area of the gastrointestinal tract due to blunting of the villi

(handwritten notes next to Q4: "with organ function; liver, kidney, CVS, CNS")

32

Match each US Food and Drug Administration (FDA) pregnancy safety category with its corresponding description.

6. _____ Category A d

7. _____ Category B b

8. _____ Category C e

9. _____ Category D a

10. _____ Category X c

a. Possible fetal risk in humans is reported; however, the potential benefits may, in selected cases, outweigh the risks and warrant the use of these drugs in pregnant women.

b. Studies indicate no risk to animal fetuses; information on humans is not available.

c. Fetal abnormalities are reported, and positive evidence of fetal risk in humans has been found by animal/human studies.

d. Studies indicate no risk to the fetus.

e. Adverse effects are reported in animal fetuses; information on humans is not available.

Critical Thinking and Application

Answer the following questions on a separate document.

11. A nurse works at a community clinic frequented by a number of older adult patients. Annie comes to the clinic complaining of dizziness and nausea. As her medication history is being taken, she shows the nurse her "pillbox." Inside are almost a dozen different pills, all to be taken at noon. How could this happen, and how could she possibly need so many medications at the same time?

12. The physician confirms that Elaine's "new symptoms," as she refers to them, are a result of polypharmacy. She protests, telling the nurse, "My dear, I've got news for the doctor. I've had to take lots of drugs at the same time all my life. It never bothered me before. Why would it now when I'm even more used to it?" Explain at least three physiological changes that occur with aging and how these changes affect pharmacokinetics and pharmacodynamics.

Case Study

Read the scenario and answer the following questions on a separate document.

The nurse is performing telephone triage in a pediatric clinic. A mother calls about her 28-month-old toddler, who has had chicken pox for 2 days. She wants to give him acetylsalicylic acid because his fever is 38.3°C (100.9°F), but she is unsure because her toddler "hates to take pills."

1. Should the mother use acetylsalicylic acid for this fever? (Check a drug reference, if needed, for developmental considerations in this situation.)

2. The mother states that her husband is going to the drugstore for some medicine. What should the nurse tell her about the dosage form of an antipyretic for her toddler?

3. When the husband returns from the drugstore, he shows the mother the bottle of Children's Acetaminophen Suspension Cherry Flavour that was recommended by the store's pharmacist. She wonders why the pharmacist needs to know her child's weight before suggesting this medication. Explain.

4. The toddler receives a dose of 5 mL per the directions according to his weight of 12.7 kg. Later, when his 5-year-old sister needs a dose, she receives 7.5 mL because of her weight of 20.4 kg. If the drug contains 160 mg per 5 mL, how much medication did the 5-year-old receive in her dose?

5. What should the parents look for when evaluating their children's response to a dose of acetaminophen?

CHAPTER 5

Gene Therapy and Pharmacogenomics

Chapter Review and Examination Preparation

Select the best answer for each question.

1. The nurse is reviewing concepts of gene therapy. Which of the following correctly describes a possible approach to gene therapy? *(Select all that apply.)*
   a. Replacing a mutated gene with a healthy copy of the gene
   b. Preventing an immature gene from growing into a mature gene
   c. Inactivating a mutated gene that is functioning improperly
   d. Introducing a new gene into the body to help fight a disease
   e. Causing the body to produce new genes

2. The nurse is explaining concepts of ethical issues related to gene therapy in Canada. Which of the following statement(s) correctly reflects safety regulations in Canada? *(Select all that apply.)*
   a. Health Canada must review and approve all human clinical gene therapy trials according to the Food and Drug Regulations.
   b. Gene therapy research poses little risk to the subjects who participate in studies.
   c. Eugenics therapy is currently part of gene therapy research in the United States.
   d. Genetic therapy is exempt from approval by an institutional review board.
   e. Health Canada's Biologics and Genetics Therapies Directorate oversees gene therapy.

Match each definition with its corresponding term (not all terms are used).

3. _____ A structure in the nucleus that contains a linear thread of deoxyribonucleic acid (DNA) that transmits genetic information

4. _____ A term for all of the chromosomal material within a cell

5. _____ The complete set of genetic material of any organism

6. _____ The study of genomes, including the way genes and their products work in both health and disease

a. Chromosome

b. Chromatin

c. Genome

d. Genomics

e. Gene

f. Chromosome

Case Study

Read the scenario and answer the following questions on a separate document.

Riley, a 27-year-old construction worker, fell off a roof 2 months ago. As a result, Riley needs to have surgery on his ankle. The nurse preparing him for the surgery conducts a health history. Riley mentions that he is a bit nervous because his cousin had surgery and had a "terrible reaction" to the medications.

1. Is this information about his cousin significant? Explain.

2. What priority questions should the nurse ask?

3. When obtaining a genetic history, how many generations back should the nurse ask about?

4. What considerations should the health care providers involved in surgery prioritize with regard to Riley's medications?

CHAPTER 6

Medication Errors: Preventing and Responding

Chapter Review and Examination Preparation

Provide the best answer for each of the following:

1. A(n) _medication error_ is any preventable adverse drug event that involves the use of inappropriate medication by a patient or health care provider. It may or may not cause harm to the patient.

2. A(n) _adverse X_ [_idiosyncratic_] reaction is an abnormal and unexpected response to a medication, other than an allergic reaction, that is peculiar to an individual patient.

3. A(n) _idiopathic_ [X _allergic reaction_] is an immunological reaction resulting from an unusual sensitivity of a patient to a particular medication.

4. A(n) _adverse drug reaction_ is a type of adverse drug event that is defined as any unexpected, unintended, or excessive response to a medication.

5. A(n) _adverse drug event_ is an undesirable occurrence related to the administration of or failure to administer a prescribed medication.

6. True or false: High-alert medications are involved in more errors than other drugs. Explain why. _F_

7. True or false: All adverse drug events are caused by medication errors. Explain why. _F_

8. Identify strategies to avoid medication errors. _5 rights_

9. Name at least four of the classes of medications that are considered "high-alert" drugs.

10. The Institute for Safe Medication Practices Canada recommends that certain abbreviations be written out in full. Write out the meaning of each abbreviation that appears in boldface below.

digoxin 250 **mcg** PO now	_microgram_
furosemide 40 mg IV **qd**	_every day_
d/c all meds	_discontinue_
NPH insulin 8 **u SQ ac** breakfast **qd**	_units subcutaneous before daily_
Garamycin otic drops 2 **gtts AD** bid	_drops_ _right ear_

β blocker

11. The prescriber orders "Metoprolol 25 mg PO bid. Hold if systolic blood pressure is less than 95 mm Hg." Today the pharmacy supplied 50 mg tablets because there were no 25 mg tablets in stock.
    a. How many tablets will the nurse administer per dose? *0.5*
    b. The nurse gives the patient the entire tablet. How many milligrams does the patient receive? *50*
    c. What will the nurse do next? *monitor the pt's VS esp. BP, HR   report to physician*
       report med error according to policy

a 12. The order reads, "Give levothyroxine (Synthroid) 50 mcg PO every morning." How is this dose expressed in
b   milligrams (mg)?
    a. .05 mg
    b. 0.05 mg
    c. 0.050 mg
    d. 50,000 mg

13. The order reads, "Give furosemide 50 mg per gastrostomy tube every morning." The medication is available in liquid form, 10 mg/1 mL. Calculate how much medication the nurse will administer. *5 mL*

14. Mark the medication cup with the answer you obtained for Question 13.

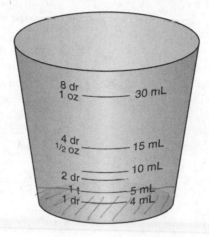

Case Study

Read the scenario and answer the following questions on a separate sheet of paper.

A nursing student discovers that she has given her patient two acetylsalicylic acid (Aspirin) tablets instead of the one-tablet daily dose that was ordered for antiplatelet effects. She is upset and talks with her fellow students, who tell her to keep quiet about it. "One extra Aspirin will not hurt your patient," they tell her.

1. What should the nursing student do first? Describe other appropriate actions after this.

2. How could the student have prevented this error?

3. Should the patient be told about it? Explain your answer.

4. If the patient was not hurt by this incident, is it considered a medication error? Explain.

5. The student has decided to inform her instructor. The instructor helps the student complete a report to the Canadian Medication Incident Reporting and Prevention System. Explain the reason for this report. Will the student's name be reported?

CHAPTER 7

Patient Education and Drug Therapy

Chapter Review and Examination Preparation

Select the best answer for each question.

1. An educational session focused on the safe administration of medication is being prepared. Which of the following is the best example of a cognitive domain-based learning activity?
   a. Having the patient demonstrate the self-administration of nasal spray
   b. Teaching a patient the skill of measuring the apical pulse before taking digoxin
   c. Giving the patient the list of foods to avoid while taking oral anticoagulants
   d. Having a family member show the patient how to give an injection

2. The nurse is developing a discharge plan regarding a patient's medications. When is the ideal time to begin discharge planning?
   a. When family members are near the patient (to allow for discussion)
   b. Just before the patient leaves the hospital (to ensure compliance)
   c. Immediately following the patient's pain medication (to alleviate symptoms)
   d. As soon as possible, allowing the patient to determine when he or she is ready

3. The nurse is providing discharge teaching for a patient who has a new colostomy following a partial colectomy. The patient is very upset and anxious because of the colostomy. Which statement about this anxiety is true?
   a. It may be an obstacle to learning at this time.
   b. It means that a family member needs to be taught instead of the patient.
   c. It will have no effect on the patient's ability to learn.
   d. It may result in the patient having an increased motivation to learn.

4. A nurse has completed an education session on self-administration of insulin injections. Which statement(s) or action describe(s) successful learning in the affective domain? (Select all that apply.)
   a. The patient states, "I am feeling more confident about insulin self-injection."
   b. The patient states, "It is important to check my blood sugar before I take the insulin."
   c. The patient states, "Insulin works to lower my blood sugar levels."
   d. The patient measures the correct amount of insulin in the syringe for the injection.
   e. The patient injects himself with insulin using the correct technique.

5. A patient has been instructed to take 25 mg of diphenhydramine (Benadryl) oral syrup twice a day as treatment for a severe case of poison ivy. The medication comes in a bottle that contains 12.5 mg/5 mL. The nurse will be teaching the patient how to measure a dose of the medication. How many millilitres will the nurse measure for each dose?

6. During a teaching session, the nurse demonstrates how to draw up insulin into a syringe. The patient then provides a return demonstration and draws up 17 units of insulin. Mark on the syringe the correct dose of 17 units.

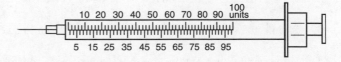

38

Copyright © 2017 Elsevier Canada, a division of Reed Elsevier Canada, Ltd.

Critical Thinking and Application

Answer the following questions on a separate document.

7. The nurse is to present information regarding antihypertensive drug therapy to two patients, a 40-year-old and a 72-year-old. Describe the different teaching strategies the nurse should use with each patient regarding possible alterations in thought processes and sensory-perceptual status.

8. The nurse is to instruct a mother and her 8-year-old child in using a metered-dose inhaler. Neither mother nor child speaks English. Outline specific strategies to use in developing an effective teaching plan for this patient.

9. The nurse's patient has been taking oral antihyperglycemics for 1 month, and her blood glucose readings are still high. On assessment, the nurse discovers a possible reason for these high readings. Develop a nursing diagnosis for this patient based on the following:

   a. The patient says that no one has ever told her about required dietary restrictions.

   b. The patient tells the nurse that she takes the medication only if she feels ill.

10. Develop a patient teaching plan for a 55-year-old patient who will be receiving warfarin sodium (Coumadin) therapy after discharge. Refer to the appropriate chapter in the text for information. Include the following:

   a. Assessment—objective and subjective data that would be needed

   b. Nursing diagnosis

   c. Planning—measurable goal and outcome criteria

   d. Implementation—specific educational strategies

   e. Evaluation—means for evaluating that learning had occurred

Case Study

Read the scenario and answer the following questions on a separate document.

A 77-year-old man, accompanied by his wife, visits the family health clinic for a physical checkup. He has been treated for hypertension and has a history of angina. While in the clinic, he pulls a small bottle of sublingual nitroglycerin spray from his pants pocket and states, "I never go anywhere without this." He says he "gets along okay" with his medicines at home and that it "doesn't hurt anything" if he misses a day or two of his medications. His blood pressure today is 130/92 mm Hg, pulse rate is 88 beats per minute, and respiratory rate is 12 breaths per minute. Previously, his blood pressure readings have been 160/98, 152/92, and 148/94 mm Hg.

After the patient is evaluated by the physician, new medication orders are written as follows:

- hydrochlorothiazide (Apo-Hydro) 25 mg tablet, once a day
- potassium chloride (Slow-K), 600 mg (1 tablet) daily
- diltiazem (Diltiazem-60) 60 mg tablet, three times a day
- lansoprazole (Apo-Lansoprazole), 15 mg capsule, before breakfast and dinner
- nitroglycerin (Mylan-Nitro sublingual spray), as needed for chest pain

1. Based on your assessment, what priority nursing diagnosis would you suggest for this situation?

2. State a goal and outcome criteria for your nursing diagnosis.

3. Describe the teaching strategies the nurse would use when teaching this patient how to take his medications correctly.

4. How would the nurse evaluate the education process in this situation?

CHAPTER 8

Over-the-Counter Drugs and Natural Health Products

Double Puzzle

Unscramble each of the clue words. Take the letters that appear in circles and unscramble them for the final message. [Hint: the use of herbs to treat health conditions]

LAIREANV

RCGIAL

FEFREEVW

TS. NOJH'S TWRO

KONIGG

WAS OLTATPEM

NISGGNE

NAAHICCEE

LAOE

SOADELNEGL

[grid boxes with B] [grid boxes with Y]

Chapter Review and Examination Preparation

Choose the best answer for each of the following:

1. What classes of drugs are commonly used as over-the-counter (OTC) remedies? (Select all that apply.)
   a. Nonsteroidal anti-inflammatory drugs
   b. Cold remedies
   c. Antibiotics
   d. Smoking-deterrent systems
   e. Topical antiviral ointments
   f. Histamine-2 (H_2) blockers

2. What is the direct advantage of using OTC medications?
   a. Costs are more manageable for patients who are without drug insurance plans.
   b. Patients can feel better faster when self-medicating.
   c. Fewer drug interactions exist with low-potency medications.
   d. Patients can self-treat minor ailments, reducing health care visits.

3. What is Health Canada's key role in the manufacturing of natural health products?
   a. To enforce standards of quality and safety for natural health products
   b. To require manufacturers of natural health products to prove efficacy
   c. To set standards for quality control and consumer satisfaction
   d. To define natural health products as dietary supplements in order to promote safety

4. The nurse prioritizes readiness for enhanced self-health management as the most appropriate nursing diagnosis for a patient. What patient behaviour best exemplifies this nursing diagnosis?
   a. Patient takes anticoagulant medication as instructed to decrease development of blood clots.
   b. Patient asks about taking omega-3 fatty acids to reduce risks for coronary artery disease.
   c. Patient requests a meeting with the dietitian to understand the role of food in growth and development.
   d. Patient increases dietary intake of protein supplements to increase muscle mass.

5. The nurse is admitting a patient who has a diagnosis of right lower lobe pneumonia. Upon assessment, the nurse learns that the patient is wearing a herbal aromatherapy pack on her chest. What should the nurse do first?
   a. Remove the pack immediately.
   b. Report the pack to the physician.
   c. Ask the patient about the herbal pack.
   d. Document the presence of the herbal pack.

6. A construction worker is treating himself with acetaminophen after an injury on the job. After 2 days, he comes to the urgent care facility because he thinks his hand is broken. He tells the nurse that he has been taking two "extra-strength" acetaminophen tablets 8 times a day but that he still has pain. Each tablet is 500 mg. How many milligrams per day has he taken?

7. Is there a concern regarding the acetaminophen intake of the construction worker in question 6? Explain your answer.

8. The nurse is caring for a patient who is preparing to undergo anticoagulant medication therapy. What natural health products should the nurse tell the patient to avoid? (Select all that apply.)
   a. Chamomile
   b. Cranberry
   c. Garlic
   d. *Ginkgo biloba*
   e. Ginger root
   f. Grapefruit

9. What is the nurse's rationale for avoiding the natural health products listed under question 8 when a patient is taking an anticoagulant?

Case Study

Read the scenario and answer the following questions on a separate document.

A 30-year-old woman is in the clinic for her yearly gynecological checkup. She is not pregnant but would like to have children soon and states that she and her husband are trying to conceive. She states that she is "concerned" about her health and watches her diet and exercises regularly to stay in shape. She has a family history of heart disease but no other conditions. Her physical assessment revealed no abnormalities or health problems.

On her medical history sheet, she writes that she takes several drug and natural health products, as follows:

"*Echinacea*, from September to March, to prevent influenza"
"Adult Aspirin, one tablet every day, to prevent a heart attack"
"Garlic tablets twice a day for my heart"
"Kava tea as needed for relaxation"
"Valerian capsules for sleep as needed (usually three or four times a week)"

1. Are there any drug or natural health drug interactions in this listing?

2. Do any of these products have a potential for problems if used over the long term?

3. Is there any specific information on which the nurse should focus in taking the patient's history or performing an assessment, given that the patient is using these drugs and natural health products?

4. The patient tells the nurse that she thinks the natural health products are safe because the government would not allow them to be sold if they were not. Is this true?

5. What would the nurse emphasize when teaching this patient about the use of natural health products and OTC drugs?

CHAPTER 9

Vitamins and Minerals

Chapter Review and Examination Preparation

Match each definition with its corresponding term.

1. _____ Specialized protein that catalyzes chemical reactions in organic matter

2. _____ A deficiency of cyanocobalamin

3. _____ A nonprotein substance that combines with a protein molecule to form an active enzyme

4. _____ A condition caused by a vitamin D deficiency that is characterized by soft, pliable bones

5. _____ An inorganic substance ingested and attached to enzymes or other organic molecules

6. _____ An organic compound essential in small quantities for normal physiological and metabolic functioning in the body

7. _____ A condition resulting from an ascorbic acid deficiency that is characterized by weakness and anemia

8. _____ An essential organic compound that can be dissolved and stored in the liver and fatty tissues

9. _____ Biologically active chemicals that make up vitamin E compounds

10. _____ A disease of the peripheral nerves caused by an inability to assimilate thiamine

11. _____ An essential organic compound that can be dissolved in water but is not stored in the body for long periods of time

12. _____ A disease resulting from a niacin or a metabolic defect that interferes with the conversion of tryptophan to niacin

a. Beriberi

b. Coenzyme

c. Enzyme

d. Fat-soluble vitamin

e. Mineral

f. Pellagra

g. Pernicious anemia

h. Rickets

i. Scurvy

j. Tocopherols

k. Vitamin

l. Water-soluble vitamin

44

Choose the best answer for each of the following:

13. When giving vitamins, the nurse needs to remember that certain vitamins can be toxic if consumed in excess amounts. These include which of the following? (Select all that apply).
    a. Vitamin A
    b. Vitamin C
    c. Niacin
    d. Vitamin D
    e. Vitamin K
    f. Folic acid

14. A patient is planning to increase vitamin C supplement doses. What priority information should the nurse provide to the patient?
    a. They are usually nontoxic because vitamin C is water soluble.
    b. They can produce nausea, vomiting, headache, and abdominal cramps.
    c. They can lead to scurvylike symptoms.
    d. They may cause dangerous heart dysrhythmias.

15. A patient ingested excessive amounts of water-soluble vitamins. What is the nurse's priority action?
    a. Record weight changes. (The body will store water-soluble vitamins in muscle and fat tissue until needed.)
    b. Observe for jaundice. (The vitamins are stored in the liver until needed.)
    c. Obtain blood profile. (The vitamins circulate in the blood, bound to proteins until needed.)
    d. Monitor urinary output. (Excess amounts are excreted by the kidneys.)

16. While reviewing the diet of a patient who has a calcium deficiency, the nurse recalls that efficient absorption of calcium in the diet requires adequate amounts of which substance?
    a. Magnesium
    b. Intrinsic factor
    c. Coenzymes
    d. Vitamin D

17. A 5-year-old patient is prescribed a new medication that reads, "Administer vitamin K (phytonadione) 1 mg subcutaneously now." The medication is available in a 2 mg/1 mL ampule. How many millilitres will the nurse draw up for the injection?

Critical Thinking and Application

Answer the following questions on a separate document.

18. A patient developed vitamin D deficiency as the result of long-term use of lubricant laxatives. She is advised to take supplements for vitamin D deficiency. However, the physician also advises her to get vitamin D through more natural sources, both dietary and endogenous. The patient inquires, "What did he mean by 'endogenous?'" What explanation should the nurse provide the patient concerning endogenous sources? Develop a list of foods that contain a high vitamin D content.

19. A patient had undergone an ileal resection for a condition affecting digestive functions. The patient is experiencing signs of malabsorption. Routine laboratory tests reveal mild anemia.

    a. What type of anemia does the nurse expect?

    b. Considering the patient's condition, what is the primary contributing factor to this deficiency?

    c. Create a handheld patient education card for this patient, focusing on diet. Be sure to include a list of foods that contain the vitamin or vitamins from which she is most likely to suffer a deficiency.

20. A patient is hospitalized with severe hypocalcemia. The nurse's colleague, Jeffrey, recommends immediately beginning a rapid infusion of intravenous calcium. The physician's order requires infusion of 1% procaine. Refute or defend the rationales of both Jeffrey and the physician. In either case, what should the nurse watch out for most when administering intravenous calcium? Support your response with your own data.

21. A patient will be taking iron for treatment of anemia, and the physician instructs that it be taken with orange juice. The patient asks the nurse for an explanation of this. What information should the nurse provide the patient?

Case Study

Read the scenario and answer the following questions on a separate document.

A patient with a history of alcoholism was admitted to the Critical Care Unit with arrhythmias and increased confusion. The initial magnesium level is 0.067 mmol/L.

1. Considering normal serum magnesium, what is the priority treatment for this patient? Explain your answer.

2. What is your priority when assessing the patient during intravenous magnesium infusion?

3. Twelve hours later, you note that the patient's respirations are 10 breaths per minute and that his Achilles tendon reflexes are diminished. What will you do next?

4. What is the antidote for magnesium toxicity?

CHAPTER 10

Principles of Drug Administration

Chapter Review and Examination Preparation

Choose the best answer for each of the following:

_b_ 1. A nurse is preparing an intramuscular medication. After drawing fluid from an ampule with the needle pointing up, what is the best way to expel air bubbles?
   a. Draw back slightly on the plunger, tap the side of the syringe to cause bubbles to rise toward the needle, and push the plunger upward to eject air.
   b. Tap the side of the syringe to cause bubbles to rise toward the needle, draw back slightly on the plunger, and push the plunger upward to eject air.
   c. Tap the side of the syringe to cause bubbles to rise toward the needle, draw back slightly on the plunger, push the plunger upward to eject air, and eject a small amount of fluid.
   d. Draw back slightly on the plunger, tap the side of the syringe to cause bubbles to rise toward the needle, and push the plunger upward to eject air; do not eject fluid.

_c_ 2. What is the nurse's priority action when administering intradermal injections?
   a. Massage the site lightly after the injection.
   b. Have the patient massage the site until the pain diminishes.
   c. Avoid massaging the site.
   d. Apply heat to the site after the injection.

_d_ 3. When administering medication through intravenous push, what is the correct way to occlude the intrave- _a_ nous line? through an IV line
   a. Pinch the tubing just above the injection port.
   b. Pinch the tubing at least 5 cm above the injection port.
   c. Fold the tubing just above the injection port.
   d. Keep the line patent without any occlusion.

_b_ 4. The nurse is adding more than one medication to a solution. Which of the following actions is most important at this time?
   a. Use an equal volume of each medication.
   b. Assess the two drugs for compatibility.
   c. Add the drugs at least 1 hour apart.
   d. Use the same needle for both medications.

_c_ 5. What is the correct procedure for the nurse to follow when administering oral medications?
   a. If a patient cannot swallow medications, crush all medications together and administer with applesauce.
   b. Give oral medications with meals to avoid gastrointestinal upset.
   c. Stay with the patient until each medication has been swallowed.
   d. Have the patient take all medications on an empty stomach to facilitate absorption.

_c_ 6. After administering eardrops, what should the nurse do next?
   a. Press a cotton ball firmly into the ear canal.
   b. Have the patient sit up and tilt the head for 2 to 3 minutes.
   c. Gently massage the tragus of the ear.
   d. Have the patient remain in the side-lying position for 20 minutes.

_c_ 7. When administering nasal drops for the frontal or _b_ maxillary sinuses, what should the nurse do to position the patient correctly?
   a. Tilt the patient's head backward and facing toward the left side.
   b. Tilt the patient's head back over the edge of the bed, with the head turned toward the side being treated.
   c. Place a pillow under the patient's shoulders, and tilt the head back. ethmoid & sphenoid
   d. Tilt the patient's head to the side opposite the side being treated.

8. What is the most correct action the nurse can take when administering medications with a nasogastric tube?
   a. Allow the fluid to flow via gravity.
   b. Use gentle but consistent pressure when forcing the fluid into the tube.
   c. Shake the tube gently to facilitate the movement of fluid in the tube.
   d. Confirm placement of the tube after the medication is given.

9. The nurse is preparing to administer an intramuscular injection using the Z-track method. When should the nurse use this technique?
   a. When there is insufficient muscle mass in the landmarked area
   b. Whenever massaging the area after medication administration is contraindicated
   c. When medications that are known to be irritating, painful, or staining to tissues are injected
   d. When any injection is administered into the dorsogluteal muscle

10. After receiving a prescription for sublingual medication, the patient asks, "What is the advantage of taking this form of medication?" What is the nurse's best response?
    a. "It is immediately absorbed."
    b. "It is excreted rapidly."
    c. "It is metabolized immediately."
    d. "It is distributed equally."

11. The dosage of available rectal suppository medication in stock is twice the dose of the prescriber's ordered medication. What is the most appropriate intervention by the nurse?
    a. Cut the suppository in half.
    b. Call the physician for clarification.
    c. Administer another type of suppository.
    d. Instruct the patient to retain the suppository for only 5 minutes.

12. When administering rectal suppositories, what priority contraindication must the nurse consider?
    a. Vomiting
    b. Fever
    c. Constipation
    d. Rectal bleeding

13. The nurse applies a transdermal patch. What is the best location for this medication?
    a. A hairy location
    b. A nonhairy location
    c. A moist location
    d. Within a skinfold

14. What should the nurse tell the patient when teaching about the instillation of nasal drops?
    a. To clear the nasal passages by blowing the nose gently before administering the medication
    b. To clear the nasal passages by blowing the nose gently after administering the medication
    c. To sit in the semi-Fowler position for 5 minutes after the instillation of the medication
    d. To place the nose dropper approximately 1 cm into the nostril when instilling drops

15. Which intervention is most appropriate when administering ophthalmic medications? (Select all that apply.)
    a. Having the patient look upward while the medication is being instilled
    b. Instilling the prescribed number of drops into the conjunctival sac
    c. Having the patient close his or her eyes tightly after the drop has been instilled
    d. Applying gentle pressure to the patient's nasolacrimal duct for 30 to 60 seconds after instilling the drops
    e. Applying ointment to the conjunctival sac, starting at the outer canthus and working toward the inner canthus

Critical Thinking and Application

Answer the following questions on a separate document.

16. Describe how the nurse assesses the injection site for each of the following:
    a. Subcutaneous injection
    b. Intramuscular injection
    c. Intradermal injection

17. Describe the proper technique of needle insertion for each of the following:
    a. Subcutaneous injection
    b. Intramuscular injection
    c. Intradermal injection

18. The nurse is administering an intramuscular injection to a patient. After the needle enters the site, the nurse grasps the lower end of the syringe barrel with the nondominant hand and slowly pulls back on the plunger to aspirate the drug. Blood appears in the syringe. What is the priority intervention at this time?

19. The nurse is preparing a liquid medication for a patient. How does the usual procedure change when the volume of medication required is less than 5 mL?

20. A patient has been prescribed a new inhaler that contains 250 doses of medication. The order specifies that the patient is to take "one puff four times a day." How many days will this inhaler last before it becomes empty?

Case Study

Read the scenario and answer the following questions on a separate document.

A mother comes to a family practice office with her 2-year-old daughter and 8-month-old son. She is planning a trip abroad and needs to obtain immunizations for herself and her children before she leaves.

1. The mother and the infant each need to be given an intramuscular immunization. How does choosing a site and giving an intramuscular injection differ in the mother and in the infant?

2. The woman's 2-year-old daughter has an ear infection, and the physician has prescribed eardrops. What should the nurse teach the mother about giving these eardrops to her child?

3. Two days later, the mother brings the infant back to the office because she has developed a high fever. The nurse prepares to give the infant a liquid oral antipyretic and discovers that the dose is 4 mL. How does the nurse measure this medication?

4. The mother wants to add the medication to her baby's bottle. How would the nurse administer this liquid medication to the infant?

CHAPTER 11

Analgesic Drugs

Chapter Review and Examination Preparation

Choose the best answer for each of the following:

b 1. During a marathon, a runner had to drop out after
   20 kilometres because of severe muscle spasms.
   What type of pain is this classified as?
   a. Persistent pain
   b. Somatic pain
   c. Visceral pain
   d. Superficial pain

d 2. A 23-year-old male has been taken to the emergency
   department because of a suspected overdose of morphine tablets. Which drug should the nurse prepare
   to treat the patient's overdose?
   a. meperidine (Demerol)
   b. naproxen sodium (Anaprox)
   c. acetylsalicylic acid (Aspirin)
   d. naloxone hydrochloride

c 3. An anticonvulsant drug has been ordered as part
   of a patient's pain management program. The patient asks, "Do I really need to take this drug? I'm
   here for pain." What is the best response by the
   nurse?
   a. "Yes, this drug will help you sleep."
   b. "No, this drug is for preventing seizures."
   c. "Yes, it helps relieve neuropathic pain."
   d. "No, it only reduces anxiety."

d 4. Moderate to severe pain is best treated with which
   of the following?
   a. Over-the-counter drugs
   b. Opioid antagonists
   c. Benzodiazepines
   d. Opioid analgesics

b,c,e 5. A nurse is preparing to administer an opioid analgesic. Choose the priority assessment(s) the nurse
   must consider before the drug is given.
   (Select all that apply.)
   a. Blood clotting times
   b. The level of pain rated on a scale
   c. Prior analgesic use (time, type, amount, and
      effectiveness)
   d. Dietary history
   e. Allergies

6. A postoperative patient is complaining of a pain
   level of 7 on a scale of 1 to 10. The nurse checks the
   drug prescription and sees that the patient can receive "morphine 6 mg PO q4h," and the patient has
   not had a dose for 8 hours. The drug comes in a 5
   mL unit dose container that is labelled 10 mg/5 mL.
   How many millilitres will the nurse administer to
   the patient? 3 ml

7. A patient is to receive a dose of fentanyl 60 mcg IV
   stat. The drug is available in vials that contain
   50 mcg/mL. How many millilitres will the nurse
   administer for this dose? 1.2 ml

8. Mark the syringe below with the answer you
   obtained for Question 7.

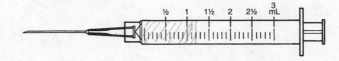

Match each type of pain with its corresponding patient description.

9. ___g___ Acute pain

10. ___f___ Persistent pain

11. ___i___ Somatic pain

12. ___h___ Visceral pain

13. ___d___ Superficial pain

14. ___b___ Vascular pain

15. ___j___ Neuropathic pain

16. ___c___ Phantom pain

17. ___e___ Central pain

a. Mr. Elias is experiencing pain that is due to psychological factors, not physical conditions or disorders.

b. Ms. Yu suggests that she has migraine headache pain.

c. Mrs. Jack feels pain where a body part has been removed.

d. Mr. Ban is experiencing pain originating from the skin and mucous membranes.

e. Mr. Kurt's pain stems from inflammation of the brain following a car accident.

f. Mr. Guramova complains of a recurring, persistent pain that has been treated by several prescribers.

g. An adolescent patient's pain occurred after a fall; the pain subsided following pain treatments.

h. Ms. Oliver's pain originates from the organs and smooth muscles.

i. An older adult feels pain that stems from the skeletal muscles, ligaments, and joints.

j. Several years ago, Mr. Vu was involved in a multi-vehicle accident that damaged his peripheral nerve fibres. He continues to experience pain.

Critical Thinking Crossword

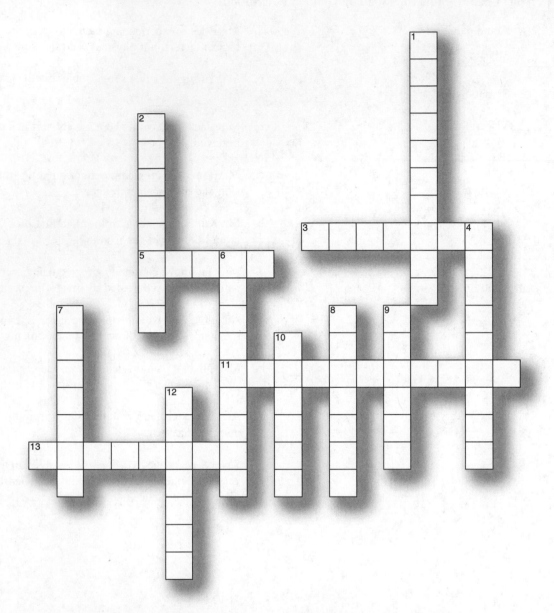

Across

3. Any drug that binds to a receptor and causes a response has _analgesic_ properties.
5. Mrs. Mitchel had breast reduction surgery yesterday and is complaining of pain around her incisions. Mrs. Mitchel is experiencing _acute_ pain.
11. Mrs. Gary is experiencing pain and itching due to a severe exposure to poison ivy on the skin of her arms and legs. She is experiencing _superficial_ pain.

Down

1. The Drug Mr. Dreary is taking binds to a receptor but prevents or blocks a response. He is taking a drug with _antagonist_ properties.
2. When a second drug is given with a primary analgesic to enhance the analgesic effect, the second drug is being used as a(n) _synergistic_ ✗ _adjuvant_ drug.
4. Mr. Polie is receiving an opioid around the clock for late-stage cancer pain. Lately, he has found that the pain drug is not working as well as it did a week ago. This is an example of opioid _tolerance_.
6. The level of stimulus needed to produce a painful sensation is referred to as the pain _threshhold_.

13. Mr. Elliot paces the floor all night, holding his side. The pain is so severe that he is nauseated. His wife brings him to the emergency department, where it is quickly discovered that Mr. Elliot has a kidney stone. The type of pain he has been experiencing is _visceral_ pain.

7. Mr. Justin twisted his ankle in a friendly basketball game with his peers after work. His wife brings him to the urgent care centre several hours later because of the pain. Mr. Justin is probably experiencing _somatic_ pain.

8. Mrs. Harlowe has experienced back pain "for years." She says that it is worse in the late afternoon and "while it's less at night, it is there all the time."

   Mrs. Harlowe is experiencing _chronic_ pain.

9. Mr. Randale is brought to the emergency department in severe pain. The emergency department team recognizes the need to immediately bring the pain under some control. After assessing that it is not contraindicated, the attending physician initiates the administration of a very strong pain reliever. This is no doubt a(n) _opioid_ analgesic.

10. This word is often used interchangeably with the term "opioid." _opiate_

12. Ms. Trundane is taking a drug that binds to part of a receptor and causes effects that are not as strong as those of a pure agonist. She is taking a(n) _partial_ agonist.

Case Study

Read the scenario and answer the following questions on a separate document.

A 52-year-old patient was admitted for surgery to remove a growth from her lower back, just under the skin. That evening she asks for pain drug. Upon assessment, the nurse finds that the patient rates her pain level as "8" and that her pain is located mainly in the immediate area around her incision. The nurse prepares to give her an intravenous dose of morphine sulphate.

1. What type of pain is the patient experiencing?

2. What nonpharmacological intervention may be used to reduce her pain?

3. Within 1 hour of receiving the morphine, the patient complains that her skin feels "itchy," but she cannot see any hives. What does the nurse tell her?

4. What serious adverse effect is possible if the patient receives too much morphine sulphate? What, if anything, can be given to treat this?

5. Two days later patient is ready to be discharged home. Her physician writes a prescription for oxycodone hydrochloride (OxyContin) and acetaminophen (Tylenol). The patient sees the label and asks why she is "also getting Tylenol" for her pain. Explain the purpose of the acetaminophen in her pain treatment.

CHAPTER 12

General and Local Anaesthetics

Chapter Review and Examination Preparation

Choose the best answer for each of the following:

d 1. Which drug classes are used as adjunctive drug with anaesthesia?
   i. Sedative–hypnotics
   ii. Anticonvulsants
   iii. Anticholinergics
   iv. Inhaled gas
   v. Opioid analgesics
   a. i, ii, iii
   b. i, ii, iv
   c. i, iii, iv
   d. i, iii, v

b 2. The nurse is preparing lidocaine. What type of anaesthesia can the nurse expect?
   a. Spinal anaesthesia
   b. Local anaesthesia
   c. Intravenous anaesthesia
   d. General anaesthesia

a 3. The patient's medication treatment includes a neuromuscular blocking drug (NMBD). What priority concern should the nurse monitor when a patient is on this treatment?
   a. Respiratory arrest
   b. Headache
   c. Bradycardia
   d. Hypertension

b 4. To decrease the possibility of a headache after spinal anaesthesia, what will the nurse instruct the patient to do?
   a. Sit in high Fowler position.
   b. Maintain strict bedrest.
   c. Limit fluids.
   d. Walk in the hall several times a day.

b,c,e 5. The nurse is reviewing the institutional policy for local anaesthesia. What procedures are most appropriate for this type of anaesthesia? (Select all that apply.)
   a. Cardioversions
   b. Suturing skin lacerations
   c. Diagnostic procedures
   d. Long-duration surgery
   e. Dental procedures

c 6. The nurse suspects malignant hyperthermia in a patient. What clinical manifestation can the nurse expect in this patient?
   a. Normal temperature change after surgery
   b. Sudden decrease in blood pressure
   c. Sudden elevation in temperature following surgery
   d. Rapid heart rate elevation followed by a decrease in temperature

c *d* 7. During a procedure, the nurse is monitoring a patient who has received dexmedetomidine (Precedex) for moderate sedation. The nurse will observe for which potential adverse effect?
   a. Respiratory depression
   b. Tachycardia
   c. Dizziness
   d. Hypotension

8. A patient is receiving an NMBD. Indicate the order in which the following areas become paralyzed once this drug is given (1 = first, 3 = last).

   a. ____2____ Limbs, neck, trunk muscles

   b. ____3____ Intercostal muscles and diaphragm

   c. ____1____ Small, rapidly moving muscles, such as those of the fingers and eyes

54

Critical Thinking and Application

Answer the following questions on a separate document.

9. Henry is a student nurse who has assisted the anaesthesiologist in surgery on prior occasions. Today, however, he is nervous because it is a child who will undergo general anaesthesia. Why might this make Henry more nervous than usual?

10. Udonis is being administered an NMBD while he is receiving mechanical ventilation. What priority assessment should the nurse constantly monitor while the patient is on NMBD treatment?

11. Angie will undergo cardioversion this afternoon, and the anaesthesiologist has explained to her that she will not be asleep but that she will not remember the procedure. Angie asks the nurse, "How can this be?" What is the nurse's explanation?

12. A patient is in the emergency department because he accidentally put a nail into his arm with a nail gun. The emergency provider requests "lidocaine with epinephrine," but the only type of lidocaine available in the supply cart is "plain" lidocaine. What is the difference, and why does it matter which one is used?

Critical Thinking Crossword

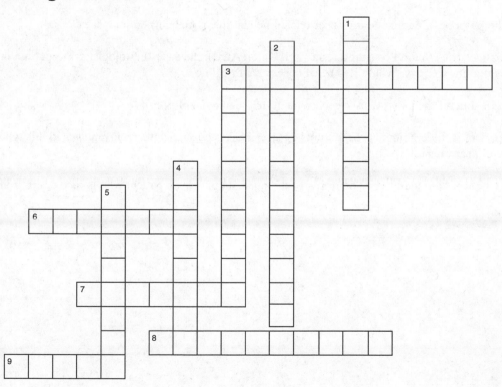

Across

3. A commonly used long-acting, nondepolarizing NMBD *Pancuronium*

6. _____*general*_____ anaesthetic drugs alter the central nervous system (CNS), resulting in loss of consciousness and deep muscle relaxation.

7. _____*local x topical*_____ anaesthetics are applied directly to the skin and mucous membranes.

Down

1. An anticholinergic drug given preoperatively to dry secretions   *Atropine*

2. A broad term for drugs that depress the CNS   *anaesthetics*

3. Anaesthetics administered directly into the CNS by various spinal injection techniques are examples of

_____*parenteral*_____ anaesthetics.

8. Drugs used in combination with anaesthetic drugs to control the adverse effects of ___adjunctive___ anaesthetics

9. Drugs that render a specific portion of the body insensitive to pain without affecting consciousness are called ___procedural X local___ anaesthetics.

4. ___balanced___ anaesthesia is the practice of using combinations of drugs, rather than a single drug, to produce general anaesthesia.

5. Another name for 9 across ___regional___

Case Study

Read the scenario and answer the following questions on a separate document.

You are a nursing student, and today you are assigned to an observation day in the operating room, with the anaesthesiologist as your contact for the day. The first case is a patient undergoing a right lower lung lobectomy to treat lung cancer. The patient has a history of paraplegia from an old automobile accident. The patient's blood pressure has been maintained at 120/72 mm Hg, and the pulse has ranged from 100 to 110 beats per minute during the surgery. The patient's body temperature has fallen to 35.7°C (96.3°F) after surgery. The patient's respirations have been maintained by ventilator.

1. Before the surgery, the anaesthesiologist explained that the patient would undergo "balanced anaesthesia." What is meant by this term?

2. What is the purpose of administering succinylcholine chloride (Quelicin) during anaesthesia?

3. As your patient goes to the Postanaesthesia Care Unit (PACU), the anaesthesiologist asks you to monitor for signs of succinylcholine toxicity. Would this be of concern at this time?

4. What can be done if the patient has received too much succinylcholine?

5. Another patient is undergoing a procedure using spinal anaesthesia. Are there advantages to this type of anaesthesia over general anaesthesia?

6. In the PACU, what are the priority concerns of the nurse monitoring a patient who is recovering from anaesthesia?

Central Nervous System Depressants and Muscle Relaxants

Chapter Review and Examination Preparation

Choose the best answer for each of the following:

1. A patient informs the nurse, "I am unable to rest. I always feel tense." What is the rationale for utilizing a low-dose hypnotic drug for this patient?
   a. It produces sleep.
   b. It slows the destruction of dopamine.
   c. It prevents nausea and vomiting.
   d. It relaxes the patient.

2. A patient who has been taking a benzodiazepine for 5 weeks has been instructed to stop the medication. What is the best way to discontinue the medication?
   a. Have the patient stop taking the medication immediately.
   b. Plan a gradual reduction in dosage.
   c. Overlap this medication with another medication.
   d. Have the patient take the medication every other day for a number of weeks.

3. A patient will be undergoing a brief surgical procedure to obtain a biopsy specimen from a superficial mass on his arm. What type of barbiturate can the nurse expect to prepare for this patient?
   a. Rapid
   b. Short
   c. Intermediate
   d. Long

4. A patient is brought to the emergency department for overdosing on barbiturates. What priority clinical manifestation must the nurse continue to monitor for this patient?
   a. Tachycardia
   b. Hypertension
   c. Dyspnea
   d. Respiratory arrest

5. A patient with back-muscle spasms is being treated with a skeletal muscle relaxant. What complementary recommendations can the nurse make to this patient to maximize the benefits for the patient?
   i. Rest
   ii. Moist heat
   iii. Physiotherapy
   iv. acetylsalicylic acid
   a. i, ii
   b. i, iii
   c. ii, iii
   d. ii, iv

6. The nurse is providing care for a patient who has accidentally taken an overdose of benzodiazepines. Which drug would be used to treat this patient?
   a. a methamphetamine
   b. a xanthine
   c. flumazenil (Anexate)
   d. naloxone hydrochloride

7. A patient will be receiving the barbiturate phenobarbital as part of treatment for seizures. The nurse assesses the patient's current list of medications. Which medication is known to cause interactions with barbiturates? (Select all that apply.)
   a. Benzodiazepines
   b. Proton pump inhibitors
   c. Oral contraceptives
   d. Anticoagulants
   e. Monoamine oxidase inhibitors (MAOIs)

8. A child will be receiving PO midazolam (Versed) orally (PO) as preoperative sedation. The child weighs 15 kg. The dose ordered is 0.5 mg/kg, and the medication is available as a syrup with a concentration of 2 mg/mL.
   a. What will be the dosage for this child? *7.5 mg*
   b. How much is the PO dose for this child in millilitres?   *3.3 mlx 3.75*

9. A patient is to receive diazepam (Valium) 10 mg twice a day through a percutaneous gastrostomy (PEG) tube. The medication comes as a liquid with a concentration of 5 mg/5 mL. How many millilitres will the nurse administer with each dose?
   10ml

10. Mark the medication cup with the amount of medication the nurse will administer for Question 9.

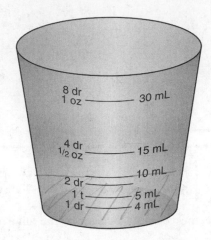

Critical Thinking and Application

Answer the following questions on a separate document.

11. A 19-year-old university student is brought to the emergency department with a suspected barbiturate overdose. What symptoms would the nurse expect to see? How is overdose treated?

12. Jackie is taking benzodiazepines to treat insomnia. Today, she visits the clinic and states that she is going to Europe for 2 months and wants a prescription that will allow her to take enough medication along for her entire stay. The physician declines. She is a little insulted and asks the nurse why the physician refused her request: "Does my doctor think I'm an addict or suicidal or something?" What does the nurse explain to her? What other options are possible for her?

13. Alice is an 81-year-old patient who weighs significantly more than her 47-year-old daughter, yet she is given a lower dose of medication for insomnia of a similar degree. Explain. Is this a dose calculation error?

14. The nurse has been asked to take a history of a patient who will be given a benzodiazepine.

    a. What conditions should the nurse ask about?

    b. What drug intake should the nurse be most concerned about?

    c. What if the patient were an infant? A great-grandfather? Would this additional information matter? Explain.

15. Jerry is recovering from an automobile crash and has received a prescription for cyclobenzaprine hydrochloride (Novo-Cycloprined) for painful muscle spasms.

    a. What should the patient be taught about this drug?

    b. What other measures should be implemented in addition to this drug therapy?

Case Study

Read the scenario and answer the following questions on a separate document.

A 51-year-old woman has had problems with insomnia "off and on for a few years" and has tried over-the-counter medications, natural health products, and prescription drugs. She likes to drink a glass of wine each night before going to bed. Today she is visiting the clinic for a checkup and requests a prescription for lorazepam (Ativan) because that was the last prescription she tried, several years ago. She says she "can't understand" why the pharmacy will not refill her prescriptions for lorazepam. The physician prescribes zopiclone (Imovane) instead.

1. Why did the physician change the patient's prescription?

2. What are the consequences of the long-term use of barbiturates?

3. What interactions should the patient be told about while she is taking zopiclone?

4. What other teachings are important for this patient?

CHAPTER 14

Central Nervous System Stimulants and Related Drugs

Chapter Review and Examination Preparation

Choose the best answer for each of the following:

1. *[handwritten: Xd / C]* A nurse administers a central nervous system (CNS) stimulant medication to a patient. What clinical manifestations can the nurse expect to observe in the patient?
   i. Increased fatigue
   ii. Decreased drowsiness
   iii. Increased respiration
   iv. Bradycardia
   v. Euphoria
   a. i, ii, iv
   b. i, iii, iv
   c. ii, iii, iv
   d. ii, iii, v

2. *[handwritten: Xd / a]* A patient has a history of cardiac dysrhythmias. What beverage or food should this patient avoid?
   i. Coffee
   ii. Tea
   iii. Diet cola
   iv. Lemon water
   v. Chocolate milk
   a. i, ii, v
   b. i, ii, iii
   c. i, ii, iii, iv
   d. i, ii, iii, v

3. *[handwritten: Xa / C]* The nurse administers a serotonin agonist medication (almotriptan malate). What is the desired therapeutic response of this medication?
   a. Controlling attention deficit hyperactivity disorder (ADHD) *[handwritten: amphetamine]*
   b. Reducing systolic pressure in hypertension
   c. Eliminating migraine headaches — *[handwritten: ↓ serotonin]*
   d. Increasing the threshold for narcolepsy
   [handwritten: dextroamphetamine]
   [handwritten: excessive daytime sleepiness]

4. *[handwritten: d]* The physician has ordered orlistat (Xenical). The nurse recognizes that this drug is used to treat which of the following?
   a. Anorexia
   b. Malnutrition
   c. Narcolepsy
   d. Obesity

5. *[handwritten: atomoxetine, modafinil]* *[handwritten: X C / b ?]* A 7-year-old child is prescribed medication to help manage ADHD. What priority instructions should the nurse give the child's caregivers?
   [handwritten: monitor moods, behaviors thoughts, feelings]
   a. Reduce blood glucose and cholesterol levels.
   b. Monitor physical growth and weight.
   c. Record grades and behaviour at school.
   d. Maintain respiratory and heart rates.

6. *[handwritten: X b, c, e]* A patient with migraine headaches is being evaluated. One potential treatment is ergotamine tablets. The nurse notes that the patient has the following conditions. Which would be a contraindication to the use of ergotamine? (Select all that apply.)
   a. Asthma   *[handwritten: cerebral, cardiac, peripheral vascular disease]*
   b. Hypertension   *[handwritten: dysrhythmias]*
   c. Glaucoma
   d. Diabetes mellitus
   e. Coronary heart disease

7. *[handwritten: b, d + c]* A patient will be taking sumatriptan (Imitrex) as part of treatment for migraine headaches. Before beginning therapy, the nurse reviews the patient's current list of medications. Which of the following medications may have an interaction with sumatriptan? (Select all that apply.)
   a. Opioids
   b. Ergot alkaloids
   c. Selective serotonin reuptake inhibitors
   d. Monoamine oxidase inhibitors
   e. Nonsteroidal anti-inflammatory drugs

60

8. A child will be taking amphetamine/dextroamphetamine (Adderall) for ADHD. He weighs 39.6 kg, and the initial dosage ordered is 2.5 mg/kg daily. How many milligrams will the nurse administer with each dose? ___99 mg___

9. The prescriber orders a medication "0.5 mg/kg IV STAT." The patient weighs 74.25 kg. How much medication will the patient receive? ___37.1 mg___

Critical Thinking and Application

Answer the following questions on a separate document.

10. Riley, aged 31 years, informs the health care provider that she falls asleep unexpectedly at work. She also indicates that she even falls asleep at her church and during social events.

    a. What health condition does Riley have?

    b. What might be the drug of choice for Riley? Describe the therapeutic effects of each drug.

    c. Develop a patient teaching plan for Riley. Offer guidelines for (i) dosage alterations and (ii) substances she might be wise to avoid.

11. George, a 14-year-old student, has been taking a medication for ADHD for 6 months. At today's follow-up visit, the physician suggests that George take a "drug holiday" on the weekends and during the school's spring break. Explain the reasoning behind "drug holidays."

Case Study

Read the scenario and answer the following questions on a separate document.

Nancy, a 44-year-old accountant, has had an increasing number of headaches in the past year. When she has these headaches, she often is nauseated and vomits. She has been to her physician, who has ordered several diagnostic tests. As a result, Nancy has been diagnosed with migraine headaches and will be given a prescription for a serotonin agonist.

1. How do serotonin agonists work in the treatment of migraine headaches?

2. What dosage form(s) would be helpful for Nancy's situation?

3. If the physician decides to write a prescription for sumatriptan succinate (Imitrex DF), Nancy's history should be assessed for which conditions?

4. What foods may be associated with the development of migraine headaches?

5. What else should be included in the therapy for Nancy's migraine headaches?

CHAPTER 15

Antiepileptic Drugs

Chapter Review and Examination Preparation

Choose the best answer for each of the following:

1. A patient is experiencing temporary lapses in consciousness that last only a few seconds. Her teachers have said that she "daydreams too much." What type of seizure can this be classified as?
   a. Simple
   b. Complex
   c. Partial
   d. Generalized

2. Which condition is a life-threatening emergency in which patients typically do not regain consciousness?
   a. Status epilepticus
   b. Tonic–clonic convulsions
   c. Epilepsy
   d. Primary epilepsy

3. Which of the following is true about the intravenous infusion of phenytoin (Dilantin)? (Select all that apply.)
   i. Phenytoin is injected quickly.
   ii. Phenytoin is injected slowly.
   iii. The injection of phenytoin is followed by an injection of sterile saline.
   iv. Phenytoin must not be infused continuously.
   v. Phenytoin is mixed with D_5W (5% dextrose and water) for the infusion.
   a. i, ii, iii
   b. i, ii, iv
   c. ii, iii, iv
   d. ii, iii, v

4. The nurse administers phenobarbital to a patient. What priority clinical manifestation should the nurse monitor as a possible adverse effect of this therapy?
   a. Constipation
   b. Gingival hyperplasia
   c. Drowsiness
   d. Dysrhythmias

5. A patient with a history of epilepsy experiences status epilepticus. What medication can the nurse expect to prepare for this condition?
   a. phenobarbital
   b. diazepam (Valium)
   c. valproic acid (Depakene)
   d. phenytoin (Dilantin)

6. A patient who is experiencing neuropathic pain tells the nurse that the physician is going to start him on a new medication that is generally used to treat seizures. The nurse anticipates that which drug will be ordered?
   a. phenobarbital
   b. phenytoin (Dilantin)
   c. gabapentin (Neurontin)
   d. lamotrigine (Lamictal)

7. Phenytoin (Dilantin) is prescribed for a patient. The nurse checks the patient's current list of medications and notes that interactions may occur with which drugs or drug classes? (Select all that apply.)
   a. Loop diuretics
   b. warfarin (Coumadin)
   c. Sulphonamide antibiotics
   d. Corticosteroids
   e. Oral contraceptives

8. A patient is unable to take oral medications and has received a loading dose of phenytoin (Dilantin) intravenously. The orders call for him to receive phenytoin 5 mg/kg per day in three divided doses. The medication comes in a vial containing 50 mg/mL. The patient weighs 90 kg.
   a. How many milligrams will the patient receive each day? For each dose? _____
   b. How many millilitres of medication will be drawn up for each dose? _____

9. Indicate on the syringe the amount of medication the nurse will draw up for each dose of the medication in Question 8.

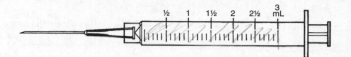

Critical Thinking and Application

Answer the following questions on a separate document.

10. Autoinduction is an important concept to consider when selecting treatment for patients. Describe autoinduction, and name one antiepileptic drug that undergoes this process.

11. Jay, an 8-year-old boy, has resisted his oral doses of topiramate (Topamax), which has made adherence to the drug regimen difficult. His mother calls and says that she has found a way to get him to take it: she crushes the tablet and sprinkles it on flavoured gelatin. How should the nurse respond?

Critical Thinking Crossword

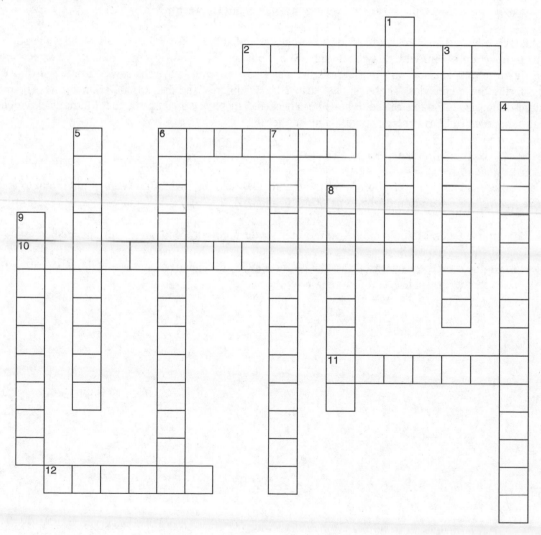

Across

2. Status epilepticus is considered a life-threatening
   _____ *emergency*

6. A type of epilepsy with an unknown cause. *primary*
10. A potentially fatal adverse effect of valproic acid
    (Depakene). *respiratory arrest* X *hepatotoxicity*
11. A brief episode of abnormal electrical activity in the
    nerve cells of the brain. *seizure*
12. Intravenously administered antiepileptic drugs
    should be delivered in this way to avoid serious
    adverse effects. *slowly*

Down

1. A type of epilepsy with a distinct cause. *secondary*
3. An involuntary spasmodic contraction of muscles
   throughout the body. *generalized seizure* X *convulsion*
4. Drugs that are considered first-line drugs for the
   treatment of status epilepticus. *benzodiazepines*
5. Another term for 6 Across. *idiopathic*
6. A barbiturate used primarily to control tonic–clonic
   and partial seizures. *phenobarbital*
7. The metabolic process that occurs when the metabolism of a drug increases over time, leading to lower-
   than-expected drug concentrations. *autoinduction*
8. Recurrent episodes of convulsive seizures. *epilepsy*
9. A first-line antiepileptic drug, the long-term use of
   which can cause gingival hyperplasia. *phenytoin*

Case Study

Read the scenario and answer the following questions on a separate document.

Four-year-old Mattie has started preschool. Today, the teacher called Mattie's mother to tell her that she noticed that Mattie seems to have a problem with "daydreaming." She explained that Mattie seemed inattentive during group work and was staring out into space several times a day. She was also worried because she saw Mattie's eyes move back and forth rapidly during these episodes. These "spells" lasted 1 to 2 minutes, and then Mattie seemed fine. The mother has brought Mattie to the pediatrician's office to have her checked. The physician suspects that Mattie is experiencing a type of seizure disorder and has ordered some diagnostic testing.

1. What type of seizure is Mattie experiencing?

2. Mattie's mother is given a prescription for a liquid antiepileptic drug for Mattie. What is important to teach the mother regarding administration of this type of medication?

3. What will the nurse teach Mattie's mother to monitor for during Mattie's therapy with this medication?

4. After a year, Mattie's mother is pleased that the seizures have "disappeared" and wants to take Mattie off the medication. What is the best response in this situation by the nurse?

CHAPTER 16

Antiparkinsonian Drugs

Chapter Review and Examination Preparation

Choose the best answer for each of the following:

1. A patient with Parkinson's disease exhibits difficulty performing voluntary movements. When documenting the patient's symptoms, what term should the nurse use to accurately describe this symptom? *d x* *b*
   a. Akinesia
   b. Dyskinesia
   c. Chorea
   d. Dystonia — *muscles contract uncontrollably*

2. Which drug may be used early in the treatment of Parkinson's disease but eventually loses effectiveness and must be replaced by another drug? *a*
   a. amantadine hydrochloride
   b. carbidopa/levodopa (Sinemet)
   c. selegiline hydrochloride
   d. entacapone (Comtan)

3. Carbidopa-levodopa therapy was initiated for a patient with Parkinson's disease. What priority instructions should the nurse give the patient concerning vitamin supplements? *c*
   a. Vitamin supplements should not be taken at this time, since the patient has increased intercellular reserves.
   b. Vitamin supplements should be taken twice a day to ensure that the patient receives enough nutrients.
   c. The patient should avoid supplements that contain vitamin B$_6$ (pyridoxine).
   d. The patient should not take more than the recommended amount of calcium.

4. A patient who is newly diagnosed with Parkinson's disease and beginning medication therapy with entacapone (Comtan), a catechol-ortho-methyltransferase (COMT) inhibitor, asks the nurse, "How soon will improvement occur?" What is the nurse's best response? *d x c*
   a. "That varies from patient to patient concerning the therapeutic response."
   b. "You should discuss that with your physician."
   c. "You should notice a difference right away."
   d. "This may take several weeks before you notice any degree of improvement."

5. A patient with Parkinson's disease is prescribed an anticholinergic drug in addition to the antiparkinsonian drug. What clinical condition does the anticholinergic drug aim to control or minimize? (Select all that apply.) *b*
   i. Drooling
   ii. Constipation
   iii. Muscle rigidity
   iv. Bradykinesia
   v. Dry mouth
   a. a, b
   b. a, c
   c. a, d
   d. a, e

6. The nurse is providing information to a patient undergoing COMT inhibitor therapy. What symptom should the nurse teach the patient to monitor as a common adverse effect of this therapy? *a x* *b*
   a. Dizziness
   b. Urine discolouration
   c. Leg edema
   d. Visual changes

7. Carbidopa/levodopa (Sinemet) is prescribed for a patient with Parkinson's disease. What priority adverse effects should the nurse tell the patient to monitor closely? (Select all that apply.) *b,c,e*
   a
   a. Palpitations
   b. Insomnia → *dopamine modulator*
   c. Hypotension
   d. Urinary frequency *retention*
   e. Gastro-intestinal distress *dyskinesia*

8. The medication order reads, "Give benztropine 2.5 mg PO every morning." The medication is available in 1 mg tablets. How many tablets will the nurse administer? ___*2.5 tablets*___

Critical Thinking and Application

Answer the following questions on a separate document.

9. Howard is on a carbidopa/levodopa/entacapone (Stalevo) treatment regimen.

   a. What are the advantages of combining the three drugs in Howard's treatment regimen? Are there any disadvantages?

   b. What problems are avoided when carbidopa is given with levodopa?

   c. How does carbidopa work to avoid the problems in question b, above?

10. Hayley is a 35-year-old new mother who experiences slowing movements, cogwheel rigidity, and pill-rolling tremor. She has been diagnosed with Parkinson's disease, a somewhat rare occurrence in someone her age. In addition to the usual history questions, what must the nurse ask in anticipation of dopaminergic therapy in Hayley's specific situation?

11. Sharon is a 45-year-old patient taking benztropine mesylate along with a dopaminergic drug for Parkinson's disease. Her 76-year-old neighbour comments that he cannot take benztropine because it is too risky for his heart and kidneys. Sharon phones and asks why this is not a concern in her case. How should the nurse answer Sharon?

Case Study

Read the scenario and answer the following questions on a separate document.

Adam is a 54-year-old man who was diagnosed with Parkinson's disease and is about to start drug therapy. His symptoms are mild, yet he has some akinesia that interferes with his ability to type at work. The physician explains that Adam may have to take a variety of drugs as the disease progresses.

1. What is the underlying pathological defect of Parkinson's disease?

2. What is the aim of drug therapy for Parkinson's disease?

3. The first drug prescribed for Adam is amantadine hydrochloride, to be taken along with levodopa/carbidopa (Sinemet CR). What is the purpose of his taking amantadine at this time?

4. Adam is informed by the prescriber that amantadine will need to be changed after the early stages. Explain.

5. How does the carbidopa affect the "on-off phenomenon" that may occur with the use of levodopa?

CHAPTER 17

Psychotherapeutic Drugs

Chapter Review and Examination Preparation

Choose the best answer for each of the following:

b 1. A patient is on clozapine (Clozaril) therapy for 2 months. What beverage(s) should the nurse instruct the patient to avoid?
   i. Grapefruit juice
   ii. Apple juice
   iii. Cola
   iv. Caffeinated tea
   v. Fruit mix beverage of apple, mango, and grapefruit
   a. i, ii
   b. i, v
   c. iii, iv
   d. iii, v

a, c, d 2. The nurse is administering clozapine (Clozaril).
b, c What long-term monitoring that is associated with this medication should the nurse prioritize? (*Select all that apply*)
   a. Mood swings
   b. Agranulocytosis
   c. Weight gain
   d. Postural hypotension

b 3. A patient is on selective serotonin reuptake inhibitor
c medication therapy. What possible adverse effect should the nurse instruct the family to monitor as a priority?
   a. Visual disturbances
   b. Tardive dyskinesia
   c. Suicidal thoughts
   d. Bleeding tendencies

c 4. The caregiver of a patient who has started on antidepressant therapy asks the nurse, "How long will it take for him to feel better?" What is the best response by the nurse?
   a. "Well, depression rarely responds to medication therapy."
   b. "He should be feeling better in a few days."
   c. "It may take 4 to 6 weeks before you see an improvement."
   d. "You may not see any effects for several months."

a, c, d 5. A patient was started on an antipsychotic drug that results in extrapyramidal effects. What clinical manifestations should the nurse monitor for? (Select all that apply.)
   a. Tremors *akathisia* *pseudoparkinsonism*
   b. Elation and a sense of well-being *acute dystonia* *tardive dyskinesia*
   c. Painful muscle spasms
   d. Motor restlessness
   e. Bradycardia

c 6. A patient has been taking antipsychotic medication for years, and his wife has noticed that he has had some new physical symptoms. She describes him as having odd facial movements, sticking out his tongue, and having movements of his arms that he cannot seem to control. The nurse suspects that the patient is exhibiting signs of which condition?
   a. Hypomania
   b. Serotonin syndrome
   c. Tardive dyskinesia
   d. Neuroleptic malignant syndrome

7. A patient will be receiving benztropine mesylate 1.5 mg PO daily. The medication comes in 0.5 mg tablets. How many tablets will the nurse administer per dose? _____3_____

8. A patient is to receive lithium carbonate 1800 mg per day in two divided doses. The medication is available in 300 mg capsules. How many milligrams of lithium will the patient receive for each dose? _900 mg_

How many capsules per dose? ___3___

Match each term with its corresponding definition or description.

9. _l_ buspirone

10. _f_ Tyramine

11. _c xg_ Tricyclics

12. _b X o_ Psychosis

13. _o X b_ Mania

14. _i_ diazepam (Valium)

15. _j_ amitriptyline (Elavil)

16. _k_ risperidone (Risperdal)

17. _c_ Benzodiazepines

18. _n_ lithium

19. _a_ Anxiety

20. _d_ Affective disorders

21. _h_ Depression

22. _e_ Bipolar affective disorder

23. _m_ Extrapyramidal

a. The unpleasant state of mind in which real or imagined dangers are anticipated or exaggerated or both

b. A state characterized by an expansive emotional state (including symptoms of extreme excitement and elation) and hyperactivity

c. A group of psychotropic drugs prescribed to alleviate anxiety

d. Emotional disorders characterized by changes in mood

e. A major psychological disorder, characterized by episodes of mania or hypomania, cycling with depression

f. Patients taking monoamine oxidase inhibitors (MAOIs) need to be taught to avoid foods that contain this substance.

g. An older class of antidepressant drugs

h. An abnormal emotional state characterized by exaggerated feelings of sadness, melancholy, and worthlessness out of proportion to reality

i. A long-acting benzodiazepine

j. The most widely used tricyclic antidepressant

k. An atypical antipsychotic drug used to treat schizophrenia

l. A nonbenzodiazepine drug used to treat anxiety

m. Term for the symptoms or adverse effects that often occur with antipsychotic medications

n. Medication used to treat mania

o. A type of serious mental illness that can take several different forms and is associated with being truly out of touch with reality

Critical Thinking and Application

Answer the following questions on a separate document.

24. Carl, a 26-year-old unemployed electrician, is brought to the emergency department by his sister. He is extremely drowsy and confused, and his breathing is slow and shallow. The sister tells the nurse that Carl has been seeing a psychiatrist for his "anxiety" and that he "takes pills" for his anxiety.

    a. Considering his health status and history, what do you suggest is wrong with this patient?

    b. How will he likely be treated?

25. David is a 49-year-old restaurant owner who was just prescribed the MAOI phenelzine sulphate. After the prescriber leaves the room but before the nurse has a chance to discuss David's medication regimen with him, David turns to his wife and says, "I'm sure this medicine will work. Let's have a bottle of wine tonight and watch television."

    a. What priority health instructions should the nurse give David?

    b. A few weeks later, David is brought to the emergency department with a severe headache, stiff neck, sweating, and elevated blood pressure. His wife says his symptoms started a few minutes after they ate at their restaurant. What is wrong with David, and what probably caused it?

26. Brian has been diagnosed with depression. Why might the physician prescribe a second-generation antidepressant instead of a first-generation antidepressant?

27. A young adult has been admitted to the emergency department with a suspected overdose of a tricyclic antidepressant. What is the rationale for closely monitoring his cardiac status?

Case Study

Read the scenario and answer the following questions on a separate document.

George, a 38-year-old businessperson, mentions during a checkup that he has felt anxious and upset over the past few months. He discusses the pressures of his business and states that he has had trouble sleeping at night, which makes him more irritable. Lately, he has been worried over a contract proposal that will take place in a few months. The physician gives him a prescription for alprazolam (Xanax) 0.25 mg three times a day.

1. George is concerned about the potential adverse effects of this medication. What should the nurse tell him?

2. What other measures should be taken for George at this time?

3. After 3 months, George is back in the office for a follow-up appointment. He is upset because a friend told him about another friend who was on the same medication but who died due to an overdose. George wants to stop taking alprazolam immediately. Is this recommended? If not, why not?

4. What are the symptoms of alprazolam overdose, and what is the antidote, if any?

5. Six months later, George is no longer taking alprazolam but comes back to the office because he still feels anxious. The physician gives him a prescription for buspirone hydrochloride. George questions why he is given a different drug. What are the advantages, if any, of his taking buspirone instead of alprazolam?

CHAPTER 18

Substance Misuse

Chapter Review and Examination Preparation

Choose the best answer for each of the following:

a, b, c, d, f   *acetaldehyde syndrome*

1. A patient who has been taking disulfiram (Antabuse) for 3 months has been off the therapy for 2 days. The patient decides to go out with friends to have a beer. What effects may he experience? (Select all that apply.) *pulsating*
   CNS throbbing head & neck, headache
   a. Diaphoresis *marked uneasiness, weakness, vertigo*
   b. Diarrhea *blurred vision, confusion*
   GI c. Vomiting *N, thirst*
   d. Euphoria
   e. Drowsiness
   CVS
   f. Facial flushing *vasodilation, orthostatic syncope,*
   chest pain

x b 2. When conducting a health teaching session about drug abuse, what information should the nurse provide concerning the most common manifestation of *d* opioid abuse?
   a. Hallucinations and fear
   b. Sleep and lethargy
   c. Stimulation and anxiety
   d. Relaxation and euphoria

c, e 3. The nurse is assisting a patient who is experiencing *t b* opioid withdrawal. The nurse anticipates the possible use of which medications? (Select all that apply.)
   a. disulfiram (Antabuse)— *alcohol abuse treatment*
   b. clonidine (Catapres)
   c. Methadone
   d. bupropion (Zyban)
   e. Naltrexone

a x 4. What condition that can lead to death may result *c* from the interactions of benzodiazepines with ethanol or barbiturates? *sedative*
   a. Cardiac dysrhythmia
   b. Convulsions
   c. Respiratory arrest
   d. Stroke

b 5. A patient with a known history of chronic excessive ingestion of ethanol has developed memory problems and comes to the health clinic with hard-to-believe stories of what has happened to him. The nurse recognizes that these symptoms are associated with which disorder?
   a. Cerebrovascular accident
   b. Korsakoff's psychosis
   c. Narcolepsy
   d. Bipolar disorder

6. A patient is to receive flumazenil 0.2 mg IV push over 30 seconds as initial treatment for a possible benzodiazepine overdose. The medication is available in a 0.1 mg/mL vial. How many millilitres of medication will the nurse draw up into the syringe for this dose? _____ *2 ml*

Match each drug with its corresponding description.

7. ___*h*___ cocaine

8. ___*i*___ methamphetamine

9. ___*b x f*___ ecstasy

10. _____ heroin *c*

a. A nicotine-free treatment for nicotine dependence

b. A drug known as the "date rape drug"

c. The source plant for heroin

d. The addictive chemical in tobacco products

11. _____g_____ disulfiram (Antabuse)

12. _____d_____ nicotine

13. _____a ×__ i__ naltrexone

14. _____j__ × a__ bupropion (Zyban)

15. _____c_____ opium

16. _____b_____ roofies—flunitrazepam treat severe insomnia

e. An opioid that is injected by "mainlining" or "skin popping"

f. A drug usually prepared in home laboratories and known for its popularity at all-night parties, such as raves— large dancing party

g. A medication that is used to deter the use of alcohol during alcohol dependence treatment

h. A stimulant that is either "snorted" through the nasal passages or injected intravenously

i. A substance commonly manufactured from the over-the-counter decongestant pseudoephedrine

j. An opioid antagonist used for opioid misuse or dependence

Critical Thinking and Application

Answer the following questions on a separate document.

17. How is nicotine used to ease withdrawal from nicotine use? How is bupropion (Zyban) used in smoking cessation programs?

18. How is medication therapy different for mild, moderate, and severe alcohol withdrawal?

19. A woman brings her teenage daughter into the emergency department. The teen is lethargic, dizzy, and has been vomiting. While the teen is being examined and stabilized, the mother tells the nurse that her daughter told her that she and her friends used cough syrup to get high. The mother states, "How could cough syrup do this?" What is the nurse's best answer?

Case Study

Read the scenario and answer the following questions on a separate document.

Fahim, a 21-year-old male, is admitted to the emergency department after he collapsed at a party. The paramedics state that there were beer-drinking contests at the party, and it is unknown how much Fahim had ingested. His friend says that Fahim was upset over losing his girlfriend, and he was worried about how heavily Fahim has been drinking in the past 2 weeks. Fahim is semiconscious and unable to answer questions coherently, and his speech is slurred. His blood pressure is 100/58 mm Hg, his pulse rate is 110 beats per minute, and his breathing is heavy, with a respiratory rate of 16 breaths per minute. He vomited on the way to the hospital.

1. Is ethanol considered a central nervous system stimulant or depressant?

2. What are the effects of severe alcoholic intoxication on the cardiovascular and respiratory systems?

3. Fahim is admitted to the medical unit for observation. What should the nurse monitor at this time?

4. The next evening Fahim is more alert but still unsteady with his gait. He says he wants to go home, but the nurse notices fine tremors of his hands. Should he be discharged at this time? Explain.

5. If Fahim continues his pattern of heavy drinking, what effects could the chronic ingestion of ethanol have on his body?

CHAPTER 19

Adrenergic Drugs

Chapter Review and Examination Preparation

Choose the best answer for each of the following.

d 1. What is a synonymous term for adrenergic drugs?
   a. Anticholinergic drugs
   b. Parasympathetic drugs
   c. Central nervous system drugs
   d. Sympathomimetic drugs

a,c,d
b,d 2. When administering adrenergic drugs, what possible effect should the nurse monitor for? (Select all that apply.) *CNS—HA, restlessness, tremors, nervousness, dizziness,*
   a. Urinary retention *insomnia, euphoria. CNS— chest pain,*
   b. ? Hypotension *hypertension vasoconstriction, tachycardia,*
   c. Decreased respiratory rate *fluctuations in BP, palpitations,*
   d. Increased heart rate *dysrhythmias*
   anorexia dry mouth, nausea, vomiting,
   taste changes (rare) sweating, muscle cramps

a,b,d 3. The nurse is aware that adrenergic drugs may be used to treat which of the following conditions? (Select all that apply.)
   a. Asthma
   b. Open-angle glaucoma
   c. Hypertension
   d. Nasal congestion
   e. Seizures
   f. Nausea and vomiting

a 4. A patient has an allergy to bees. What medication should the patient have at all times to address an allergic reaction?
   a. epinephrine
   b. formoterol fumarate dihydrate
   c. phenylephrine (Neo-Synephrine)
   d. norepinephrine (Levophed)

c 5. A 13-year-old adolescent has a positive history of asthma. Today, her physician wants to start salmeterol xinafoate administered via inhaler. What priority health instructions must the nurse provide when teaching the patient and the family about the pharmacokinetics of this medication?
   a. "It should be taken at the first sign of an asthma attack; this will help you breathe better immediately."
   b. "The dosage is two puffs every 4 hours; this should also be supplemented with one puff during attacks."
   c. "Don't use this for an asthma attack; it is supposed to help with long-term management of your symptoms."
   d. "Be sure to use your steroid inhaler first; this medication complements the relief of asthma attacks."

a,b,e 6. The nurse is reviewing the medication orders of a newly admitted patient who has an infusion of the adrenergic drug dopamine. Which of these drugs may cause an adverse interaction? (Select all that apply.)
   a. Tricyclic antidepressants
   b. Monoamine oxidase inhibitors
   c. Anticoagulants
   d. Corticosteroids
   e. Antihistamines

7. An infant is having an allergic reaction and is to receive two doses of epinephrine 10 mcg/kg subcutaneously. The infant weighs 5 kg. How many micrograms of medication will the infant receive with each dose? *25× 50*

8. The nurse is to administer epinephrine 0.5 mg subcutaneously. The ampule contains 1 mL of medication and is labelled "Epinephrine 1:1000." How many millilitres of epinephrine will the nurse give?
   0.0005 ml × 0.5ml

   1 g per /1000 ml

Critical Thinking and Application

Answer the following questions on a separate document.

9. The father of a 3-year-old is giving the child phenylephrine (Neo-Synephrine) drops as a nasal decongestant.

   a. How does this medication help with nasal congestion?

   b. The child's father comes back to the clinic and complains that after a week his child's congestion is worse, not better. What possible explanation can the nurse offer?

10. Luke has had a history of problems with a hormonal imbalance (secondary to pheochromocytoma). He has been admitted for septic shock, and the physician prescribes dopamine. Upon checking the patient's history, the nurse questions the prescription. What possible contraindication of dopamine is the nurse's priority concern?

11. Graham and Connor are both on dopamine infusions. Graham's infusion is at a low infusion rate, and Connor's is at a high infusion rate. Why might these infusion rates be different?

12. A patient in the critical care unit (CCU) received a dose of epinephrine that is too high. What effects of the drugs should the nurse monitor for? What should the nurse expect to do for this patient?

13. Derryl is a 49-year-old construction worker who presents in the urgent care centre for treatment of a leg laceration. Just after receiving an intravenous antibiotic, he starts to wheeze and says, "Oh, I just remembered. I'm allergic to penicillin!"

    a. What is happening?

    b. What should the nurse do first?

    c. What drug do you think will be given in this situation?

Case Study

Read the scenario and answer the following questions on a separate document.

Sixteen-year-old Maureen, who plays soccer on her high-school team, has been treated for asthma for a year. Her symptoms have been controlled with an inhaled steroid and occasional use of a salbutamol metered dose inhaler. This afternoon, though, her mother brings her into the Urgent Care Centre because Maureen has had trouble "getting her breath" after a particularly rough game. Maureen complains of a feeling of "tightness" in her chest and wants to sit up. She appears anxious and has a nonproductive cough. Her respiratory rate is 28 breaths per minute, and her peak expiratory flow is 70% of normal. Chest auscultation reveals a short inspiratory period with prolonged expiratory wheezing in both lungs.

1. The physician orders salbutamol via nebulizer. What should the nurse assess before, during, and after giving this medication?

2. Why is salbutamol given via inhalation rather than orally?

3. After the nebulizer medication treatment is completed, Maureen complains of feeling "shaky and jittery." What does the nurse tell her?

4. The physician gives Maureen a prescription for a salmeterol xinafoate inhaler. What is important to teach Maureen and her mother about this medication?

CHAPTER 20

Adrenergic-Blocking Drugs

Chapter Review and Examination Preparation

Choose the best answer for each of the following:

a,b
+d 1. What physiological effect(s) can the nurse expect to find in patients taking an adrenergic blockade (interacting at the site of α-adrenergic receptors)? (Select all that apply.)
   a. Vasodilation
   b. Decreased blood pressure
   c. Increased blood pressure *orthostatic hypotension*
   d. Constriction of the pupils *edema,*
   e. Tachycardia

x d 2. The nurse discovers that the intravenous infusion of
a a patient who has been receiving an intravenous vasopressor has infiltrated. The nurse will expect which drug to be used to reverse the effects of the vasopressor in the infiltrated area? *IMIV*
   a. phentolamine mesylate (Rogitine) *— treat HTN*
   b. prazosin hydrochloride (Minipress) *— treat BPH* *PO*
   c. bisoprolol fumarate *PO*
   d. metoprolol tartrate *— β-blocker, treat HTN, angina, MI* *PO, IV*

d 3. A patient has a new prescription for a beta-blocker as part of treatment for hypertension. What specific health instruction concerning drug interactions must the nurse give the patient?
   a. Allow 2 hours before taking thyroid medications.
   b. Stop taking any antibiotic while on this medication.
   c. Avoid caffeinated products.
   d. Do not ingest any alcohol-containing substances.

b 4. A patient has been given an alpha-blocker as treatment for benign prostatic hyperplasia. Which instruction is important for the nurse to include when teaching the patient about the effects of this medication?
   a. Avoid foods and drinks that contain caffeine.
   b. Change to sitting or standing positions slowly to avoid a sudden drop in blood pressure.
   c. Watch for a weight loss of 9 kg within a week.
   d. Take extra supplements of calcium.

d 5. A patient who has been taking a beta-blocker for almost 6 months tells the nurse that she wants to stop taking this medication. What is the nurse's best response to the patient?
   a. "There are no ill effects if this medication is stopped."
   b. "There should be only minimal effects if you stop taking this medication."
   c. "You may experience orthostatic hypotension if you stop this medication abruptly."
   d. "If you stop this medication suddenly, there is a possibility you may experience chest pain or rebound hypertension."

C 6. A patient has been taking tamsulosin (Flomax) for about a year. During today's office visit, he asks the nurse about taking a drug for erectile dysfunction. How should the nurse respond?
   a. "These drugs are safe to take together; I haven't heard of any interactions."
   b. "You can take them together, but the dosage of the Flomax will need to be reduced."
   c. "Taking these two drugs together may lead to dangerously low blood pressure."
   d. "You will be able to try taking these two drugs together, but watch for adverse effects."

7. An admission order reads, "Start IV of 0.9% normal saline and infuse 1 L over the next 12 hours." To what rate will the nurse set the infusion pump?

    83.3 ml/h

8. A patient is to receive labetalol hydrochloride (Trandate) 20 mg IV push over 10 minutes STAT. The medication is available in a vial that contains 5 mg/mL. How many millilitres will the nurse administer for this dose?

    4 ml

Critical Thinking and Application

Answer the following questions on a separate document.

9. Sarah, admitted to a cardiac intensive care unit, is receiving a dopamine intravenous infusion. During the first night, the nurse indicates that Sarah is "fine, vital signs stable, head-to-toe within normal limits." After 4 hours, the nurse observes that the intravenous line has dislodged and the infusion has infiltrated. What could happen as a result? What kind of treatment would you recommend? Describe the unusual injection process and its rationale.

10. Liam has had a myocardial infarction (MI). He is told that he will be prescribed a "cardioprotective drug." He asks the nurse to explain. Why can some beta-blockers be said to "protect" the heart?

11. Anna has been prescribed a beta-blocker. She is about to be released from hospital, but first her nurse gives her instructions on taking her apical pulse for 1 full minute, as well as her blood pressure. Why? What should Anna be looking for? Is there anything she should be instructed to report to her physician?

12. Trevor has a new prescription for tamsulosin (Flomax) because of a new diagnosis of benign prostatic hyperplasia. What concern, if any, is there with this drug? What instructions will he need?

Case Study

Read the scenario and answer the following questions on a separate document.

Bruce, a 58-year-old accountant, is in hospital after experiencing a myocardial infarction (MI). The physician has told him that damage to his heart was minimal, and Bruce has started post-MI rehabilitation and education. Bruce has discussed having to "mend his ways" because, in addition to the MI, he has had asthma for years that has been managed poorly. The physician discusses starting Bruce on a beta-blocker to "protect his heart" and gives him a prescription for atenolol (Tenormin).

1. What type of beta-blocker is appropriate for Bruce, and why?

2. Discuss how atenolol helps in this situation.

3. What adverse effects should Bruce be taught about when this medication is begun?

4. At his 3-month checkup, Bruce tells the nurse that he wants to stop taking the medication. Should this medication be stopped abruptly?

CHAPTER 21

Cholinergic Drugs

Chapter Review and Examination Preparation

Match each definition with its corresponding term. (Not all terms are used.)

1. ___h___ Antidote for overdose of a cholinergic drug

2. ___g___ Cholinergic drugs that act by making more acetylcholine (ACh) available at the receptor site, which allows ACh to bind to and stimulate the receptor

3. ___f___ Cholinergic drugs that bind to cholinergic receptors and activate them

4. ___b___ Receptors located postsynaptically in the effector organs (smooth muscle, cardiac muscle, glands) supplied by the parasympathetic fibres

5. ___i x j___ Receptors located in the ganglia of the parasympathetic nervous system (PSNS) and the sympathetic nervous system (SNS)

6. ___e___ A description of the action of the PSNS

7. ___j x i___ The neurotransmitter responsible for the transmission of nerve impulses to the effector cells in the PSNS

8. ___a___ The enzyme responsible for breaking down ACh

a. cholinesterase

b. muscarinic

c. catecholamine

d. "fight-or-flight"

e. "rest and digest"

f. direct-acting cholinergic drugs

g. indirect-acting cholinergic drugs

h. atropine

i. acetylcholine

j. nicotinic

Choose the best answer for each of the following:

x a 9. The desired effects of cholinergic drugs come from
c   stimulation of which receptors?
    a. Cholinergic
    b. Nicotinic
    c. Muscarinic
    d. Ganglionic

b 10. The undesired effects of cholinergic drugs come from stimulation of which receptors?
    a. Cholinergic
    b. Nicotinic
    c. Muscarinic
    d. Ganglionic

direct-acting

X C 11. When a patient mentions bethanechol chloride
b (Duvoid) when asked about medication history, the
nurse recognizes that this drug is used for the treatment of which condition?
   a. Diarrhea
   b. Urinary retention *relax sphincter*
   c. Urinary incontinence
   d. Bladder spasms *increased tone & motility*

X C 12. When caring for a patient with a diagnosis of
d myasthenia gravis, the nurse can expect to have
the prescriber order which medication to treat the
symptoms of this condition?
   a. bethanechol chloride (Duvoid) — *urinary retention*
   b. galantamine (Reminyl) — *Alzheimer's*
   c. donepezil hydrochloride (Aricept) — *dementia → Parkinsons*
   d. pyridostigmine bromide (Mestinon) — *diagnose myasthenia gravis*

C 13. A 62-year-old female patient started taking donepezil hydrochloride (Aricept) for early stages of Alzheimer's disease. Her daughter expresses relief that
"there is finally a pill to cure Alzheimer's disease."
What is the most therapeutic response by the nurse?
   a. "She should expect reversal of symptoms
      within a few days."
   b. "The dosage should be increased if no improve-
      ment is noted."
   c. "This drug may help to improve symptoms, but
      it is not intended as a cure."
   d. "Yes, it has been a great help for many patients."

b,c,d,X,f 14. A patient has received an inadvertent overdose of a
cholinergic drug. What early manifestations of a
cholinergic crisis should the nurse monitor for? (Select all that apply.)
   a. Dry mouth
   b. Salivation
   c. Flushing of the skin
   d. Abdominal cramps *↑ tone*
   e. Constipation *relax sphincter diarrhea*
   f. Dyspnea

a 15. The nurse will prepare to give which drug to a patient who is experiencing a cholinergic crisis?
   a. atropine sulphate
   b. memantine hydrochloride (Ebixa)
   c. donepezil (Aricept)
   d. physostigmine salicylate

16. An intravenous piggyback medication is ordered to
be infused over 1 hour. The volume of the medication bag is 100 mL; the tubing drop factor is 10 gtts/
mL. What is the rate for a gravity infusion of this
medication? ___17 gtt/min___

17. The order reads, "Give pyridostigmine (Mestinon)
0.25 mg/kg IV now." The patient weighs 106 kg.
How many milligrams of medication will the patient
receive? (Record answer using one decimal place.)
___26.5 mg___

Critical Thinking and Application

Answer the following questions on a separate document.

18. What are the effects of cholinergic poisoning that are listed by the acronym SLUDGE?

19. Sandra recently had abdominal surgery. Although she feels well rested, she is unable to void urine. She has some distention in her lower abdomen over the symphysis pubis.

   a. What drug is likely to be the drug of choice?

   b. Sandra is still unable to void her urine. Her urinary retention worsens and becomes painful, and she begins to exhibit signs of a renal stone, which is confirmed by radiography. How much can the prescriber increase her dosage?

21. Kevin has been determined to have a high potential for a negative reaction to the cholinergic prescribed to him. However, his physician believes that the potential benefits are worth the risk.

   a. The nurse will closely monitor Kevin for what reaction?

   b. In addition to close monitoring, what else can the nurse do to prepare?

22. Bea has recently been diagnosed with myasthenia gravis and is taking medication for the treatment of symptoms associated with the disease. She asks the nurse, "How much success can I expect?"

    a. How should the nurse respond?

    b. What kind of negative effects should Bea report to her physician?

Case Study

Read the scenario and answer the following questions on a separate document.

Carol is a 68-year-old retired banker who has been diagnosed with early-stage Alzheimer's disease. She has remained active in her church activities and plays tennis every week. She is in the family health clinic today with her son and is asking about "new drugs that are available to reverse Alzheimer's disease." Her son is concerned because Carol was also diagnosed with Parkinson's disease 6 months ago (controlled with medications).

1. What drugs are available to "reverse" Alzheimer's disease? Explain.

2. The physician is considering prescribing either galantamine hydrobromide (Reminyl) or rivastigmine hydrogen tartrate (Exelon) for Carol. Is there anything in this patient's history that may influence the choice of drugs used?

3. Describe the different mechanisms of action of direct-acting and indirect-acting cholinergic-blocking drugs.

4. Carol is given a prescription for Exelon. What possible adverse effects should she monitor for? What are the strategies to help manage the occurrence of adverse effects?

5. Carol has difficulty swallowing tablets. What should the prescriber suggest?

CHAPTER 22

Cholinergic-Blocking Drugs

Chapter Review and Examination Preparation

Choose the best answer for each of the following:

a, c, f 1. Before giving an anticholinergic drug, the nurse should check the patient's history for which conditions? (Select all that apply.)
   a. Glaucoma
   b. Osteoporosis
   c. Acute asthma
   d. Thyroid disease
   e. Diabetes mellitus
   f. Benign prostatic hyperplasia

a, c, d 2. Adverse effects to expect from anticholinergic drugs include which of the following? (Select all that apply.)
   a. Dilated pupils
   b. Constricted pupils
   c. Dry mouth
   d. Urinary retention
   e. Urinary frequency
   f. Diarrhea

b 3. In reviewing the medication orders for a newly admitted patient, the nurse recognizes that atropine sulphate is an indication for which condition?
   a. Myasthenia gravis
   b. Reduction of secretions preoperatively
   c. Tachycardia due to sinoatrial node defects
   d. Narrow-angle glaucoma

✗a
c 4. During patient teaching a 70-year-old man who will be taking an anticholinergic drug, the nurse should re-inforce the point that this medication places the patient at higher risk for which problem?
   a. Angina *↑HR, dysrhythmias,*
   b. Fluid overload *xerostomia, constipation*
   c. Heat stroke *↓ sweating*
   d. Hypothermia

b 5. A 28-year-old patient is preparing to take a cruise and has asked for medication for motion sickness. The prescriber orders transdermal scopolamine patches. What must the nurse say to this patient regarding the proper use of the patches?
   a. "The patch can be applied anywhere on the upper body."
   b. "Apply the patch 4 to 5 hours before travel."
   c. "Apply the patch just before boarding the ship."
   d. "Be sure to change the patch daily."

✗c 6. A patient has a new prescription for tolterodine
d L-tartrate (Detrol). Which condition, if present, would make it necessary to reduce the usual dosage of this drug?
   a. Coronary artery disease
   b. Diabetes mellitus
   c. Hypertension
   d. Cirrhosis of the liver

7. The preoperative orders read, "Give atropine 0.6 mg IV push, 30 minutes before the procedure." The medication comes in a 1 mg/mL vial. How much medication will the nurse administer? *0.6 mL*

8. A 14-month-old toddler is in the preoperative area, and the medication order reads, "Give glycopyrrolate 4 mcg/kg IV now." The toddler weighs 10 kg.
   a. How many micrograms of medication will the toddler receive for this dose? *40 mcg*
   b. The medication is available in a vial that contains 0.2 mg/mL. How many millilitres will the nurse draw up into the syringe for this dose?
      200 m/X 0.2 ml

Critical Thinking and Application

Answer the following questions on a separate document.

9. A patient is given atropine sulphate before surgery. Describe how this drug is helpful during the perioperative period. What other drug can be used for this purpose?

10. A male patient is brought into the emergency department conscious but with an overdose of a cholinergic blocker.

    a. Describe how this patient will be treated.

    b. How should the nurse respond if this patient begins having hallucinations related to the overdose?

11. Harry is taking dicyclomine hydrochloride (Bentylol) for irritable bowel syndrome. He calls the clinic and tells the nurse that he would like to get his doctor's permission to take an antihistamine for his cold. What drug interactions might Harry expect?

12. How does atropine work in the following situations?

    a. A patient is experiencing severe bradycardia, with a heart rate of 38 beats per minute, and he is losing consciousness.

    b. A pilot has been exposed to an organophosphate insecticide in an industrial accident.

Case Study

Read the scenario and answer the following questions on a separate document.

Sashima, aged 62 years, is in the outpatient clinic today for a routine annual health assessment. During history taking, she admits to having a "terrible problem" with her bladder. She describes having sudden urges to urinate and is "ashamed to say" that at times, she has lost control of her bladder. She has had no other health issues except for "some eye problems" off and on for the past year. The physician is considering starting Sashima on tolterodine L-tartrate (Detrol).

1. What are the contraindications for this medication? Are there any potential concerns, given Sashima's history?

2. What are the advantages of using tolterodine? Why is this considered the drug of choice?

3. Sashima enjoys working outside in her yard. What special precautions should she take?

4. After a week of therapy, she calls the clinic to complain of a dry mouth. She says she did not think this was supposed to happen with this drug. What advice should the nurse provide?

CHAPTER 23

Antihypertensive Drugs

Chapter Review and Examination Preparation

Choose the best answer for each of the following:

c 1. A 46-year old male patient has been taking clonidine hydrochloride (Catapres) for 5 months. For the last 2 months, his blood pressure has been normal. During this office visit, he tells the nurse that he would like to stop taking the drug. What is the nurse's best response?
   a. "I'm sure the doctor will stop it; your blood pressure is normal now."
   b. "Your doctor will probably have you stop taking the drug for a month, and then we'll see how you do."
   c. "This drug should not be stopped suddenly; let's talk to your doctor."
   d. "It's likely that you can stop the drug if you exercise and avoid salty foods."

bt
X d,e,f 2. When administering angiotensin-converting enzyme (ACE) inhibitors, the nurse keeps in mind that adverse effects include which of the following? (Select all that apply.)
   a. Diarrhea
   b. Fatigue
   c. Restlessness
   d. Headaches
   e. A dry cough
   f. Tremors

X 3.ᶜ A patient with type 2 diabetes mellitus has developed hypertension. What is the blood pressure goal for this patient?
   a. Less than 110/80 mm Hg
   b. Less than 120/80 mm Hg
   c. Less than 130/80 mm Hg
   d. Less than 140/90 mm Hg

a 4. A patient is being treated for a hypertensive emergency. The nurse expects which drug to be used?
   a. sodium nitroprusside (Nipride)
   b. losartan potassium (Cozaar)
   c. captopril (Capoten)
   d. prazosin hydrochloride (Minipress)

d 5. Julie, who is in her eighth month of pregnancy, has pre-eclampsia. Her blood pressure is 210/100 mm Hg this morning. This type of hypertension is classified as which of the following?
   a. Primary
   b. Idiopathic
   c. Essential
   d. Secondary

at
c,d,e 6. A β-blocker is prescribed for a patient with heart failure and hypertension. Which adverse effects, if present, may indicate that a serious problem is developing while the patient is on this medication? (Select all that apply.)
   a. ? Edema
   b. Nightmares
   c. Shortness of breath
   d. Nervousness
   e. Constipation

7. The order reads, "Give captopril 25 mg PO every 8 hours." The available tablets are at a strength of 12.5 mg. How many tablets will the nurse administer per dose? ___2___

8. The order reads, "Give enalapril (Vasotec) 5 mg IV push over 5 minutes now." The medication is available in a vial with the strength of 1.25 mg/mL. How many millilitres will the nurse administer for this dose? ___4 mL___

Critical Thinking and Application

Answer the following questions on a separate document.

9. Nasim, aged 61 years, comes to the emergency department with symptoms of a severe hypertensive emergency. The emergency department physician on call initiates therapy with sodium nitroprusside (Nipride). The patient is transferred to the Intensive Care Unit and monitored. Hours later, his blood pressure falls to 100/60 mm Hg, and he is lethargic and complaining of feeling dizzy. What priority action should the nurse take?

10. Indicate which ACE inhibitor would be best for the following patients. Explain your answers.

    a.   Irene, who has liver dysfunction, has high blood pressure, and is seriously ill

    b.   Kory, who has a history of poor adherence to his medication regimen

11. Lance will be starting prazosin hydrochloride (Minipress) for hypertension. What should he be taught before he takes the first dose of this medication?

12. White and Black patients are known to react differently to antihypertensive agents.

    a.   Which antihypertensives are considered more effective in White patients than in Black patients?

    b.   Which antihypertensives are considered more effective in Black patients than in White patients?

Critical Thinking Crossword

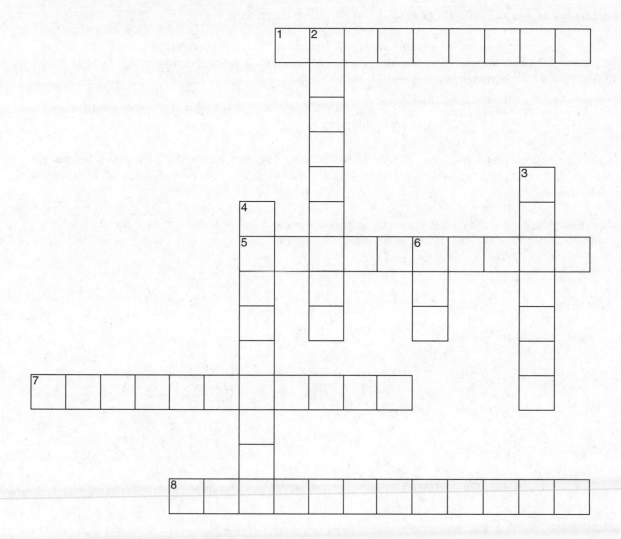

Across

1. High blood pressure associated with diseases such as renal, pulmonary, endocrine, and vascular disease is known as ___systemic___ *secondary* hypertension.
5. Another term for 3 Down.
7. A common adverse effect of adrenergic drugs that involve a sudden drop in blood pressure when patients change position is known as __orthostatic__ hypotension.
8. Drugs that are used in the management of hypertensive emergencies. *vasodilators*

Down

2. Another term for 3 Down. *essential*
3. Elevated systemic arterial pressure for which no cause can be found is known as *primary* __idiopathic__ hypertension.
4. The primary effect of these drugs, which is to decrease plasma and extracellular fluid volumes. *diuretics*
6. Drugs that are often used as first-line drugs in the treatment of both heart failure and hypertension are known by the acronym-including term ___ACE___ inhibitors.

Case Study

Read the scenario and answer the following questions on a separate document.

John is a 44-year-old Black man who has been seen twice in the last month for "blood pressure problems." At his first visit, his blood pressure was 144/90 mm Hg; at the second visit, his blood pressure was 154/96 mm Hg. The physician is preparing to start John on antihypertensive therapy.

1. What initial drug therapy would be appropriate for John? What factors are considered when choosing which drug to use?

2. John tells you that he hopes this medication will not "slow him down" because he likes to "jump out of bed and get started" with his day. What priority health teaching should the nurse provide for this patient to help adjust his blood pressure medication?

3. John also mentions that he likes to go to the gym three times a week and visit with his friends in the sauna after a good workout. What teaching will the nurse emphasize for this patient?

CHAPTER 24

Antianginal Drugs

Chapter Review and Examination Preparation

Choose the best answer for each of the following:

c 1. The purpose of antianginal drug therapy is to do which of the following? (Select the best response.)
   a. To increase myocardial oxygen demand
   b. To increase blood flow to peripheral arteries
   c. To increase blood flow to ischemic cardiac muscle
   d. To decrease blood flow to ischemic cardiac muscle

c 2. A patient is on nitroglycerin therapy. Which of the following common adverse effects is it a priority to teach the patient about?
   a. Blurred vision
   b. Dizziness
   c. Headache
   d. Weakness

a, c 3. A patient who has a history of dysphagia is placed on nitroglycerin therapy. What available form of nitroglycerin is appropriate for this patient? (Select all that apply.)
   a. Continuous intravenous drip
   b. Intravenous bolus
   c. Sublingual spray
   d. Oral dosage forms
   e. Topical ointment
   f. Rectal suppository

d 4. In regard to a patient using transdermal nitroglycerin patches, the nurse knows that the prescriber will order which of the following procedures for preventing tolerance?
   a. Leaving the old patch on for 2 hours after applying a new patch
   b. Applying a new patch every other day
   c. Leaving the patch off for 24 hours once a week
   d. Removing the patch at night for 8 hours, and then applying a new patch in the morning

a
c 5. Which important specific information should be given to a patient taking β-blockers for angina?
   a. These drugs are for long-term prevention of angina episodes.
   b. These drugs must be taken as soon as angina pain occurs.
   c. These drugs will be discontinued if dizziness is experienced.
   d. These drugs need to be carried with the patient at all times in case angina occurs.

b 6. A patient with coronary artery spasms will be most effectively treated with which type of antianginal medication?
   a. β-blockers
   b. Calcium channel blockers
   c. Nitrates
   d. Nitrites

a 7. During his morning walk, a man begins to experience chest pain. He sits down and takes one nitroglycerin sublingual tablet. After 5 minutes, the chest pain is worsening. What action would be the priority in this situation?
   a. Call 911 (emergency medical services).
   b. Take another nitroglycerin tablet.
   c. Take two more nitroglycerin tablets at the same time.
   d. Sit quietly to wait for the pain to subside.

8. The order reads, "Give isosorbide dinitrate 80 mg twice a day." The medication is available in 40 mg capsules. How many capsules will the patient receive for each dose? _____ 2 _____

Critical Thinking and Application

Answer the following questions on a separate document.

9. The order reads, "Nitroglycerin transdermal patch, 0.2 mg/hr; apply one patch in the morning and remove every evening at 10 p.m." The pharmacy has supplied a transdermal patch that supplies 0.4 mg/hr. What will the nurse do in order to administer this drug?

10. While playing racquetball at a community centre, a nurse notices a commotion at a gathering of senior citizens in a nearby room. The nurse rushes in to find a man lying unconscious on the floor. Several people say that he is having a heart attack. One man hands the nurse a pill bottle and asks, "Would it help to give him one of my heart pills?" A woman agrees, saying, "Yes! Can't you put it under his tongue?" The nurse sees that the medication bottle is labelled isosorbide dinitrate. What does the nurse know about this medication, and what needs to be done next?

11. Victoria is a 70-year-old patient seen in the emergency department for a laceration to her thumb. During the assessment, Victoria tells the nurse that she has been tired and depressed and has been having nightmares since her physician prescribed heart medicine for her angina. Which drug does the nurse suspect Victoria is taking and why?

12. During a nurse's home visit with Taylor, she shows the nurse a journal entry describing the duration, time of onset, and severity of a recent angina attack. She reports no adverse effects from her nitroglycerin and shows the nurse where she keeps the tablets: in a clear plastic pillbox on the kitchen windowsill. What will the nurse discuss with Taylor?

Case Study

Read the scenario and answer the following questions on a separate document.

While playing handball, 59-year-old Gideon experiences chest pain. He has had angina before and carries sublingual nitroglycerin in his gym bag.

1. What type of angina is he experiencing?

2. What should he do to treat this episode of angina?

3. After he takes the nitroglycerin tablets, the chest pain does not subside. He wants his handball partner to drive him to the hospital. Is this what he should do at this time?

4. Other than nitroglycerin, which class of drugs is typically good for this type of angina?

CHAPTER 25

Heart Failure Drugs

Chapter Review and Examination Preparation

Choose the best answer for each of the following.

b 1. A patient has started digoxin therapy. What is this medication's serum therapeutic level for which the nurse must monitor?
   a. 0.1 to 0.5 ng/mL
   b. 0.8 to 2.0 ng/mL
   c. 2.0 to 5.0 ng/mL
   d. 5.0 to 8.4 ng/mL

cXd 2. A patient is experiencing digitalis toxicity. What antidote medication should the nurse begin to prepare to address the toxicity?
   a. vitamin K
   b. atropine
   c. digoxin immune Fab Digibind
   d. potassium

b 3. Before giving oral digoxin, the nurse discovers that the patient's radial pulse is 55 beats/min. What priority action must the nurse do next to address the pulse?
   a. Give the dose.
   b. Delay the dose until later.
   c. Hold the dose, and notify the physician.
   d. Check the apical pulse for 1 minute.

a 4. Which statement regarding digoxin therapy and potassium levels is correct?
   a. Low potassium levels increase the chance of digoxin toxicity.
   b. High potassium levels increase the chance of digoxin toxicity.
   c. Digoxin reduces the excretion of potassium in the kidneys.
   d. Digoxin promotes the excretion of potassium in the kidneys.

b 5. When infusing milrinone, the nurse will keep which consideration in mind?
   a. The patient must be monitored for hyperkalemia.
   b. The patient's cardiac status must be monitored closely.
   c. The drug may cause reddish discolouration of the extremities.
   d. Hypertension is the primary effect seen with excessive doses.

+a,c
d,e,f 6. When caring for a patient who is taking digoxin, the nurse should monitor for which signs and symptoms of toxicity? (Select all that apply.)
   a. Anorexia
   b. Diarrhea
   c. Visual changes blurred, yellow-tinged vision, halos
   d. Nausea and vomiting
   e. Headache
   f. Bradycardia

c,e,f 7. A patient who has heart failure will be started on an oral angiotensin-converting enzyme inhibitor. While monitoring the patient's response to this drug therapy, which laboratory tests would be a priority? (Select all that apply.)
   a. White blood cell count
   b. Platelet count
   c. Serum potassium level
   d. Serum magnesium level
   e. Creatinine level
   f. Blood urea nitrogen

8. A patient is to receive an initial dose of digoxin (Lanoxin) 0.5 mg intravenous (IV) push, followed by an oral maintenance dose of 0.25 mg orally (PO) daily, starting the next day. The medication is available in ampules that contain 0.25 mg/mL. How many millilitres will the patient receive for the IV dose?_____2_____

9. Mark the syringe with the correct amount of digoxin the patient will receive for the IV dose in Question 8.

10. Convert the 0.25 mg dose to micrograms. _____250_____

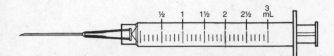

Critical Thinking and Application

Answer the following questions on a separate document.

11. The nurse is caring for Charlotte, who is undergoing cardiac glycoside therapy. She begins to vomit and complains of a headache and fatigue. Diagnostic studies reveal short episodes of ventricular tachycardia on the electrocardiogram and a serum potassium level of 6 mmol/L. What action might the nurse expect to be taken?

12. While monitoring Fredrick after oral digoxin (Lanoxin) administration, the nurse notes increased urinary output, decreased dyspnea and fatigue, and constipation. Fredrick complains that if he were allowed to eat bran as often as he used to, he wouldn't be constipated. What do the nurse's findings indicate? How will the nurse response to Fredrick?

13. Micha is experiencing heart failure that has not responded well to diuretic and digoxin therapy. The physician changes his medication to milrinone.

    a. What effect does milrinone have on cardiac muscle contractility and on the blood vessels?

    b. What advantage does this phosphodiesterase inhibitor have over the cardiac glycosides?

    c. What is the primary adverse effect of milrinone?

Case Study

Read the scenario and answer the following questions on a separate document.

A 68-year-old woman is admitted to the hospital with a diagnosis of mild left-sided heart failure. She is comfortable at rest, but she has noticed that she has symptoms when she tries to get dressed or do simple housework. She becomes short of breath with activity, tires easily but cannot sleep at night, and feels "generally irritable." She also has diffuse bilateral crackles (that do not clear with coughing) and a third heart sound. She has slight pedal edema. The physician has ordered therapy with intravenous digoxin.

1. Explain the meaning of each of the following several effects of digoxin:
    a. Positive inotropic effect
    b. Negative chronotropic effect
    c. Negative dromotropic effect

2. As a result of these effects, what would the nurse expect to see with regard to each of the following?
    a. Stroke volume
    b. Venous blood pressure and vein engorgement
    c. Coronary circulation
    d. Diuresis

3. After 3 days of therapy, the patient complains of feeling nauseated and has no appetite. She also wonders why the lights are so bright and blurry. Her radial pulse rate is 52 beats per minute. When the result of the patient's laboratory work is checked, the nurse notes that the woman's digoxin level from that morning was 3.5 ng/mL. What should the nurse do?

CHAPTER 26

Antidysrhythmic Drugs

Chapter Review and Examination Preparation

Choose the best answer for each of the following:

1. The nurse notes in the patient's medication history that the patient is receiving a lidocaine infusion. Based on this finding, the nurse interprets that the patient has which disorder?
   a. Atrial fibrillation
   b. Bradycardia
   c. Complete heart block
   d. Ventricular dysrhythmias

2. When monitoring a patient who is taking quinidine, the nurse recognizes that the possible adverse effects of this drug include which of these conditions? (Select all that apply.)
   a. Weakness
   b. Tachycardia
   c. Gastro-intestinal upset
   d. Tinnitus
   e. Ventricular ectopic beats

3. A patient has started amiodarone hydrochloride (Cordarone) therapy. What priority adverse effect should the nurse should monitor for?
   a. Pulmonary toxicity
   b. Hypertension
   c. Urinary retention
   d. Visual halos

4. A nurse is assisting a colleague with administering a dose of verapamil hydrochloride. The nurse notes that his medication is used to treat which of the following health conditions?
   a. Cardiac asystole
   b. Heart block
   c. Ventricular dysrhythmia, including premature ventricular contractions
   d. Recurrent paroxysmal supraventricular tachycardia (PSVT)

5. A patient is experiencing a rapid dysrhythmia, and the nurse is preparing to administer adenosine (Adenocard). What is the correct way to administer this drug?
   a. It should be given as a fast intravenous push.
   b. It should be given intravenously, slowly over 5 minutes.
   c. It should be taken with food or milk.
   d. It should be given as an intravenous drip infusion.

6. If a drug has a prodysrhythmic effect, what should the nurse monitor the patient for?
   a. Decreased heart rate
   b. New dysrhythmias
   c. A decrease in dysrhythmias
   d. Reduced blood pressure

7. **Match the site to its correct intrinsic rate:**
   a. Sinoatrial node   (1) 40 to 60 beats/min
      _____
   b. Atrioventricular node (2) 40 or fewer beats/min
      _____
   c. Purkinje fibres   (3) 60 to 100 beats/min
      _____

8. A patient will be starting therapy with quinidine. Which of the drugs is a contraindication for quinidine? (Select all that apply.)
   a. cimetidine
   b. amiodarone
   c. digoxin
   d. warfarin (Coumadin)
   e. erythromycin

9. A patient with sustained ventricular tachycardia will be receiving a lidocaine infusion following a bolus dose. The order reads, "Give a bolus of 1.5 mg/kg, then start a drip at 2 mg/min." The lidocaine is available as 20 mg/mL, and the patient weighs 99 kg. How many milligrams of lidocaine will be given in the bolus dose? _____

10. A patient is to receive adenosine (Adenocard) as initial treatment for PSVT. The dose is 6 mg IV push. The medication is available in a vial that contains 3 mg/mL. How many millilitres will the nurse draw up into the syringe for this dose? _____

Critical Thinking and Application

Answer the following questions on a separate document.

11. Raj, who has been diagnosed with hypertension, is hospitalized after a myocardial infarction (MI).

    a. To reduce the risk of sudden cardiac death for this patient, the physician prescribes a drug from which class?

    b. How would a history of asthma in Raj affect the choice of drug?

12. Nick has a life-threatening ventricular tachycardia that has been resistant to treatment. What medication can the nurse expect to be used? What specific precautions are of priority with this medication?

13. Warrick is a 50-year-old teacher being treated with lidocaine after an MI.

    a. Warrick is upset and says that he hates injections; he wants to know why he can't just take a pill. What does the nurse tell him?

    b. If Warrick has a history of cirrhosis, how would the dosage of the lidocaine be affected?

Case Study

Read the scenario and answer the following questions on a separate document.

Jarrod, aged 39 years, has a new prescription for verapamil as part of his treatment for occasional PSVT. This is the first time he has taken this medication. He states he has no previous history of heart problems but that he does smoke one pack of cigarettes a day.

1. How do calcium channel blockers such as diltiazem work?

2. What therapeutic effects are expected?

3. Is there a possible concern with drug interactions?

4. After 4 months of therapy, Jarrod experiences dizziness, dyspnea, and a rapid heart rate, and is taken to the emergency department. He is diagnosed with sustained PSVT, and intravenous verapamil does not help. What drug may be tried next?

CHAPTER 27

Coagulation-Modifier Drugs

Chapter Review and Examination Preparation

Choose the best answer for each of the following:

1. Which health condition(s) is anticoagulant therapy used for? (Select all that apply.)
    a. Atrial fibrillation
    b. Thrombocytopenia
    c. Myocardial infarction
    d. Presence of mechanical heart valves
    e. Aneurysm
    f. Leukemia

2. During the teaching of a patient who will be taking warfarin sodium (Coumadin) at home, which statement by the nurse is correct regarding over-the-counter drug use?
    a. "Choose nonsteroidal anti-inflammatory drugs as needed for pain relief."
    b. "Aspirin products may result in an increased anticoagulant effect."
    c. "Vitamin E therapy is recommended to improve the effect of warfarin sodium."
    d. "Mineral oil is the laxative of choice while taking anticoagulants."

3. A patient is at high risk for a stroke. Which medication can the nurse expect to administer to prevent platelet aggregation?
    a. acetylsalicylic acid (Aspirin)
    b. warfarin sodium
    c. heparin sulphate (Heparin LEO)
    d. streptokinase

4. After administering subcutaneous heparin, what priority action should the nurse do next?
    a. Use the same sites for injection to reduce trauma.
    b. Use a 2.5 cm needle for subcutaneous injections.
    c. Inject the medication without aspirating for blood return.
    d. Massage the site after the injection to increase absorption.

5. During thrombolytic therapy, the nurse monitors for bleeding. Which symptoms may indicate a serious bleeding problem? (Select all that apply.)
    a. Hypertension
    b. Hypotension
    c. Decreased level of consciousness
    d. Increased pulse rate
    e. Restlessness

6. Which drug is recommended for the prevention and treatment of deep vein thrombosis (DVT) after a major surgical procedure?
    a. Antiplatelet drugs, such as acetylsalicylic acid (Aspirin)
    b. Adenosine diphosphate inhibitors, such as clopidogrel (Plavix)
    c. Anticoagulants, such as warfarin sodium
    d. Low-molecular-weight heparins, such as enoxaparin sodium (Lovenox)

7. The nurse is preparing a patient's morning medications and, upon reviewing the list of drugs, notes that the patient is to receive heparin 5,000 units and enoxaparin, both subcutaneously. What is the nurse's priority action at this time?
    a. Administer the drugs in separate sites.
    b. Hold the drugs, and clarify the order with the prescriber.
    c. Administer the enoxaparin and hold the heparin.
    d. Check the patient's activated partial thromboplastin time (aPTT).

8. A patient is to receive a bolus dose of heparin 8,000 units via IV push. The vial contains heparin 10,000 units per mL. How many millilitres of medication will the nurse draw up to administer the ordered dose?_____

9. A patient who weighs 75 kg is to receive daily doses of fondaparinux (Arixtra). According to the dosage chart for the drug below, how many milligrams will this patient receive per dose?_____

Patient weight <50 kg	5 mg daily
Patient weight 50–100 kg	7.5 mg daily
Patient weight >100 kg	10 mg daily

Match each definition with its corresponding term. (Note: Not all terms will be used.)

10. _____ A drug that prevents the lysis of fibrin, thereby promoting clot formation

11. _____ The termination of bleeding by mechanical or chemical means

12. _____ A substance that prevents platelet plugs from forming

13. _____ A drug that dissolves thrombi

14. _____ The general term for a substance that prevents or delays coagulation of the blood

15. _____ A laboratory test used to measure the effectiveness of heparin therapy

16. _____ A test used, along with another measure, to evaluate the effectiveness of warfarin sodium therapy

17. _____ A standardized measure of the degree of coagulation achieved by drug therapy with warfarin sodium

18. _____ A substance that reverses the effect of heparin

19. _____ A substance that reverses the effect of warfarin sodium

20. _____ Naturally occurring tissue plasminogen activator secreted by vascular endothelial cells

21. _____ A blood clot that dislodges and travels through the bloodstream

a. prothrombin time

b. aPTT

c. international normalized ratio (INR)

d. streptokinase

e. alteplase (Activase)

f. thrombus

g. embolus

h. vitamin K

i. protamine sulphate

j. antiplatelet drug

k. antifibrinolytic

l. thrombolytic drug

m. anticoagulant

n. hemostasis

Critical Thinking and Application

Answer the following questions on a separate document.

22. Hilary is a 60-year-old homemaker who receives subcutaneous heparin therapy for the prevention of DVT. After the nurse administers her injection, Hilary complains of pain and begins to rub the site. What priority health teaching must the nurse provide Hilary to address the rubbing of the site?

23. During cardiopulmonary bypass for heart surgery, Max is intentionally given a large dose of heparin. The surgeon then determines that the effects of the heparin need to be reversed quickly.

    a. How will this be done?

    b. How will the amount of antidote be determined?

    c. What is the most commonly used test for determining the effects of heparin therapy?

24. Following surgery, Ferdinand has a chest tube put in place. The site has been bleeding excessively. What type of drug might the physician prescribe in this situation, and why?

25. Nick, a 38-year-old writer who has von Willebrand's disease, has undergone emergency surgery after an automobile accident. What drug is used in the management of bleeding in patients such as Nick? What is its effect?

26. Tanya has been given alteplase (Activase) during treatment for acute myocardial infarction.

    a. Does the nurse expect Tanya to have an allergic reaction to the drug? Explain your answer.

    b. A few minutes later, Tanya suffers a re-infarction. What drug should Tanya receive now?

27. Ursula, an inpatient on the nurse's unit, is on anticoagulant therapy. The nurse enters the room to find that Ursula is restless and confused.

    a. Why are these findings significant?

    b. In this case, what other problems might the nurse expect to find?

    c. What should the nurse do?

28. Joanne is receiving subcutaneous heparin 5,000 units twice a day for DVT prevention. Will her anticoagulation be monitored by laboratory work? Explain.

Case Study

Read the scenario and answer the following questions on a separate document.

After experiencing transient ischemic attacks, Doug has been started on clopidogrel (Plavix). He has a history of atherosclerotic heart disease and has had problems with peptic ulcer disease.

1. He asks, "Why am I on this fancy medicine? Why can't I just take an Aspirin a day, like they say on television?" What does the nurse tell him?

2. What should he be taught to report to his health care provider while he is taking this drug?

3. What precautions should he follow while he is taking this drug?

4. What herbal products should he avoid while he is taking this drug?

CHAPTER 28

Antilipemic Drugs

Chapter Review and Examination Preparation

Choose the best answer for each of the following:

1. Patients taking cholestyramine resin (Olestyr) may experience which adverse effects?
   a. Blurred vision and photophobia
   b. Drowsiness and difficulty concentrating
   c. Diarrhea and abdominal cramps
   d. Belching and bloating

2. What instructions should the nurse include for a patient on antilipemic therapy? (Select all that apply.)
   a. Taking supplements of fat-soluble vitamins
   b. Taking supplements of B vitamins
   c. Increasing fluid intake
   d. Choosing foods that are lower in cholesterol and saturated fats
   e. Increasing the intake of raw vegetables, fruit, and bran

3. In reviewing the history of a newly admitted cardiac patient, the nurse knows that the patient would have a contraindication to antilipemic therapy if which condition is present?
   a. Liver disease
   b. Kidney disease
   c. Coronary artery disease
   d. Diabetes mellitus

4. A woman is being screened in the cardiac clinic for risk factors for coronary artery disease. Which would be considered a negative (favourable) risk factor for her?
   a. A high-density lipoprotein (HDL) cholesterol level of 0.77 mmol/L
   b. An HDL cholesterol level of 1.9 mmol/L
   c. Early menopause
   d. Age of 57 years

5. A patient who has started taking nicotinic acid (niacin) complains that he "hates the side effects." What is the best response by the nurse to address this patient's concern?
   a. "You will soon build up tolerance to these adverse effects."
   b. "You should take the niacin on an empty stomach."
   c. "You can take the niacin every other day if the adverse effects are bothersome."
   d. "Try taking a small dose of ibuprofen (Motrin) or another nonsteroidal anti-inflammatory drug 30 minutes before taking the niacin."

6. A patient asks, "What is considered the 'good cholesterol?'" Which of the following will the nurse name as an answer?
   a. Very-low-density lipoprotein (VLDL)
   b. Low-density lipoprotein (LDL)
   c. High-density lipoprotein (HDL)
   d. Triglycerides

7. The nurse is preparing to administer a newly ordered statin drug to a patient and is reviewing the patient's list of current medications. Which medications may cause an interaction with the statin drug? (Select all that apply.)
   a. warfarin (Coumadin)
   b. metformin (Glucophage)
   c. erythromycin
   d. cyclosporine
   e. gemfibrozil

8. The medication order reads, "Give lovastatin 30 mg daily at bedtime, PO." The medication is available in 20 mg tablets. How many tablets will the nurse administer to the patient? _____

9. A patient is to receive niacin (Niaspan) 1.5 g per day in two divided doses. The medication is available in 250 mg extended-release tablets. How many milligrams will the patient receive for each dose?

   How many tablets per dose? _____

Critical Thinking and Application

Answer the following questions on a separate document.

10. José is a 46-year-old business executive who travels frequently. He is slightly overweight "from all that room service," but he did quit smoking 6 years ago. During a routine checkup, José is found to have an LDL cholesterol level of 6 mmol/L. He says, "I'm a busy man! Just give me some pills. I've got a plane to catch!" Will the physician prescribe an antilipemic for José? Explain your answer.

11. Katherine has been treated with cholestyramine for type IIa dyslipidemia for the past two 2 months. She tells the nurse that she "can't stand being so irregular" and that she has developed another "embarrassing problem" as well. What is wrong with Katherine, and how can the nurse help her?

12. Jim is a 55-year-old lawyer being treated with lovastatin for dyslipidemia. His current health status includes mild hypertension and a peptic ulcer. The nurse knows that niacin (Niaspan) is frequently prescribed as an adjunct to other antilipemic drugs. Would niacin be helpful for Jim? Explain your answer.

13. The nurse is visiting Nila, a homebound patient who is being treated for dyslipidemia and hypertension. During the visit, Nila takes her antihypertensive medication and then begins to mix her dose of cholestyramine resin (Olestyr) into a glass of orange juice. What does Nila need to be taught?

Case Study

Read the scenario and answer the following questions on a separate document.

Matt is diagnosed with type IIa dyslipidemia and has been given a prescription for atorvastatin (Lipitor). He acts thrilled with the news and says, "Great! Now I don't have to worry about watching my diet, because I'm on this medicine!"

1. Is he right? What type of dietary guidelines should he follow while on this therapy?

2. What therapeutic effects does one hope to see as a result of taking this medication?

3. After two 2 months of therapy, his liver enzyme levels are slightly elevated. Is this a concern? What other laboratory values will be monitored while Matt is taking atorvastatin?

4. Matt calls the office to complain about some muscle pain. He thought he had pulled a muscle during a tennis match, but the pain has not lessened in 3 days. Is this a concern?

CHAPTER 29

Diuretic Drugs

Chapter Review and Examination Preparation

Choose the best answer for each of the following:

1. Which of the following are indications for the use of diuretics? (Select all that apply.)
   a. Increased urine output
   b. Reduced uric acid levels
   c. Hypertension
   d. Open-angle glaucoma
   e. Edema associated with heart failure

2. When advising a patient who is taking a potassium-sparing diuretic such as spironolactone (Aldactone), what dietary guidelines should the nurse recommend?
   a. No dietary restrictions
   b. Consuming foods high in potassium, such as bananas and orange juice
   c. Avoiding excessive intake of foods high in potassium
   d. Drinking 1 to 2 litres of fluid per day

3. When teaching a patient about diuretic therapy, what should the nurse recommend as the best time of day to take the required medications?
   a. Morning
   b. Midday
   c. Bedtime
   d. Time of day does not matter

4. When monitoring a patient for hypokalemia related to diuretic use, the nurse looks for which possible symptoms?
   a. Nausea, vomiting, and anorexia
   b. Diarrhea and abdominal pain
   c. Orthostatic hypotension
   d. Lethargy and muscle weakness

5. A patient with severe heart failure has been started on therapy with a carbonic anhydrase inhibitor, but the nurse mentions that this medication may be stopped in a few days. What is the rationale for this short treatment?
   a. Carbonic anhydrase inhibitors (CAIs) result in respiratory alkalosis within a few days.
   b. Metabolic acidosis develops 2 to 4 days after therapy is started.
   c. CAIs can dramatically reduce the fluid overload related to heart failure.
   d. Allergic reactions to CAIs are common.

6. A patient has a new order for daily doses of spironolactone (Aldactone). Which of the following conditions may be a contraindication to this drug therapy? (Select all that apply.)
   a. Heart failure
   b. Renal failure
   c. Diabetes mellitus
   d. Deep vein thrombosis
   e. Hyperkalemia

7. A patient is to receive furosemide (Lasix) 120 mg every morning via a percutaneous endoscopic gastrostomy (PEG) tube. The medication is available in a liquid form (40 mg/5 mL). Mark on the medication cup how many millilitres the patient will receive for this dose.

8. A patient is to receive 30 g of mannitol (Osmitrol) intravenously. The medication on hand is mannitol 20% in a 500 mL bag. How many millilitres will the patient receive? _____

Match each term with its corresponding definition.

9. _____ Diuretics

10. _____ Potassium-sparing diuretics

11. _____ Kaliuretic diuretics

12. _____ Osmotic diuretics

13. _____ Thiazides

14. _____ Ascites

15. _____ CAI

16. _____ Loop diuretics

17. _____ Nephron

18. _____ Glomerular filtration rate

a. Potent diuretics that act along the ascending limb of the loop of Henle (e.g., furosemide [Lasix])

b. An index of how well the kidneys are functioning as filters

c. Drugs that accelerate the rate of urine formation

d. The main structural unit of the kidney

e. Diuretics that cause the body to lose potassium

f. Diuretics that result in the diuresis of sodium and water and in the retention of potassium (e.g., spironolactone [Aldactone])

g. Diuretics that act on the distal convoluted tubule, where they inhibit sodium and water resorption (e.g., hydrochlorothiazide [Apo-Hydro])

h. Abbreviation for a class of diuretics that inhibit the enzyme carbonic anhydrase (e.g., acetazolamide)

i. Drugs that induce diuresis by increasing the osmotic pressure of the glomerular filtrate, resulting in a rapid diuresis (e.g., mannitol)

j. An abnormal intraperitoneal accumulation of fluid

Critical Thinking and Application

Use a separate document to answer the following questions.

19. Madison is a 62-year-old retired teacher who is being treated for diabetes and open-angle glaucoma. The prescriber ordered a diuretic as an adjunct drug in the management of Madison's glaucoma.

    a. Which diuretic drug was probably prescribed?

    b. What undesirable effect of the drug does the prescriber need to consider?

20. The nurse is about to administer mannitol to a patient who is in early acute renal failure.

    a. What is the significance of this patient's kidney blood flow and glomerular filtration in this situation?

    b. By what means does the nurse administer the mannitol? What special guidelines should the nurse follow?

    c. The patient later complains of headache and chills. Should the mannitol therapy be ended? Explain your answer.

21. Jeff has been admitted to the nurse's unit for treatment of ascites. He also has some kidney impairment and a history of heavy drinking.

    a. Which diuretic drug will the nurse expect to be administered to Jeff?

    b. What monitoring will be performed frequently? Why?

22. Byron is a 39-year-old bricklayer taking a thiazide for hypertension. During a follow-up visit, he tells the nurse that he thinks the drug is affecting his "love life."

    a. To what adverse effect of thiazide therapy is Byron probably referring?

    b. While talking to Byron, the nurse notices a package of licorice in Byron's coat pocket. Byron tells the nurse that he eats the candy for "energy," especially because he has been feeling so tired the past couple of days. What will the nurse tell Byron?

23. The nurse receives a call from Barbara, who recently started diuretic therapy for hypertension. Barbara is concerned because her neighbour, who also takes medication for hypertension, told her not to eat a lot of bananas or other foods containing potassium. Barbara says, "But you told me to eat foods high in potassium. What's going on?" What is the nurse's response to Barbara?

24. Paula will be started on diuretic therapy for hypertension, but she also has moderate renal failure. Which diuretic—a loop diuretic or a thiazide diuretic—would be more effective for Paula? Explain your answer.

Case Study

Read the scenario and answer the following questions on a separate document.

Lenore has been taking furosemide (Lasix) for 3 months as part of her treatment for heart failure. Now she is complaining that she is feeling tired and that she has muscle weakness and no appetite. Her blood pressure is 100/50 mm Hg.

1. What do her symptoms suggest? How did this condition occur?

2. What dietary measures could have prevented these problems?

    The physician switches Lenore's medication (see above) to spironolactone (Aldactone).

3. How does this drug differ from furosemide?

4. For what drug interactions should the nurse check before Lenore begins taking spironolactone?

CHAPTER 30

Fluids and Electrolytes

Chapter Review and Examination Preparation

Choose the best answer for each of the following:

a,b,d,e

1. What are the common uses of crystalloids? (Select all that apply.)
   a. Fluid replacement
   b. Promotion of urinary flow
   c. Transport of oxygen to cells
   d. Replacement of electrolytes
   e. As maintenance fluids
   f. Replacement of clotting factors

c 2. The intravenous order for a newly admitted patient calls for "Normal saline to run at 100 mL/hr." The nurse will choose which concentration of normal saline?
   a. 0.33%
   b. 0.45%
   c. 0.9%
   d. 3.0%

b 3. A patient has been admitted with severe dehydration after working outside on a very hot day. What intravenous fluid should be administered for rapid fluid replacement?
   a. Albumin
   b. Hetastarch
   c. Fresh frozen plasma
   d. 0.9% sodium chloride

c 4. When giving intravenous potassium, which of the following is important for the nurse to remember?
   a. Intravenous doses are preferred over oral dosage forms.
   b. Intravenous solutions should contain at least 50 mmol/L.
   c. Potassium must always be given in diluted form.
   d. Potassium should be given by slow intravenous bolus.

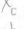 *c* 5. A patient is receiving blood products. What priority
b assessment should the nurse monitor for to determine a possible transfusion adverse reaction?
   a. Subnormal temperature and hypertension
   b. Apprehension, restlessness, fever, and chills
   c. Decreased pulse and respiration and fever
   d. Headache, nausea, and lethargy

b 6. A patient with a blood disorder requires a replacement product that contains clotting factors. Which product can the nurse expect to administer?
   a. Plasma protein fraction
   b. Fresh frozen plasma
   c. Packed red blood cells
   d. Albumin

7. The following intravenous (IV) is to be given: 1,000 mL 5% dextrose in water (D_5W) with 20 mEq potassium chloride (KCl) over the next 24 hours. The tubing drop factor is 15. At what rate will the KCl be administered? ___42 mL/h___

8. An IV antibiotic needs to infuse over 30 minutes. The intravenous piggyback bag contains 50 mL. Calculate the setting for the infusion pump.
   ___100 mL/h___

100

Critical Thinking and Application

Answer the following questions on a separate document.

9. List the advantages and disadvantages of using crystalloids to replace fluid in patients with dehydration.

10. Some fluids are known as oxygen-carrying resuscitation fluids.

    a. Which class of fluids is given this designation?

    b. Why are these fluids able to carry oxygen?

    c. Why is their origin a potential problem for a recipient?

11. Natasha is a 16-year-old student who is brought to the clinic by her mother. Her mother says that Natasha has been on "some sort of fad diet." The mother is concerned because Natasha is tired and weak. During assessment, Natasha admits that she has been using laxatives and eating little during the past few weeks.

    a. What electrolyte imbalance is this patient experiencing?

    b. What interventions can the nurse expect to correct the imbalance?

12. Samuel, a 45-year-old postal carrier, has come to the emergency department sweating profusely and complaining of stomach cramps and diarrhea. He says that he has been "miserable" from the heat the past few days. His serum sodium level is 128 mmol/L.

    a. What electrolyte imbalance does the nurse suspect?

    b. The health care provider prescribes oral sodium tablets. What adverse effect of sodium may be of special concern for Samuel?

13. Vanessa is receiving a transfusion of a blood product.

    a. The nurse observes Vanessa, knowing that an adverse reaction to the transfusion may be manifested by what signs and symptoms?

    b. Vanessa's husband is crying and says, "People get AIDS [acquired immune deficiency syndrome] from transfusions. What happens if Vanessa gets AIDS?" How should the nurse best respond to this patient and her husband?

    c. Forty-five minutes after the transfusion is started, Vanessa is restless with an increased pulse rate. What are the nurse's next priority actions?

Case Study

Read the scenario and answer the following questions on a separate document.

An older adult man is admitted to the unit with hypoproteinemia caused by chronic malnutrition. You note that he has some edema over his body, and his total protein level is 48 g/L.

1. What is the relationship between his serum total protein level and the edema you have noted?

2. You are preparing to give him 1 unit of 5% albumin. How does albumin work in this situation?

3. What advantages does albumin have over crystalloids in this situation?

4. What adverse effects will you monitor for while he is receiving albumin?

CHAPTER 31

Pituitary Drugs

Chapter Review and Examination Preparation:

1. When administering vasopressin, what is the priority vital sign to monitor?
   a. Temperature
   b. Pulse
   c. Respirations
   d. Blood pressure

2. A nurse is administering octreotide (Sandostatin) to a patient who has a metastatic carcinoid tumour. The patient asks about the purpose of this drug. Which statement best responds to the patient's concern?
   a. "This drug helps to reduce the size of your tumour."
   b. "This drug works to prevent the spread of your tumour."
   c. "Octreotide is given to reduce the nausea and vomiting you are having from the chemotherapy."
   d. "This drug helps to control the flushing and diarrhea that you are experiencing."

3. Which nursing diagnosis is most appropriate for a patient who is receiving a pituitary drug?
   a. Constipation
   b. Disturbed body image
   c. Impaired physical mobility
   d. Impaired skin integrity

4. What priority instruction(s) should the nurse provide a patient taking desmopressin acetate (DDAVP Spray) nasal spray for the treatment of diabetes insipidus to obtain maximum benefit from the drug? (Select all that apply.)
   a. Clear the nasal passages before spraying the drug.
   b. Clear the nasal passages after spraying the drug.
   c. Take an over-the-counter preparation to control mucus production.
   d. Administer the nasal spray at the same time every day.

5. During assessment, the nurse discovers that a patient on corticotropin therapy is experiencing tremors and slight tetany. The nurse recognizes that these findings may indicate the development of which of the following?
   a. Hypokalemia
   b. Hyperkalemia
   c. Hypocalcemia
   d. Hypernatremia

6. When assessing a patient who is receiving octreotide therapy, the nurse will closely monitor which assessment finding?
   a. Blood glucose levels
   b. Pulse
   c. Weight
   d. Serum potassium levels

7. A child who weighs 20 kg (44 pounds) and is experiencing growth failure is to receive growth hormone therapy. The dosage ordered is 0.3 mg/kg per week, to be given as a series of one injection per day for 6 days.
   a. What is the total dose per week that this child will receive?
   b. What is the dose per injection?

8. The order reads, "Give octreotide (Sandostatin) 50 mcg IV bid." The drug is available in a strength of 0.1 mg/mL. How many millilitres will the nurse draw up for this dose? (Indicate your answer on the syringe.)

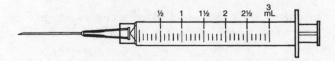

9. **Complete the following table:**

Hormone	Function	Mimicking Drug(s)
Adrenocorticotropic hormone (ACTH, corticotropin)	Targets adrenal gland; mediates adaption to stressors; promotes synthesis of the following three hormones: **a.**	**b.**
Growth hormone	**c.**	**d.**
e.	Increases water resorption in the distal tubules and collecting duct of nephron; concentrates urine; potent vasoconstrictor	**f.**
Endogenous oxytocin	**g.**	**h.**

ACTH, adrenocorticotropic hormone

Critical Thinking and Application

Answer the following questions on a separate document.

10. A nurse started working in a specialized endocrinology clinic. The nurse's first patient is a grade-2 student who is not growing at the expected rate. The physician determined that this patient is a candidate for somatropin (Humatrope) therapy. The parents are nervous about giving injections to the patient. What should be emphasized when teaching the parents about giving this drug?

11. A patient is being assessed for possible adrenocortical insufficiency. The physician orders a dose of cosyntropin. The patient, upon hearing that he will be receiving an injection, states, "Oh, good! The doctor has already found something to cure me!" How will the nurse respond?

Case Study

Read the scenario and answer the following questions on a separate document.

Colin has been experiencing severe thirst, which "of course, makes me go to the bathroom all the time, it seems." He is also dehydrated despite the amount of water he has been drinking. He is diagnosed with diabetes insipidus.

1. What two drugs may be used to treat this patient's diabetes insipidus?

2. What are priority cautions that the nurse should follow when taking these drugs?

3. The physician decides that Colin should do well with vasopressin therapy. Indicate how you would describe the treatment and its therapeutic effects (that is, how it mimics the natural hormone) to the patient.

4. Following your explanation, Colin says, "Okay, okay, but what does it do for me?" Explain the physical improvements Colin should be able to see.

CHAPTER 32

Thyroid and Antithyroid Drugs

Chapter Review and Examination Preparation

Choose the best answer for each of the following:

1. A patient was started on levothyroxine (Eltroxin) therapy. The patient asks the nurse, "When will this drug take effect?" What the is nurse's best response?
   a. Immediately
   b. Within a few days
   c. Within a few weeks
   d. Within a few months

2. A patient wants to switch brands of levothyroxine. Which response best addresses the patient's concern?
   a. "If you do this, you should reduce the dosage of your current brand before starting the new one."
   b. "Levothyroxine has been standardized, so there is only one brand."
   c. "It shouldn't matter if you switch brands; they are all very much the same."
   d. "You should check with your physician before switching brands."

3. What specific food products should the patient avoid when on antithyroid therapy?
   a. Soy products and seafood
   b. Bananas and oranges
   c. Dairy products
   d. Processed meats and cheese

4. Which information needs to be included in the nurse's teaching of patients taking thyroid drugs? (Select all that apply.)
   a. Keeping a log or journal of individual responses and a graph of pulse rate, weight, and mood would be helpful.
   b. The drug will be discontinued if the adverse effects become too strong.
   c. The drug needs to be taken at the same time every day.
   d. Nervousness, irritability, and insomnia may be a result of a dosage that is too high.
   e. Take thyroid replacement drugs after meals.

5. A patient is scheduled for a radioactive isotope study. This patient indicates daily use of levothyroxine. Which patient instructions should the nurse provide the patient prior to the study?
   a. Continue to take the drug as ordered.
   b. Skip the drug on the morning of the test.
   c. Stop the drug about 4 weeks before the test.
   d. Reduce the dosage 1 week before the test.

6. The nurse has been providing patient education regarding thyroid hormone replacement therapy. Which statement by the patient reflects a need for further teaching?
   a. "I will take this pill in the mornings."
   b. "Sometimes this medicine can make my heart skip beats, but that's a normal side effect."
   c. "I need to take this pill on an empty stomach and wait about 30 to 60 minutes before eating."
   d. "I will be sure to go to the clinic to have my thyroid levels tested regularly."

7. Levothyroxine (Synthroid) 88 mcg PO (orally) is ordered. What is 88 mcg expressed as in milligrams? _____

8. The order reads, "Give levothyroxine (Synthroid) 150 mcg IV now." The vial of drug, once reconstituted, contains 0.1 mg/mL. How many millilitres will the nurse draw up for this dose?

_____

Answer the following questions on a separate document.

9. Abby, aged 43 years, comes into the clinic complaining of hair loss, lethargy, and constipation. "I just can't eat anything," she says. As the nurse takes her blood pressure, the nurse notices that Abby's skin feels thickened; she also seems to have a lump in her neck. The primary health care provider diagnosed her with hypothyroidism. Suggest several possible appropriate drugs. Which of those is generally preferred? Why?

10. After undergoing a thyroidectomy as treatment for a thyroid tumour that turned out to be benign, a patient is given a prescription for levothyroxine (Eltroxin). "I thought I would be cured after this surgery!" she exclaims. "Why do I have to take a pill every day?" What priority health information should the nurse provide the patient?

11. A 32-year-old patient is prescribed propylthiouracil as part of treatment for Graves' disease. What laboratory tests are important to assess before she begins this drug?

Critical Thinking Crossword

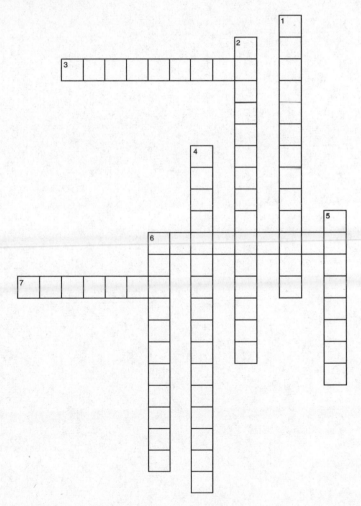

Across

3. The type of hypothyroidism that results from insufficient secretion of thyroid-stimulating hormone (TSH) from the pituitary gland
6. The principal thyroid hormone that influences the metabolic rate
7. The type of hypothyroidism that is due to the inability of the thyroid gland to perform a function

Down

1. The most commonly prescribed synthetic thyroid hormone
2. Excessive secretion of thyroid hormones
4. A drug used to treat hyperthyroidism
5. The type of hypothyroidism that stems from reduced secretion of TSH from the hypothalamus
6. Another name for thyroid-stimulating hormone

Case Study

Read the scenario and answer the following questions on a separate document.

Gwen, a 38-year-old teacher, has come to the clinic complaining of having "no energy or appetite," yet her weight has increased by 6.8 kg in the last month. The nurse notes that Gwen's hair is thin and that her skin is dull. Laboratory work reveals an elevated level of TSH.

1. What do these symptoms suggest? What drug does the nurse expect to be ordered for Gwen?

2. Explain the concept of "euthyroid" as it would relate to this patient's condition.

3. One month after therapy has begun, Gwen calls the office to complain that she can't sleep at all since she started taking the drug. She says she tries to take it at the same time every morning but often forgets and takes it at dinnertime. What teaching, if any, does she need to help her with this problem?

CHAPTER 33

Antidiabetic Drugs

Chapter Review and Examination Preparation

Choose the best answer for each of the following:

1. What is the most immediate and serious adverse effect of insulin therapy?
   a. Hyperglycemia
   b. Hypoglycemia
   c. Bradycardia
   d. Orthostatic hypotension

2. A dose of long-acting insulin has been ordered at bedtime for a diabetic patient. The nurse expects to give which type of insulin?
   a. regular (Novolin)
   b. lispro (Humalog)
   c. NPH (neutral protadine Hagedorn) (Novilin ge)
   d. glargine (Lantus)

3. A patient is to be placed on an insulin drip to control his high blood glucose levels. Which type of insulin will be used for this intravenous infusion?
   a. regular (Novolin)
   b. lispro (Humalog)
   c. NPH (Novilin ge)
   d. glargine (Lantus)

4. While monitoring a patient who is receiving insulin therapy, the nurse observes for which signs of hypoglycemia?
   a. Decreased pulse and respiratory rates and flushed skin
   b. Increased pulse rate and a fruity, acetone breath odour
   c. Weakness, sweating, and confusion
   d. Increased urine output and edema

5. When giving oral acarbose (Glucobay), the nurse should administer it at what time?
   a. 15 minutes before a meal
   b. 30 minutes before a meal
   c. With the first bite of a meal
   d. 1 hour after eating

6. A patient taking rosiglitazone (Avandia) tells the nurse, "There's my insulin pill!" The nurse describes the action of rosiglitazone by explaining that this drug is not insulin but that it works by a certain mechanism of action. Which of the following correctly describes how rosiglitazone acts?
   a. It acts by stimulating the cells of the pancreas to produce insulin.
   b. It acts by decreasing insulin resistance.
   c. It acts by inhibiting hepatic glucose production.
   d. It acts by decreasing the intestinal absorption of glucose.

7. The nurse will monitor for significant interactions if sitagliptin (Januvia) is given with which of the following?
   a. Corticosteroids
   b. Sulphonylureas
   c. Thyroid drugs
   d. Nonsteroidal anti-inflammatory drugs

8. The sliding-scale insulin order reads, "Glucose testing before meals. For glucose results of over 8.3 mmol/L, administer regular insulin (Humulin R) insulin, 1 unit for every 1.1 mmol/L over 8.3 mmol/L." If the blood glucose level is 13.2 mmol/L, how much insulin (in units) will the patient receive?

9. A patient will be receiving NPH insulin 30 units combined with 7 units of regular insulin. Mark the illustrated insulin syringe at the line that indicates the combined dose of insulin.

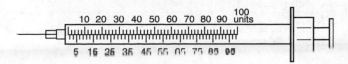

Critical Thinking and Application

Answer the following questions on a separate document.

10. What is the mechanism of action of each of the following drugs?

    a. sitagliptin (Januvia)

    b. metformin (Glucophage)

11. Alisa occasionally experiences hypoglycemia as a result of her diabetes drug therapy.

    a. The nurse will teach Alisa about what signs and symptoms of hypoglycemia?

    b. The nurse knows that one of the early signs of hypoglycemia is irritability. Why is this true?

    c. If Alisa experiences hypoglycemia at home, what are the treatment options?

12. A new graduate nurse is in the drugs room preparing a dose of Humulin-R to administer to a patient.

    a. Before the nurse administers the drug, how will the nurse's co-worker verify the order?

    b. After examining the syringe, the nurse's co-worker tells the graduate nurse that the syringe must be discarded because the insulin is cloudy. The new graduate states, "Insulin is supposed to look this way." Who is right, the new nurse or the co-worker?

    c. The nurse examines the vial. A date on the label indicates that it has been on the shelf in this room for 2 months. Is this a problem?

13. Alec, a 20-year-old university student, has been diagnosed with type 1 diabetes. The health care provider determines that the best treatment for this patient is with an insulin product that has an onset of 1 or 2 hours and a duration of 10 to 18 hours.

    a. What type of insulin does Alec require?

    b. What cultural considerations must the health care provider consider when choosing a specific drug for Alec?

14. Francine is 5 feet tall and weighs 81 kg. Laboratory studies from a routine physical indicate an elevated fasting blood glucose level and a hemoglobin A_{1C} level of 6.6%. The nurse's assessment reveals that Francine is a smoker with mild hypertension. The physician suspects type 2 diabetes. What initial treatment is indicated for Francine? Explain your answer.

15. Nadine is taking insulin every morning, with sliding-scale coverage. The specified dosages are (1) NPH (Novolin ge NPH) insulin, 20 units every morning before breakfast, and (2) regular (Novolin ge) insulin, sliding-scale coverage, before meals and at bedtime, as follow:

Blood glucose less than 11.1 mmol/L:	no additional coverage
Blood glucose 11.1 to 13.8 mmol/L:	2 units regular insulin
Blood glucose 13.9 to 16.6 mmol/L:	4 units regular insulin
Blood glucose more than 16.7 mmol/L:	6 units regular insulin
Blood glucose more than 19.4 mmol/L:	call for orders

How much insulin will Nadine receive in the following circumstances?

    a.   Before breakfast if her blood glucose level is 15.3 mmol/L

    b.   Before lunch if her blood glucose level is 10.9 mmol/L

    c.   Before dinner if her blood glucose level is 18.2 mmol/L

16. A patient who has been taking metformin (Glucophage) for type 2 diabetes mellitus needs to have a radiology examination with contrast dye. What is the nurse's best action regarding the metformin?

17. For each symptom listed below, specify whether it is associated with hyperglycemia or hypoglycemia.

    a.   Irritability

    b.   Fatigue

    c.   Polydipsia

    d.   Tremors

    e.   Sweating

Case Study

Read the scenario and answer the following questions on a separate document.

The health care provider is planning to prescribe glipizide (Glucotrol) for Deepak, a 50-year-old financial advisor with a history of renal failure and type 2 diabetes. In particular, Deepak requires treatment for the short-term elevation in blood glucose level that occurs after he eats.

1. Are there specific guidelines for when this drug needs to be taken?

2. At a visit 3 months later, during a blood draw for fasting laboratory tests, Deepak tells the nurse, "I've been good for the past few days, so I'm sure my fasting levels are okay. But thankfully the doctor won't know how I've been sneaking snacks." What laboratory test will be ordered to monitor Deepak's diabetes, and what will this test indicate?

3. A few weeks later, Deepak comes down with gastro-enteritis. He is vomiting and has been unable to eat all day. What should he do, and why?

CHAPTER 34

Adrenal Drugs

Chapter Review and Examination Preparation

Choose the best answer for each of the following:

1. A 35-year-old patient takes prednisone (Winpred) for the management of asthma. This patient notices that the dosage of the drug has decreased in the past week and asks the nurse, "Why can't I just stop taking the drug? I'm breathing better." Which of the following should the nurse tell this patient?
   a. Sudden discontinuation of this drug may cause an adrenal insufficiency.
   b. Abrupt discontinuation may result in withdrawal symptoms.
   c. Cushing's syndrome may develop as a reaction to a sudden drop of serum cortisone levels.
   d. Absence of asthmatic symptoms is an indication to stop the drug.

2. The nurse is reviewing the use of oral glucocorticoids. Which of the following is the preferred oral glucocorticoid for anti-inflammatory or immunosuppressant purposes?
   a. fludrocortisone (Florinef)
   b. dexamethasone
   c. prednisone
   d. hydrocortisone (Solu-Cortef)

3. When monitoring a patient who is taking corticosteroids, what adverse effects should the nurse watch for? (Select all that apply.)
   a. Fragile skin
   b. Increased glucose levels
   c. Nervousness
   d. Hypotension
   e. Weight loss
   f. Drowsiness

4. The nurse expects which of the following drugs to be used to inhibit the function of the adrenal cortex in the treatment of Cushing's syndrome?
   a. fludrocortisone
   b. dexamethasone
   c. prednisone
   d. hydrocortisone

5. A patient who has been taking corticosteroids has developed a "moon face" and facial redness and has many bruises on her arms. What is the most appropriate nursing diagnosis for this patient?
   a. Risk for infection
   b. Imbalanced nutrition (less than body requirements)
   c. Deficient fluid volume
   d. Disturbed body image

6. Corticosteroids have the ability to retain sodium. Which health condition should the nurse closely monitor as a priority when administering corticosteroids?
   a. Diabetes mellitus
   b. Seizure disorders
   c. Heart failure
   d. Hyperthyroidism

7. The order reads, "Give dexamethasone 1.5 mg, twice a day." The drug is available in 3 mg tablets. How many tablets will the nurse give for each dose?

   _____

8. An infant is to receive methylprednisolone (Solu-Medrol) 0.5 mg/kg intravenously every 6 hours. The infant weighs 6.3 kg. How many milligrams of drug will this infant receive per dose? (Record answer using one decimal place.) _____

Critical Thinking and Application

Answer the following questions on a separate document.

9. Rachel, a 30-year-old hospital receptionist, is receiving glucocorticoid therapy following a kidney transplant. The nurse is reviewing Rachel's drug regimen with her when Rachel mentions that she frequently uses acetylsalicylic acid (Aspirin) or ibuprofen (Motrin) to treat problems such as headaches or menstrual cramps. She also says that she enjoys walking for exercise and likes to visit sick children on the hospital's pediatric ward when she has time. Considering Rachel's lifestyle, what issues does the nurse discuss with her?

10. Peter, a 21-year-old mechanic, has developed a severe skin rash after a camping trip. The health care provider recommends prednisone therapy. The nursing assessment reveals that Peter has type 1 diabetes.

    a. Does that finding affect the prescription of prednisone? Explain your answer.

    b. To help minimize gastro-intestinal effects, what suggestions would the nurse have for someone taking an oral form of the systemic adrenal drugs?

11. The nurse is watching a student nurse prepare to apply a topical glucocorticoid to a patient's skin rash. After putting on gloves, the student places some of the drug on her finger. Should the nurse intervene, or is the student nurse doing fine so far? What other consideration is involved in determining the technique for applying a topical drug?

12. Lila is prescribed a steroid drug delivered via inhaler. What special instructions does the nurse give her?

Case Study

Read the scenario and answer the following questions on a separate document.

Julia, a 17-year-old patient, presents in the Urgent Care Centre because of an exacerbation of asthma. She is usually able to control it with inhaled bronchodilators, but the physician decides to give her a short course of prednisone in a dose that starts high and then tapers down over a week's time.

1. Why is the dose tapered instead of just discontinued after a week?

2. What are potential effects of long-term therapy?

3. Is this drug a glucocorticoid or a mineralocorticoid? Explain the difference.

4. What time of day should Julia take this drug? Explain.

CHAPTER 35

Women's Health Drugs

Chapter Review and Examination Preparation

Choose the best answer for each of the following:

1. When reviewing the health history of a patient who wants to begin taking oral contraceptives, what are the contraindications to this drug therapy? (Select all that apply.)
   a. Multiple sclerosis
   b. Pregnancy
   c. Thromboembolic disorders
   d. Breast cancer
   e. Abnormal vaginal bleeding
   f. Estrogen-dependent cancers

2. When teaching patients about postmenopausal estrogen replacement therapy, which statement is the most correct?
   a. "The smallest dose that is effective will be prescribed."
   b. "Oral forms should be taken on an empty stomach for best absorption."
   c. "Estrogen therapy should be long term to prevent menopausal symptoms."
   d. "If estrogen is taken, supplemental calcium will not be needed."

3. When combination oral contraceptives are used to provide postcoital emergency contraception, the nurse should remember which fact?
   a. They are not effective if the woman is already pregnant.
   b. They should be taken within 12 hours of unprotected intercourse.
   c. They are given in one dose.
   d. They are intended to terminate pregnancy.

4. When reviewing an order for dinoprostone (Prostin E2) cervical gel, the nurse recalls that this drug is used for which purpose?
   a. To induce abortion during the third trimester
   b. To improve cervical inducibility ("ripening") near term for labour induction
   c. To soften the cervix in women who are experiencing infertility problems
   d. To reduce postpartum uterine atony and hemorrhage

5. A pregnant woman is experiencing contractions. During what time are pharmacological measures to stop contractions used?
   a. Before the twentieth week of gestation
   b. Between the twentieth and thirty-seventh weeks
   c. After the thirty-seventh week
   d. At any time during the pregnancy if delivery is not desired

6. What patient teaching is appropriate for a patient taking alendronate (Fosamax)? (Select all that apply.)
   a. Take it on an empty stomach.
   b. Take it at night just before going to bed.
   c. Take with an 8-ounce (240 mL) glass of water.
   d. Take with a sip of water.
   e. Take first thing in the morning upon arising.
   f. Do not lie down for at least 30 minutes after taking.

7. A patient is beginning a new prescription of raloxifene (Evista). The nurse will teach the patient to expect which potential adverse effects? (Select all that apply.)
   a. Leg cramps
   b. Loss of appetite
   c. Diarrhea
   d. Hot flashes
   e. Drowsiness

8. The patient is to receive medroxyprogesterone (Depo-Provera) 500 mg weekly on Mondays for 4 weeks. The drug is available in vials of 400 mg/mL. How many millilitres will the nurse administer with each injection? (Record answer using one decimal place.) _____

    Mark the syringe with the correct amount the nurse will draw up for this injection.

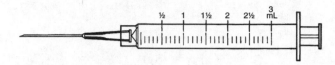

9. A patient is to receive megestrol (Megace) 400 mg each morning as an appetite stimulant. The drug is available in an oral suspension with a concentration of 40 mg/mL. How many millilitres will the nurse administer for this dose? _____

Critical Thinking and Application

Answer the following questions on a separate document.

10. Osvalda is a 48-year-old woman exhibiting symptoms of menopause. Assessment of Osvalda reveals a history of depression and mild arthritis.

    a. What priority question(s) should the nurse ask this patient and why?

    b. The health care provider decides to prescribe estrogen therapy. At this time, what does the nurse know about the dose and the length of time the estrogen will be administered?

11. Brenda is a 25-year-old patient with type 2 diabetes that is controlled by oral drugs. She is at the Family Health Clinic today because her menstrual periods have ceased. The nurse practitioner has decided to prescribe a hormonal drug.

    a. Which drug will the nurse practitioner likely prescribe?

    b. What adjustments to Brenda's existing drug regimen might need to be made?

12. Joyce receives a prescription for combined norethindrone–ethinyl estradiol (Alesse) for birth control purposes. At a follow-up visit 4 months later, she tells the nurse, "I am really messing up. I take the pills for 3 weeks, but when I'm off them for a week, sometimes I don't remember to start again."

    a. What might the nurse suggest to help Joyce?

    b. Joyce expresses concern that her menstrual bleeding, now that she is on birth control pills, is "nothing compared with what it used to be." She asks whether she is okay. What does the nurse tell Joyce?

13. Salema, a sales associate in a bookstore, is being treated for fertility problems. She is currently on a drug regimen that includes chorionic gonadotropin and menotropins.

    a. Why is Salema taking two fertility drugs?

    b. After the first course of treatment, Salema does not become pregnant. Describe her next course of treatment.

14. Ilsa has been taking estrogen therapy for several weeks. During a routine checkup, she tells the nurse that she has not been able to quit smoking. She also mentions that she is going to Aruba for a vacation the following month. What patient teaching does Ilsa require?

15. Vee, aged 33 years, comes in for her yearly gynecological examination, and the health care provider recommends alendronate (Fosamax) 5 mg daily. Vee experienced early menopause last year and asks the nurse, "Why did the doctor wait until now to start me on estrogen? I didn't need it before."

    a.   What does the nurse explain about the purpose of this drug?

    b.   What risk factors might Vee have to support therapy with alendronate?

16. Paul is receiving 400 mg of megestrol (Megace). This drug is a progestin, a female hormone. Why is a male patient receiving this drug?

Case Study

Read the scenario and answer the following questions on a separate document.

Olivia, a 34-year-old patient, is having mild contractions. She is in the thirtieth week of gestation, and the health care provider determines that she is experiencing premature labour.

1.   What nonpharmacological treatment is the health care provider likely to recommend?

2.   In Canada, are there other strategies that may be used to delay preterm labour?

CHAPTER 36

Men's Health Drugs

Chapter Review and Examination Preparation

Choose the best answer for each of the following:

1. An 18-year-old athlete asks the nurse about taking steroids to "beef up" his muscles. Which of the following statements is the most correct?
   a. There should be no problems as long as he does not exceed the recommended dose.
   b. Long-term use may cause a life-threatening liver condition.
   c. He would need to be careful to watch for excessive weight loss.
   d. These drugs also tend to increase sperm count.

2. For which health conditions or purposes would androgens be prescribed for a woman? (Select all that apply.)
   a. Development of secondary sex characteristics
   b. Fibrocystic breast disease
   c. Ovarian cancer
   d. Treatment of endometriosis
   e. Prevention of postmenopausal osteoporosis
   f. Metastatic breast cancer

3. A patient will be receiving testosterone therapy for male hypogonadism and has a new prescription for transdermal testosterone (Androderm) patches. What priority health teaching should the nurse convey?
   a. Apply the patch only on the scrotum.
   b. Apply the patch to the chest or back.
   c. If the adverse effects become bothersome, the patient should stop using the patch.
   d. The patch should be applied to a different area of the upper body each day.

4. Before a patient begins therapy with finasteride (Proscar), what laboratory test should be performed?
   a. Blood glucose level
   b. Complete blood count
   c. Urinalysis
   d. Prostate-specific antigen (PSA) level

5. A patient is taking finasteride (Proscar) for the treatment of benign prostatic hypertrophy. His wife, who is 3 months pregnant, is worried about the adverse effects that may occur with this drug. Which of the following statements by the nurse is the most important at this time?
   a. "Gastric upset may be reduced if he takes this drug on an empty stomach."
   b. "You should notice therapeutic effects of increased libido and erection within 1 month."
   c. "This drug should not be handled by pregnant women because it may harm the fetus."
   d. "He may experience transient hair loss while taking this drug."

6. Which drug is used, in low doses, for androgenic alopecia in both men and women?
   a. finasteride (Propecia)
   b. vardenafil (Levitra)
   c. danazol
   d. minoxidil

7. A patient has a new prescription for finasteride (Proscar). The nurse will instruct the patient about which potential adverse effects? (Select all that apply.)
   a. Loss of erection
   b. Gynecomastia
   c. Headaches
   d. Increased libido
   e. Ejaculatory dysfunction

8. A patient is to receive testosterone cypionate (Depo-Testosterone) 300 mg every 2 weeks as an intramuscular injection. The drug is available in two strengths: 100 mg/mL and 200 mg/mL.
   a. Which is the most appropriate strength?

   _____

   b. How many millilitres will the nurse administer per injection? _____

Critical Thinking and Application

Answer the following questions on a separate document.

9. Manuel is being treated for hypogonadism. He has been taking intramuscular injections of testosterone cypionate but has complained about the pain caused by the injections. Today he will be switched to an oral dosage form. He expects to get "testosterone pills." However, the nurse remembers the poor performance of the drug when given via that route, and she tells him that this oral form will probably not be testosterone itself.

   a. Manuel is skeptical of switching drugs and asks for more information. Explain why oral testosterone does not work well.

   b. What can the nurse expect Manuel to receive instead?

   c. Discuss potential contraindications that might apply to this patient.

10. Ky, a recent immigrant to Canada, is living temporarily with his sister and her two small children. He has been diagnosed with male hypogonadism and has been prescribed testosterone in the AndroGel pump form, which comes as a 60 actuation metered-dose pump.

    a. English is a second language for Ky. Describe to him what "60 actuation metered dose" means and what its implications are in terms of drug dosing.

    b. What specific instructions should Ky receive about the use of the pump?

11. Walter has been prescribed finasteride (Proscar) for his benign prostatic hyperplasia. He asks, "How does it work?" The nurse explains that it will cause his prostate to decrease in size and will alleviate discomfort. He is concerned about taking this new drug. What are the most important things for the nurse to include in his patient teaching plan?

12. Compare the application methods of the following forms of testosterone: Testoderm patch, Androderm patch, and AndroGel.

Case Study

Read the scenario and answer the following questions on a separate document.

Abu, aged 72 years, has asked the physician for "help with a private matter." He tells the physician that he would like to try "that drug that helps with a certain problem" (i.e., sildenafil).

1. What assessment findings may contraindicate the use of sildenafil for Abu?

2. If Abu is a candidate for therapy with sildenafil citrate (Viagra), what should he be told about it?

3. What concerns would there be about his liver function? About his vision?

4. When should he take this drug?

CHAPTER 37

Antihistamines, Decongestants, Antitussives, and Expectorants

Chapter Review and Examination Preparation

Choose the best answer for each of the following:

1. A patient requests information about antihistamine use. What health teaching should the nurse include for this patient? (Select all that apply.)
   a. Antihistamines are best tolerated when taken with meals.
   b. The patient can suck on hard candy or chew gum if dry mouth is experienced.
   c. The main adverse effect of antihistamines is drowsiness.
   d. Over-the-counter drugs are generally safe to use with antihistamines.
   e. The patient should avoid drinking alcoholic beverages while taking antihistamines.

2. A patient asks the nurse for advice about one of the newer antihistamines that does not cause drowsiness. Which is the most appropriate drug?
   a. desloratadine (Aerius)
   b. diphenhydramine hydrochloride (Benadryl)
   c. dimenhydrinate
   d. clemastine

3. Which drugs are considered first-line drugs for the treatment of nasal congestion? (Select all that apply.)
   a. Antihistamines such as diphenhydramine hydrochloride
   b. Decongestants such as oxymetazoline (Vicks Sinex)
   c. Antitussives such as dextromethorphan (Benylin)
   d. Expectorants such as guaifenesin (Robitussin Liquid)
   e. Inhaled corticosteroids such as beclomethasone

4. When giving an antitussive, the nurse should remember that they are used primarily for what reason?
   a. To relieve nasal congestion
   b. To thin secretions to ease the removal of excessive secretions
   c. To stop the cough reflex when the cough is nonproductive
   d. To suppress productive and nonproductive coughs

5. The nurse is preparing to administer an expectorant drug. What priority patient instructions must the nurse teach the patient?
   a. Avoid fluids for 30 to 35 minutes after the dose.
   b. Drink plenty of fluids, unless contraindicated, to aid in expectoration of sputum.
   c. Avoid operating heavy machinery or driving while taking this drug.
   d. Expect the secretions to become thicker.

6. A patient has been self-medicating with diphenhydramine to help her sleep. She calls the clinic nurse to ask, "Why do I feel so tired during the day after I take this pill? I get a good night's sleep!" Which is the most appropriate statement by the nurse?
   a. "You are probably getting too much sleep."
   b. "You are taking too much of the drug."
   c. "This drug is not really meant to help people sleep."
   d. "This drug often causes a 'hangover effect' during the day after taking it."

7. A patient is to receive guaifenesin 300 mg via a nasogastric tube. The available drug is syrup, 100 mg/5mL.
   a. How many millilitres will the nurse administer?
   b. Mark the drug cup with your answer.

8. A 5-year-old child is to receive a one-time dose of diphenhydramine (Benadryl) 6.25 mg orally (PO). The drug is available in a syrup form with a concentration of 12.5 mg/5 mL. How many millilitres will the nurse administer for this dose? _____

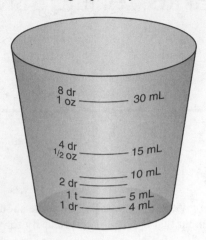

Critical Thinking and Application

Answer the following questions on a separate document.

9. Ling was seen in the office several days ago with a common cold. She has been on decongestant therapy with oxymetazoline hydrochloride since then. Today, she calls to say, "I thought I was getting over this, but suddenly my nose is more stuffed up than ever." Does Ling possibly need a stronger dosage of decongestant? Explain your answer.

10. Keith has been using a topical nasal decongestant for the past few days. He calls the family health clinic to report that he is feeling nervous and dizzy and that his heart seems to be racing. What might be the cause of Keith's symptoms?

11. How does dextromethorphan differ from other antitussive drugs in its mechanism of action? What about its drug interaction profile?

12. Lisa is a 5-year-old patient who has bronchitis accompanied by a nonproductive cough. The health care provider prescribed guaifenesin for the cough. Lisa's father tells the nurse that his 11-year-old son was prescribed Robitussin AC several months ago for a severe cough. He asks whether his son's cough medicine would help Lisa, since "there is plenty left in the bottle." What does the nurse tell him?

13. Britney gave birth recently and is breastfeeding her baby. She calls the pediatrician's office because she wants to take an over-the-counter antihistamine for her allergies. "It's okay now that I've given birth, right?" What is the nurse's best answer?

Case Study

Read the scenario and answer the following questions on a separate document.

James, a 35-year-old electrician, is seen in the emergency department with a rash on his arms and hands that appeared after he was working in his yard. The nurse suspects that the physician will prescribe topical diphenhydramine (anti-itch cream), but during the nursing assessment, James says that he has diabetes.

1. How does James's diagnosis of diabetes affect his possible treatment with diphenhydramine?

2. If James does receive a topical diphenhydramine, what other drug might be found in combination with it?

The topical drug did not help his rash, and James has been switched to oral diphenhydramine. He tells the nurse that he expects to return to work tomorrow and hopes this drug "does the trick."

3. What cautions, if any, should James be aware of while taking this drug?

4. Are there any concerns with drug interactions?

CHAPTER 38

Respiratory Drugs

Chapter Review and Examination Preparation

Choose the best answer for each of the following:

1. The nurse is teaching a group of patients about the use of bronchodilators. It is important to remind them that using bronchodilators too frequently may cause which adverse effects? (Select all that apply.)
    a. Blurred vision
    b. Increased heart rate
    c. Decreased heart rate
    d. Nausea
    e. Nervousness
    f. Tremors

2. A patient is on leukotriene antagonist therapy. What health teaching must the nurse provide this patient about this class of drugs?
    a. If a dose is missed, the patient may take a double dose to maintain therapeutic blood levels.
    b. The patient should gargle or rinse his or her mouth after taking the drug.
    c. The drug should be taken at the first sign of bronchospasm.
    d. Improvement should be seen within 1 week of use.

3. Which drug acts by blocking leukotrienes, thus reducing inflammation in the lungs?
    a. salbutamol sulphate (Ventolin)
    b. methylprednisolone (Solu-Medrol)
    c. theophylline (Theolair)
    d. montelukast

4. A patient is experiencing status asthmaticus. What priority drug should the nurse prepare to administer?
    a. salbutamol sulphate (Ventolin)
    b. epinephrine
    c. theophylline (Theolair)
    d. montelukast

5. When a patient is taking parenteral xanthine derivatives, such as aminophylline, the nurse should monitor for which adverse effect?
    a. Decreased respirations
    b. Hypotension
    c. Tachycardia
    d. Hypoglycemia

6. A patient who is taking a ß-adrenergic agonist for bronchodilation may also take which type of inhaled drug for its anti-inflammatory effects?
    a. Corticosteroid
    b. Anticholinergic
    c. Xanthine derivative
    d. Antileukotriene

7. A patient has a new prescription for an ipratropium bromide/albuterol sulphate (Combivent) metered-dose inhaler. The patient is to take two puffs four times a day. The inhaler contains 200 puffs. After how many days should the patient replace the inhaler? _____

8. A 6-year-old child is to receive salbutamol sulphate (Airomir) 0.1 mg/kg orally (PO) three to four times a day. The child weighs 18 kg. How many milligrams will the child receive per dose? (Record answer using one decimal place.) _____

Critical Thinking and Application

Answer the following questions on a separate document.

9. Tom, a 70-year-old retiree who smoked for 40 years, has been diagnosed with chronic obstructive pulmonary disease (COPD); the treatment regimen prescribed includes theophylline (Theolair). After a few weeks, Tom tells the nurse that he is experiencing nausea and "bad heartburn at night." The laboratory studies show the level of theophylline in his blood to be 130 mcmol/L. What might be wrong with Tom, and how can it be corrected?

10. Willie is a 9-year-old boy who is brought to the emergency department by his aunt because he is having an acute asthma attack. The physician orders epinephrine to be administered subcutaneously. How does the nurse calculate the dosage for Willie?

11. Sylvia has come to the clinic today complaining of nausea, palpitations, and anxiety. She says that her heart feels "as if it's going to fly out" of her chest. Physical examination confirms an increased heart rate. Sylvia's records indicate that she has asthma, for which she uses a salbutamol (Ventolin) inhaler. What does the nurse suspect might be wrong with Sylvia, and what suggestions does the nurse have for her?

12. Roberta, a 65-year-old office manager, has arthritis, glaucoma, and emphysema. The health care provider is planning prophylactic treatment for her emphysema.

    a. What three types of drugs might be considered for a patient with COPD?

    b. What factor must the physician keep in mind when determining the best drug for Roberta?

13. Several months ago, the health care provider prescribed an orally administered corticosteroid for Jonathan, who has chronic bronchial asthma.

    a. What are the disadvantages of administering the corticosteroids orally?

    b. Today the physician adds beclomethasone dipropionate (QVAR) to Jonathan's drug regimen and also reduces the dosage of the oral corticosteroid. Is that safe?

14. Sam is a 10-year-old girl who is to be treated with Advair for asthma.

    a. What drugs are contained in Advair? Explain why they would be used in Sam's case.

    b. What other drug would be an important component of Sam's daily routine? Explain.

15. Justin calls the nurse at the office because he experiences "palpitations and a racing heart" every morning after breakfast. He is taking theophylline as part of his treatment for asthma. Upon questioning, he states that he has been drinking an extra cup of coffee in the morning "to get going" because his coughing has kept him from sleeping well. What could be his problem?

Case Study

Read the scenario and answer the following questions on a separate document.

Jennie has been treated for adult-onset asthma for 3 years. The health care provider started her taking one daily 10 mg tablet of montelukast.

1. How does this drug differ from traditional antiasthma drugs?

2. Jennie says, "I hope this medicine works better than the other one I took when I had an asthma attack." How should the nurse respond?

3. Jennie takes ibuprofen (Advil) on occasion for arthritic pain. What should the nurse advise about taking this drug with montelukast?

4. After 3 months, Jennie stops taking the montelukast. She says that her symptoms are "better" and "I don't want to take medicine unless I need it." Is this appropriate?

CHAPTER 39

Acid-Controlling Drugs

Chapter Review and Examination Preparation

Choose the best answer for each of the following:

1. A patient with kidney failure wants to take an antacid for "sour stomach." The nurse needs to consider that some antacids may be dangerous when taken by patients with kidney failure. Thus, which of the following types of antacid should be recommended?
   a. Activated charcoal
   b. Aluminum-containing antacids
   c. Calcium-containing antacids
   d. Magnesium-containing antacids

2. A patient with peptic ulcer disease will be starting drug therapy. He tells the nurse that he smokes and wonders if that will affect his treatment. What is the nurse's best response?
   a. "Smoking has no effect on these drugs."
   b. "The actions of antacids are less potent when the patient smokes."
   c. "Smoking has been shown to decrease the effectiveness of H_2 blockers."
   d. "Smoking has been shown to increase the adverse effects of H_2 blockers."

3. Which drug class would be used as first-line therapy for gastro-esophageal reflux disease that has not responded to customary medical treatment?
   a. H_2 blockers
   b. Antacids
   c. Mucosal protectors
   d. Proton pump inhibitors

4. A nurse administers a proton pump inhibitor drug for several patients. What important information must the nurse know about this drug? (Select all that apply.)
   a. It should be taken 1 hour before taking antacids.
   b. It should be taken 30 to 60 minutes before meals.
   c. It should be taken with meals.
   d. It is part of the treatment of patients with *Helicobacter pylori* infections.
   e. There are few adverse effects with proton pump inhibitors.

5. A pregnant woman asks the nurse about taking an antacid for indigestion. What is the nurse's best response?
   a. "You won't be allowed to take an antacid while you are pregnant."
   b. "Let's check with your obstetrician to see what is recommended."
   c. "Go ahead and use an aluminum-based antacid."
   d. "Sodium bicarbonate would be the safest choice."

6. A patient is to receive cimetidine 300 mg by intravenous piggyback (IVPB) twice a day. The drug is available in a concentration of 150 mg/mL. How many millilitres will the nurse draw up to prepare

   for the IVPB dose? _____

7. The patient is to receive pantoprazole (Protonix) 40 mg mixed in 100 mL of 5% dextrose in water (D_5W), intravenously over 30 minutes. The nurse

   will set the infusion pump to what rate? _____

123

Critical Thinking and Application

Answer the following questions on a separate document.

8. Veronica is advised to take omeprazole (Losec) to treat her severe case of gastro-esophageal reflux disease; nothing else has worked. Develop a patient teaching plan that will instruct Veronica in how this drug should be taken.

9. Kurt has called to ask which antacid he should take. He has been to the store and is confused by the great variety on the shelves. He says he needs something for "occasional heartburn" when he eats something too spicy. He has a history of heart failure and is taking antihypertensive drugs. What type of antacid should he take, and what other instructions would he need?

10. Vlad is taking enteric-coated Aspirin for mild arthritis symptoms. He tells the nurse that he plans to take Aspirin with his favourite antacid, Maalox, because he does not want any stomach problems. What should the nurse tell him?

11. Frank has been diagnosed with a peptic ulcer caused by *Helicobacter pylori*. He has been told that he will be started on drug therapy for this disease. What does this therapy involve?

12. The nurse is caring for a patient who has been transferred to the step-down unit after spending a week in the Critical Care Unit after a myocardial infarction. The nurse notices that the patient's drug list includes a proton pump inhibitor, but there is no mention of any gastro-intestinal disorders on his chart. What is the reason for this drug?

Match each definition with its corresponding term. (Note: Some definitions may have more than one answer; some terms may be used more than once.)

13. _____ Drugs that block all acid secretion in the stomach

14. _____ Generic name for a cytoprotective drug

15. _____ Antacids that have constipating effects

16. _____ The cause of many peptic ulcers

17. _____ Drugs used to relieve the painful symptoms associated with gas

18. _____ A type of antacid that may contribute to the development of kidney stones

19. _____ A highly soluble antacid form with a quick onset but short duration of action

a. Aluminum-containing antacids

b. Calcium-containing antacids

c. Magnesium-containing antacids

d. Antiflatulents

e. Proton pump inhibitors

f. *Helicobacter pylori*

g. Sodium bicarbonate

i. Sucralphate

Case Study

Read the scenario and answer the following questions on a separate document.

Eda, aged 78 years, has been treating herself with antacids for "heartburn" for 6 months. After an endoscopy of her upper gastro-intestinal tract, she was diagnosed with gastro-esophageal reflux disease. The decision has been made to start treatment with cimetidine. Eda has been generally healthy except for a history of asthma. She says that she does not smoke but that she enjoys going to a bingo session every Saturday for a few hours, where there is smoking, beer, and pizza.

1. When Eda sees the prescription for cimetidine, she asks, "Why do I need a prescription? I can buy this over the counter." What does the nurse say in reply?

2. How will the cimetidine work to help gastro-esophageal reflux disease?

3. What cautions, if any, are associated with the use of cimetidine?

4. Will staying in a smoke-filled room affect Eda's therapy? Explain.

CHAPTER 40

Antidiarrheal Drugs and Laxatives

Chapter Review and Examination Preparation

Choose the best answer for each of the following:

1. A nurse is preparing to administer bismuth subsalicylate (Pepto-Bismol). Which of the following patients is most appropriate choice for this drug?
   a. A 7-year-old child who has chickenpox
   b. A 23-year-old woman who has severe abdominal pain
   c. A 45-year-old man who is complaining of constipation
   d. A 58-year-old man who developed diarrhea after travelling outside of the country

2. The nurse will teach a patient who is self-treating with bismuth subsalicylate to avoid which drug because of the possibility of toxicity?
   a. acetylsalicylic acid
   b. acetaminophen
   c. calcium supplements
   d. vitamin tablets

3. A patient asks for a drug that will provide rapid relief of constipation. After ruling out possible contraindications, which drug would the nurse recommend?
   a. psyllium
   b. methylcellulose
   c. docusate sodium (Colace)
   d. magnesium hydroxide (Milk of Magnesia)

4. A patient has been given polyethylene (Pegalax) in preparation for a colonoscopy. He begins to have diarrhea after about 45 minutes. Two hours later, he tells the nurse that the diarrhea has not stopped yet. What should the nurse do?
   a. Give him an antidiarrheal drug, such as diphenoxylate (Lomotil).
   b. Give him another dose of the polyethylene glycol (PEG) 3350 to finish cleansing his bowel.
   c. Remind him that it may take up to 4 hours to completely evacuate the bowel.
   d. Report this to the health care provider.

5. A 79-year-old woman visits the clinic today and tells the nurse that her "bowels just aren't right." She wants advice on the best laxative to take so that she can have a bowel movement every day. Which of the following is appropriate for the nurse to tell this patient? (Select all that apply.)
   a. "A normal bowel pattern does not necessarily mean that you will have a bowel movement every day."
   b. "Try taking Metamucil with sips of water."
   c. "You can try taking Milk of Magnesia every other day; it's a mild laxative."
   d. "Let's talk about increasing fluids and fibre in your diet."
   e. "Mineral oil would be safe for long-term use if needed."

6. The order for a child with severe diarrhea reads, "Give diphenoxylate with atropine (Lomotil) 0.3 mg/kg/day in 4 divided doses." The drug is available in an oral solution with a concentration of 2.5 mg/5 mL. The child weighs about 20 kg.
   a. How many milligrams will the child receive per dose? _____
   b. How many millilitres will the child receive per dose? _____

7. The order for a child reads, "Give lactulose 5 g, PO daily after breakfast." The drug is available as an oral solution in a unit-dose package that contains 10 g/15 mL. How many millilitres will the nurse administer per dose? _____

Critical Thinking and Application

Answer the following questions on a separate document.

8. Anna has called the health clinic in a panic. She says that she has been taking Pepto-Bismol for diarrhea and noticed this morning that her tongue is "a funny colour." She asks, "Have I overdosed on this stuff? What should I do?" How should the nurse respond to Anna?

9. Martina is a 55-year-old store manager with osteoporosis and glaucoma. She has recently developed diarrhea, and the health care provider is considering antidiarrheal therapy. Martina tells the nurse that her husband recently "had a bout of diarrhea" for which he was prescribed a belladonna alkaloid. Martina wonders whether the same drug would help in her case. What should the nurse tell her?

10. Hillary has come to the health care provider's office complaining of constipation. During the nursing assessment, Hillary mentions that she recently started graduate school and has not had time lately to keep up her usual exercise regimen and that her diet is a "disaster." She says that on some days, all she has time to do is grab a milkshake at the student union. She also tells the nurse that she has been taking antacids for "heartburn." What might be causing Hillary's constipation?

11. Ira, a 45-year-old accountant, has chronic constipation.

    a. What are the advantages of bulk-forming laxatives for treating Ira's problem?

    b. The health care provider prescribes psyllium. What instructions does the nurse give Ira regarding its administration?

12. Drake is a 5-year-old boy with constipation. The health care provider has ordered treatment with glycerin suppositories.

    a. Why is glycerin a good choice for Drake?

    b. For what adverse effects will the nurse monitor?

Critical Thinking Crossword

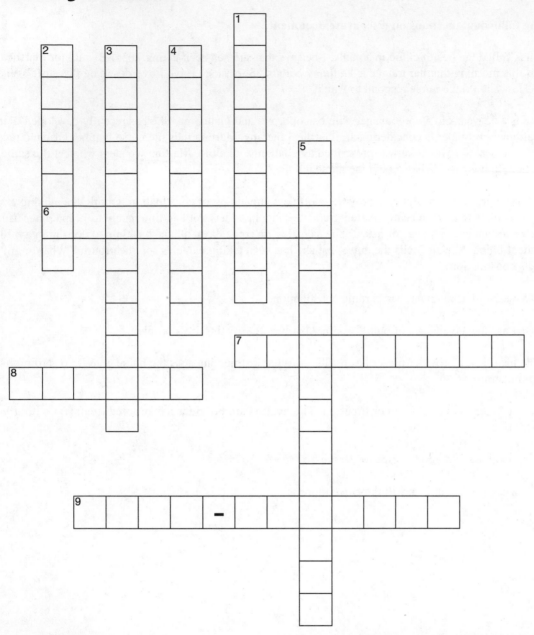

Across

6. A type of laxative that softens the stool
7. Another term for intestinal flora modifier
8. One type of laxative that increases osmotic pressure in the small intestine, increasing water content and resulting in distention
9. Laxatives that absorb water into the intestine, increasing the volume and distending the bowel (two words)

Down

1. Antidiarrheal drug that acts by coating the walls of the gastro-intestinal tract and binding to causative bacteria or toxins to allow elimination via the stool
2. Drugs that decrease bowel motility
3. A type of laxative that increases fecal water content in the large intestine, resulting in distention, increased peristalsis, and evacuation
4. A laxative that stimulates the nerves that supply the intestine, resulting in increased peristalsis
5. Antidiarrheal drug that acts by decreasing peristalsis and muscular tone of the intestine, thus slowing the movement of substances through the gastro-intestinal tract

Case Study

Read the scenario and answer the following questions on a separate document.

Charles, aged 54 years, recently completed a 2-week course of antibiotic therapy for pneumonia. He is now experiencing severe diarrhea.

1. What is the probable cause of his diarrhea?

2. What antidiarrheal is indicated for him?

3. How does this antidiarrheal work?

4. Is this antidiarrheal considered to be a drug or a dietary supplement? Explain.

CHAPTER 41

Antiemetic and Antinausea Drugs

Chapter Review and Examination Preparation

Choose the best answer for each of the following.

1. A patient requests drug to reduce symptoms of nausea. What antiemetic drug(s) can the nurse expect to prepare that is (are) known to cause drowsiness and a drying of secretions? (Select all that apply.)
   a. Antihistamines
   b. Antidopaminergic drugs
   c. Serotonin blockers
   d. Tetrahydrocannabinoids
   e. Anticholinergics

2. A nurse is reviewing chemotherapy with a newly hired nurse on the Oncology Unit. Which antinausea drug or drug class is indicated for preventing chemotherapy-induced nausea and vomiting? (Select all that apply.)
   a. Antihistamines
   b. Neuroleptics
   c. Serotonin blockers
   d. Anticholinergics
   e. Tetrahydrocannabinoids

3. When reviewing the drugs used for nausea and vomiting, which drug is a synthetic derivative of the major active substance in marijuana?
   a. ondansetron (Zofran)
   b. metoclopramide hydrochloride
   c. prochlorperazine
   d. dronabinol

4. A patient is undergoing chemotherapy. When giving antiemetics, the nurse will remember that these drugs are most effective against nausea when given at what time?
   a. Before meals
   b. At bedtime
   c. Before chemotherapy begins
   d. Just after chemotherapy begins

5. When giving dronabinol to a patient with acquired immune deficiency syndrome (AIDS), the nurse knows that in addition to reducing nausea, this drug may also have what effect?
   a. Euphoria
   b. Enhanced appetite
   c. Reduced pain
   d. Enhanced sleep

6. The order reads, "Give prochlorperazine 10 mg IM every 4 hours as needed for nausea. Maximum of 4 doses/day." The drug is available in an ampule that contains 5 mg/mL. Mark the syringe with the amount the nurse will administer for each dose.

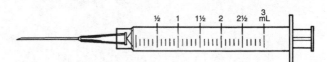

7. A patient is about to receive his first chemotherapy treatment with a drug that is known to cause nausea and vomiting. One of the premedication orders reads, "Give ondansetron (Zofran) PO 24 mg one-half hour before chemotherapy begins." Because the patient does not like to take pills, the drug is ordered in a syrup that contains 4 mg/5 mL. How many millilitres of drug will the nurse administer for this dose? _____

Critical Thinking and Application

Answer the following questions on a separate document.

8. Petra has gastro-esophageal reflux disease, and the health care provider has ordered oral metoclopramide four times a day for 2 weeks.

   a. What instructions should the nurse give Petra for administration of the drug?

   b. A few days later, Petra calls to say that she thinks the drug is "too strong." She also mentions that her evening routine includes "a couple of glasses of wine." What does the nurse tell Petra?

9. Nellie is prescribed prochlorperazine through an intramuscular injection. She is on nil per os (NPO) (i.e., nothing by mouth) status and has no intravenous access at this time. The nurse is preparing the injection when Nellie says, "I hate shots. Can't I just take it by mouth?" What alternatives are there for administering this drug, and what should the nurse do?

10. Chuck, a 33-year-old who is in a later stage of AIDS, has lost much weight and has no appetite. The health care provider prescribes dronabinol. When Chuck finds out that this drug is derived from marijuana, he becomes upset. "Why am I prescribed pot?" he asks. What is the best explanation by the nurse?

Case Study

Read the scenario and answer the following questions on a separate document.

Suk is preparing for his second course of chemotherapy as part of treatment for leukemia. One of the chemotherapy premedications is ondansetron (Zofran). His chemotherapy will last daily for 1 week.

1. What are potential contraindications to the use of ondansetron?

2. Suk tells the nurse that he still has nausea. He is puzzled because "I take the medicine for nausea as soon as I feel nauseated." How should the nurse address his concerns?

3. One day, Suk complains to the nurse that he gets a headache every time the ondansetron is administered. What should the nurse do?

CHAPTER 42

Nutritional Supplements

Chapter Review and Examination Preparation

Choose the best answer for each of the following:

1. A nurse is developing a nutritional plan for a patient who is unable to ingest food orally. The health care provider prescribes peripherally administered total parenteral nutrition (TPN) for this patient. What is the maximum concentration of dextrose the nurse can administer for this patient?
   a. 10%
   b. 20%
   c. 50%
   d. 100%

2. An elderly patient is placed on an enteral supplementary diet. The dietitian recommends Ensure or Sustacal. What are these supplements examples of?
   a. Elemental or monomeric solutions
   b. Blenderized solutions
   c. Polymeric, lactose-free solutions
   d. Polymeric, milk-based solutions

3. When monitoring a patient who is receiving TPN through a central line, what priority condition must the nurse continuously assess for? (Select all that apply.)
   a. Pneumothorax
   b. Aspiration
   c. Hyperglycemia
   d. Infection
   e. Air embolus

4. What health teaching should the nurse provide a patient regarding the most common adverse effect of beginning an enteral nutritional supplement therapy?
   a. Anorexia
   b. Constipation
   c. Diarrhea
   d. Flatulence

5. When reviewing a patient's need for nutritional supplementation, the nurse remembers that peripheral TPN is most appropriate for which patients?
   a. Patients who will receive short-term TPN (for less than 2 weeks)
   b. Patients who will receive long-term delivery of TPN (for more than 2 weeks)
   c. Patients with severe nutritional problems
   d. Patients who wish to reduce their weight

6. What is the priority nursing intervention for patients receiving enteral feedings?
   a. Warm feeding-tube formulas above room temperature
   b. Starting the infusions at the maximum rate ordered
   c. Keeping the head of the bed flat
   d. Giving tube feeding formulas that are at room temperature

7. A patient will be receiving TPN. The first bag is to infuse at 50 mL per hour for 4 hours, then 75 mL per hour for 4 hours, then at 100 mL per hour thereafter. What is the intravenous intake for the TPN

   over the first 12 hours of the infusion? _____

Critical Thinking and Application

Answer the following questions on a separate document.

8. Pauline is receiving enteral feeding using a newer nasogastric tube (7 French diameter).

    a. What are the advantages and disadvantages of these newer tubes?

    b. What symptoms would Pauline develop if she were lactose intolerant?

    c. Pauline's tube feeding rate is 50 mL per hour. After 24 hours, the nurse notes that the residual amount is 120 mL. What priority intervention must the nurse initiate?

9. Ronaldo, who is on TPN therapy, has a weak pulse, hypertension, tachycardia, and decreased urinary output. He seems somewhat confused, and on examining him, the nurse notes that he exhibits pitting edema. What is happening with this patient? What priority nursing interventions must be initiated?

Critical Thinking Crossword

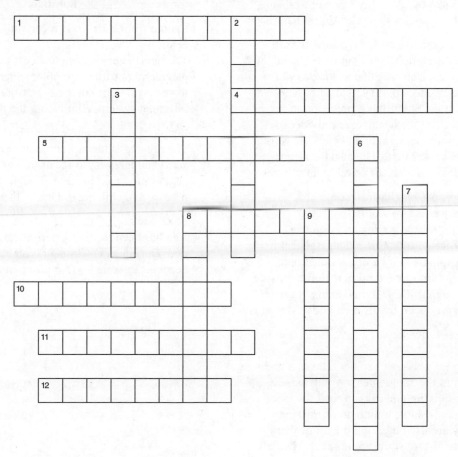

Across

1. Martin is receiving an oral antibiotic when it is determined that he is going to need nutritional supplementation as well. However, you are concerned that the nutritional supplement will decrease the absorption of the drug because of high gastric acid content or prolonged emptying time. What is the generic name of the antibiotic Martin is taking?

4. Nat needs amino acids in nutritional supplements. The main use or primary role of amino acids is

   protein synthesis, or _____.

5. Wilson is about to receive a _____, in which a feeding tube will be surgically inserted directly into his stomach.

8. Ling is worried about her husband, who has postsurgical nausea. She sees that his roommate is receiving TPN and asks the nurse, "Can't you do that for my husband just while he's so nauseated?" TPN, the nurse explains, is to be used only when enteral support is impossible or when the gastro-intestinal tract's

   _____ or functional capacity is insufficient.

10. Celia comes to the clinic when a cut on her hand "just won't heal up." She also says that as long as she is here, she would like to report symptoms of hair loss and scaly dermatitis. She wants a prescription for her skin problem, but the health care provider says, "There's something more going on here." He runs a few tests and discovers that Celia also has decreased platelets and some evidence of possible fatty liver.

    He says he suspects Celia has essential _____ deficiency. (Answer is two words.)

11. Mason is having trouble getting and digesting enough dietary forms of amino acids. His health care provider explains that he needs nutritional supplementation through enteral nutrition to ensure that he gets enough of these amino acids because they cannot be produced by his own body. Mason is

    suffering from a deficiency of _____ amino acids.

12. Craig, a third-year university student, takes a great deal of interest in the supplementary nutritional product he is receiving and asks to read the label. He says, "There are some amino acids missing from this. Why aren't you giving me all of them?" The nurse explains that some amino acids (i.e., all but eight) are manufactured in the body, using

    _____ sources.

Down

2. When Sheila asks why she needs amino acid supplemental feedings, the nurse explains that amino acids promote growth and help with wound healing. One of the principal ways they do so is by reducing or slowing the breakdown of proteins, or

   _____.

3. The Johnsons recently appeared in a television commercial for Ensure because they drink Ensure to take care of a few extra nutritional needs they have experienced with aging. Their nephew recently had surgery, and while recovering, he received nasogastric delivery of a modular formulation to supplement a polymeric feeding formulation he needed. Also, when their grandson was an infant, his parents supplemented his breastfeeding with an infant nutritional formulation. Each member of the Johnson family discussed here has received some

   form of _____ nutrition.

6. Lauren from 8 Down is receiving _____ amino acids.

7. The nurse is explaining to Zoe's family that the parenteral nutritional supplementation that is about to start will help Zoe by bypassing the entire gastro-intestinal system, eliminating the need for absorp-

   tion, _____, and excretion.

8. The nursing student, Lauren, is reviewing amino acids and is trying to recall the two amino acids that are not produced in large enough quantities during infancy and childhood. One of these is histidine; the

   other one is _____.

9. Ken has been receiving peripheral parenteral nutrition. During an assessment, you note that his vein becomes inflamed. What problem is this?

Case Study

Read the scenario and answer the following questions on a separate document.

The nurse is caring for Genevieve, who is receiving peripheral parenteral nutrition via an intravenous (IV) line in her right forearm. The nurse's assessment shows that bag number 3 is infusing at 100 mL per hour via an infusion pump, and the bag has about 300 mL remaining. The site is intact, without redness or swelling.

1. Two hours later, Genevieve calls the nurse because she accidentally pulled the IV line out of her arm. The remaining 300 mL of TPN has spilled onto the floor. The nurse has tried to restart the IV line but has not had success yet. What could occur if the nurse cannot restart the infusion?

2. At last, the IV line is re-inserted, but the nurse then discovers that bag number 4 has not yet been ordered from the pharmacy. What should the nurse hang until bag four is ready?

3. What else should the nurse monitor while Genevieve is receiving peripheral parenteral nutrition?

Antibiotics Part 1: Sulphonamides, Penicillins, Cephalosporins, Macrolides, and Tetracyclines

Chapter Review and Examination Preparation

Choose the best answer for each of the following.

1. A patient is started on penicillin medication therapy to treat an infection. What priority drug substance(s) should the nurse teach the patient to avoid to prevent drug interaction? (Select all that apply.)
   a. Alcohol
   b. Oral contraceptives
   c. digoxin
   d. Nonsteroidal anti-inflammatory drugs
   e. warfarin (Coumadin)
   f. Anticonvulsants

2. Which intervention is important for the nurse to perform before beginning antibiotic therapy?
   a. Obtain a specimen for culture and sensitivity.
   b. Give the antibiotic with an antacid to reduce gastro-intestinal upset.
   c. Monitor for adverse effects.
   d. Restrict oral fluids.

3. What priority instructions should the nurse convey to the patient when a tetracycline antibiotic is taken to aid absorption?
   a. Ingest with milk.
   b. Take with 240 mL of water.
   c. Allow 30 minutes before taking iron preparations.
   d. Use an antacid to decrease gastro-intestinal discomfort.

4. A patient is to receive antibiotic therapy with a cephalosporin. When assessing the patient's drug history, the nurse recognizes that an allergy to which type of drug may be a possible contraindication to cephalosporin therapy?
   a. Cardiac glycosides
   b. Thiazide diuretics
   c. Penicillins
   d. Macrolides

5. When asked about drug allergies, a patient says, "I can't take sulpha drugs because I'm allergic to them." Which question should the nurse ask next?
   a. "Do you have any other drug allergies?"
   b. "Who prescribed the drug for you?"
   c. "How long ago did this happen?"
   d. "What happened when you took the sulpha drug?"

6. A patient is being prepared for colon surgery and will be receiving 1 gram of cefazolin intravenously before surgery. The patient asks the nurse why this drug needs to be taken before surgery. Which of the following is the nurse's best response?
   a. "This drug helps to clear out your bowels before surgery."
   b. "This drug helps to reduce the number of bacteria in your intestines before surgery."
   c. "This drug is given to sterilize your bowel before surgery."
   d. "This drug is given to prevent an infection after surgery."

7. A patient is to receive medication through a feeding tube. The order reads, "Give amoxicillin 250 mg per feeding tube every 8 hours." When reconstituted, the concentration of the medication is 125 mg/5 mL. How many millilitres will the nurse give per dose?

_____

Critical Thinking and Application

Answer the following questions on a separate document.

8. Julian, a 50-year-old banker, is scheduled for colorectal surgery tomorrow. The health care provider is planning to administer a prophylactic antibiotic. What medication is frequently used for this purpose, and why?

9. Sean is a 19-year-old first-year university student who has been diagnosed with gonorrhea. The health care provider has prescribed doxycycline (Doxycin) therapy. During the nursing assessment, the nurse and Sean discuss his diet, which includes "lots of meat, milk, and veggies." Sean also says that he jogs frequently and is a member of the tennis team.

    a. In addition to instruction about sexually transmitted diseases, what health teaching does Sean require?

    b. A few days later, Sean calls and complains of an upset stomach and diarrhea. What does the nurse suspect might be the problem Sean is experiencing?

10. Sandra is a 59-year-old travel consultant who has bronchitis and has been taking an antibiotic for 1 week. She calls the nurse and complains of severe itching and a whitish discharge in her vaginal area. What has happened, and what caused it?

Critical Thinking Crossword

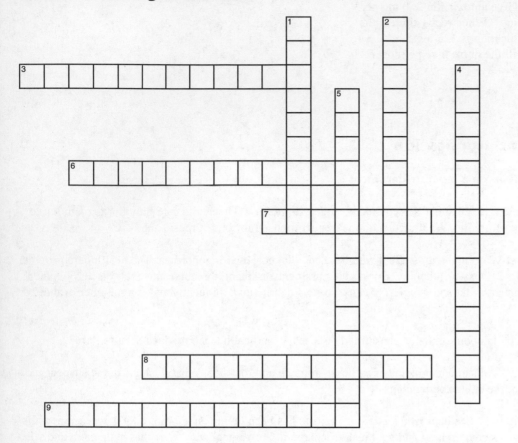

Across

3. Antibiotics taken before exposure to an infectious organism in an effort to prevent the development of infection
6. The classification for doxycycline (Doxycin)
7. An antibiotic derived from a fungus or mould often seen on bread or fruit
8. Antibiotics that kill bacteria
9. The classification for cefazolin

Down

1. The classification for erythromycin
2. The classification for sulphisoxazole
4. Antibiotics that inhibit the growth of bacteria
5. An infection that occurs during antimicrobial treatment for another infection and involves overgrowth of a nonsusceptible organism

Case Study

Read the scenario and answer the following questions on a separate document.

A 78-year-old patient, admitted to the hospital with a stroke 2 days earlier, has developed a urinary tract infection. His Foley catheter is draining urine that is cloudy and dark yellowish-orange with a strong odour. This patient is receiving a continuous intravenous heparin infusion and a comorbidity of type 2 diabetes. The health care provider orders combination sulphamethoxazole and trimethoprim.

1. What should be assessed before administering this medication?

2. Are there any potential drug interactions?

3. Why were these particular antibiotics chosen?

4. Is this antibiotic bactericidal or bacteriostatic? Explain.

CHAPTER 44

Antibiotics Part 2: Aminoglycosides, Fluoroquinolones, and Other Drugs

Chapter Review and Examination Preparation

Choose the best answer for each of the following:

1. Upon assessment, a patient on aminoglycosides drug therapy complains of tinnitus. In planning for an appropriate nursing intervention, the nurse knows that this finding is an indication of which problem?
   a. Cardiotoxicity
   b. Hepatotoxicity
   c. Ototoxicity
   d. Nephrotoxicity

2. A patient has been admitted to the unit with a stage IV pressure ulcer. After 2 days, the wound culture comes back positive for methicillin-resistant *Staphylococcus aureus* (MRSA). What drug should the nurse prepare as the drug of choice for treatment of MRSA infections?
   a. vancomycin (Vancocin)
   b. gentamicin sulphate
   c. ciprofloxacin (Cipro)
   d. dapsone

3. A patient who is receiving vancomycin (Vancocin) therapy needs to notify the nurse immediately if which effects are noted? (Select all that apply.)
   a. Ringing in the ears
   b. Dizziness
   c. Hearing loss
   d. Fullness in the ears
   e. Nausea

4. Against which of the following organisms would the use of metronidazole (Flagyl) be most effective?
   a. *Clostridium difficile*
   b. MRSA
   c. *Mycobacterium leprae*
   d. *Chlamydia*

5. The nurse is reviewing the list of drugs for a patient who will be starting antibiotic therapy with an aminoglycoside. Which of the following drugs may present a potential interaction with the aminoglycoside? (Select all that apply.)
   a. metoprolol (Lopresor), a beta-blocker
   b. furosemide (Lasix), a loop diuretic
   c. warfarin (Coumadin), an oral anticoagulant
   d. vancomycin (Vancocin), an antibiotic
   e. levothyroxine (Synthroid), a thyroid hormone

6. A patient will be taking oral neomycin before having bowel surgery. The order reads, "Give 1 g per hour for 4 doses PO" (orally). The patient cannot swallow pills, so an oral solution of 125 mg/5 mL has been ordered. How many millilitres will the nurse give for each 1 g dose?

   _____

7. The order reads, "Give colistimethate (Coly-Mycin) 2.5 mg/kg/day IVPB [intravenous piggyback]. Infuse over 5 minutes." The patient weighs 74 g. How many milligrams will the patient receive per dose? (Record answer using one decimal place.)

   _____

Critical Thinking and Application

Answer the following questions on a separate document.

8. Angie has a severe infection and is receiving an aminoglycoside once a day. She says, "They tell me I have a terrible infection. Why am I not getting the antibiotic more than once a day? I don't understand." How should the nurse respond to Angie's concern?

9. Explain the concept of "trough" levels during aminoglycoside therapy and the way in which kidney function is monitored.

10. Greg has been taking amiodarone (Cordarone) for a heart rhythm problem. He has developed an infection from an open wound, and the sensitivity report indicates that levofloxacin is the best choice of drug to fight this infection. Are there any concerns?

11. Nitrofurantoin (Macrodantin) has been ordered for a patient who has a severe urinary tract infection caused by *Escherichia coli*. Explain why this drug is used for this type of infection. What priority instructions should the nurse provide the patient to ensure that this drug does not cause renal impairment?

Case Study

Read the scenario and answer the following questions on a separate document.

Virgil has been admitted to the medical unit and placed on aminoglycoside therapy as part of treatment for a urinary tract infection with *Pseudomonas*. He is 65 years old, awake, and alert, but anxious about his problem and wants to "hurry up and get better."

1. For which two serious toxicities will the nurse monitor, what are their symptoms, and how can they be prevented?

2. The physician adds penicillin to Virgil's drug regimen. Explain the reason for this.

3. Virgil's "trough" aminoglycoside level is 3.0 mcg/mL, and his serum creatinine level is increased from 2 days earlier. Are these results a concern? What should the nurse do? Explain.

CHAPTER 45

Antiviral Drugs

Chapter Review and Examination Preparation

Choose the best answer for each of the following:

1. The nurse is administering acyclovir (Zovirax) and recalls that it is considered the drug of choice for treatment of which viral infection?
   a. Cytomegalovirus (CMV)
   b. Human immunodeficiency virus (HIV)
   c. Respiratory syncytial virus (RSV)
   d. Varicella-zoster virus (VZV)

2. When administering ganciclovir (Cytovene), the nurse keeps in mind that the main dose-limiting toxicity for this drug is which condition?
   a. Kidney failure
   b. Gastro-intestinal disturbance
   c. Peripheral neuropathy
   d. Bone marrow suppression

3. When reviewing the health history of a patient who is to receive foscarnet (Foscavir), the nurse knows that which condition would be a contraindication to its use?
   a. Renal toxicity
   b. CMV retinitis
   c. Asthma
   d. Immunosuppression

4. When reviewing the use of amantadine (Symmetrel), the nurse expects that the drug would be used most appropriately in which of the following patients?
   a. A 29-year-old man who tests positive for HIV infection
   b. A 22-year-old woman who is in her eighth month of pregnancy and tests HIV positive
   c. A heart transplant patient who is to receive prophylaxis for influenza A
   d. An older adult patient who requires prophylaxis for influenza B

5. A patient calls the clinic nurse to ask for oseltamivir (Tamiflu) "because I was exposed to the flu over the weekend at a family reunion." The nurse knows that oseltamivir is used for which of the following? (Select all that apply.)
   a. Prevention of infection after exposure to influenza virus types A and B
   b. Reduction of the duration of influenza in adults
   c. Treatment of topical herpes simplex virus infections
   d. Reduction of the severity of shingles
   e. Treatment of lower respiratory tract infections caused by respiratory syncytial virus

6. The nurse is preparing to administer the aerosol form of ribavirin. Which condition is a contraindication to this drug?
   a. Asthma
   b. Pregnancy
   c. Hypertension
   d. Type 2 diabetes

7. The order reads, "Give acyclovir, 0.25 g IVPB [intravenous piggyback] now." The drug comes in a vial that contains 1,000 mg. The label reads, "Add 20 mL of diluent for a solution that contains 50 mg/mL." The drug will be added to 100 mL D$_5$W (5% dextrose in water) for IVPB infusion. How many millilitres of reconstituted drug will the nurse add to the 100 mL bag for infusion? _____

8. The order for a 1-year-old child reads, "Give amantadine (Symmetrel) 4.4 mg/kg/day in two divided doses." The child weighs 9.9 kg. How many milligrams will the child receive per dose? _____

Critical Thinking and Application

Answer the following questions on a separate document.

9. Amy is 12 weeks into her pregnancy when she discovers that she is HIV positive. Amy is upset and says, "I won't live long enough to have this baby. We're both going to die." Is it possible to treat Amy and the fetus? Explain your answer.

10. Bailey, a 53-year-old teacher, has shingles.

    a. What drug does the nurse expect the health care provider to prescribe?

    b. Several months later, Bailey calls the office to say that the symptoms have returned. What action does the nurse expect to be taken now?

11. Brenda, 3 years old, has bronchopneumonia caused by RSV.

    a. What antiviral drug is used to treat RSV?

    b. Brenda's mother wonders whether the treatment will be completed before Brenda's birthday, which is 2 weeks away. What does the nurse tell her?

12. The nurse overhears a co-worker explaining to a student nurse the procedure for administering acyclovir (Zovirax) intravenously. After the acyclovir is diluted in sterile water, the co-worker says, "We'll administer this over at least an hour." Should the nurse intervene? Explain your answer.

13. Stacey has had symptoms of influenza for 4 days and feels miserable. She calls the nurse practitioner in the clinic to ask for "that medicine, Tamiflu, that is supposed to make the flu symptoms better." Should Stacey receive this drug at this time? Provide a thorough explanation.

Case Study

Read the scenario and answer the following questions on a separate document.

Simon, a 30-year-old stockbroker, has been diagnosed with genital herpes simplex type 2 (HSV-2) infection. The health care provider has prescribed topical acyclovir (Zovirax).

1. What does the nurse teach Simon regarding the administration of this drug?

2. Simon asks the nurse how long it will take for the acyclovir to cure his herpes. What is the nurse's best response?

3. What else should the nurse discuss with Simon, who is sexually active?

4. HSV-2 virus is closely related to which other viruses?

CHAPTER 46

Antitubercular Drugs

Chapter Review and Examination Preparation

Choose the best answer for each of the following:

1. A patient with active tuberculosis has been started on isoniazid (INH) therapy. What laboratory test must the nurse closely monitor when the patient is on this drug therapy?
   a. Liver enzyme levels
   b. Hematocrit and hemoglobin level
   c. Creatinine level
   d. Platelet count

2. What priority health information must the nurse include for a patient taking INH therapy?
   a. Urine and saliva may be reddish orange.
   b. Pyridoxine (vitamin B_6) may be needed to prevent neurotoxicity.
   c. Injection sites should be rotated daily.
   d. The drugs should be taken with an antacid to reduce gastric distress.

3. Patients who are in the initial period of treatment for tuberculosis need to be taught to do which of the following priority activities? (Select all that apply.)
   a. Wash their hands and cover the mouth when coughing or sneezing to reduce the spread of tuberculosis.
   b. Throw away dirty tissues with care.
   c. Be sure to get adequate rest, nutrition, and relaxation.
   d. Skip drug doses occasionally if gastric distress occurs.
   e. Avoid all visitors until symptoms improve.

4. A patient with newly diagnosed tuberculosis asks the nurse how long "all this medicine" will need to be taken. What is the most appropriate answer?
   a. 6 months
   b. 12 months
   c. 24 months
   d. A lifetime

5. The nurse is explaining antitubercular therapy to a patient. The patient asks, "Why do I have to take so many different drugs?" What is the nurse's best response?
   a. "It helps to prevent the tuberculosis from becoming resistant to the drugs."
   b. "It makes sure that the disease is cured."
   c. "These drugs will reduce symptoms immediately."
   d. "You will have fewer adverse effects."

6. The patient is to receive INH 0.3 g daily. The drug is available as 100 mg tablets. How many tablets will the nurse administer per dose? _____

7. The patient has new orders for pyrazinamide 30 mg/kg/day. The patient weighs 59.4 kg. How many milligrams will the patient receive per day?

   Is this dosage safe? _____

144

x

Critical Thinking and Application

Answer the following questions on a separate document.

8. Diane, a 33-year-old proofreader, has been prescribed prophylactic INH treatment.

   a. What laboratory studies should be performed before the start of therapy? Why?

   b. After Diane has taken the INH for 2 months, the physician significantly reduces her dosage of the drug. Why might that be?

9. Ina is undergoing antituberculosis therapy that includes streptomycin.

   a. How is streptomycin administered?

   b. Ina takes an oral contraceptive. Is that a concern with Ina's streptomycin therapy? Explain your answer.

10. Why would an eye examination be performed before instituting antituberculosis therapy?

11. Fabian, a 42-year-old marketing executive, is on antituberculosis therapy. During his first follow-up visit, he is evasive when the nurse asks him about his adherence to his therapy regimen. He does tell her that he has been busy lately, entertaining various clients "at everything from cocktail parties to big sit-down dinners."

   a. What issues should the nurse discuss with Fabian?

   b. Several weeks later, Fabian returns for another follow-up visit. On examination, the nurse sees no apparent signs of tuberculosis. How can Fabian's therapeutic response be confirmed?

12. Frannie is a homeless 68-year-old woman who lives in a shelter some of the time. She was diagnosed at the community health clinic with tuberculosis, and antituberculosis therapy has been instituted.

   a. What education issues are of particular concern in Frannie's case?

   b. Frannie is staying at the shelter and seems to be handling her drug regimen well, but one day she comes by the clinic to tell the nurse that she is afraid the drug may be bad for her. "Whenever I go to the bathroom, everything is reddish orange," she says. What does the nurse suspect is going on, and what does the nurse tell Frannie?

Case Study

Read the scenario and answer the following questions on a separate document.

George, a 73-year-old retired plant foreman, has been diagnosed with tuberculosis. Nursing assessment reveals a history of gout and diabetes. He also has a history of heavy drinking.

1. What considerations will the physician keep in mind when deciding on a first-line drug for George?

2. George tells the nurse that he has been told that he has a "liver problem." His medical record indicates that he is a slow acetylator. How does this affect his therapy?

3. How will his history of heavy drinking affect his therapy?

4. The nurse instructs George on how to take vitamin B_6 along with INH therapy. When George asks why taking the vitamin B_6 is necessary, what does the nurse tell him?

CHAPTER 47

Antifungal Drugs

Chapter Review and Examination Preparation

Choose the best answer for each of the following:

1. A 14-month-old infant is brought to the family health clinic for thrush. Which drug is the most effective for treating thrush in infants?
   a. amphotericin B (Abelcet)
   b. fluconazole (Diflucan)
   c. nystatin
   d. voriconazole

2. When administering an amphotericin B infusion, what clinical manifestations should the nurse monitor to determine the occurrence of an adverse effect? (Select all that apply.)
   a. Abdominal pain
   b. Fever
   c. Malaise
   d. Diarrhea
   e. Chills
   f. Rash
   g. Nausea

3. A patient calls the Gynecological Clinic because she has begun to menstruate while taking drug for a vaginal infection. She asks the nurse, "What should I do about taking this vaginal medicine right now?" Which of the following is the nurse's best answer to this patient's question?
   a. "You should stop the drug until the menstrual flow has stopped."
   b. "Just take the drug at night only."
   c. "You should stop the drug for 3 days, then start it again."
   d. "It's okay to continue to take the drug."

4. Which drug is often used as a one-dose treatment for vaginal candidiasis?
   a. ketoconazole
   b. fluconazole (Diflucan)
   c. griseofulvin
   d. imidazole

5. The nurse is administering an antifungal drug to a patient who has a severe systemic fungal infection. Which drug is most appropriate for this patient?
   a. ketoconazole (Nizoral)
   b. fluconazole
   c. griseofulvin
   d. terbinafine (Lamisil)

6. The order reads, "Give amphotericin B (Fungizone) 20 mg in 300 mL D₅W [5% dextrose in water] over 6 hours." The nurse will set the infusion pump to

   what rate? _____

7. A patient is to receive voriconazole (Vfend) as follows: 6 mg/kg q12h × 2 doses, then change to 4 mg/kg q12h. The patient weighs about 109 kg. How much will the patient receive for each 6 mg/kg

   dose? For the 4 mg/kg dose? _____

146

Critical Thinking and Application

Answer the following questions on a separate document.

8. Yun has cryptococcal meningitis, and the health care provider prescribed fluconazole (Diflucan).

   a. Why did the health care provider choose this drug rather than one of the other -azole antifungals?

   b. The results of Yun's cerebrospinal fluid culture eventually comes back negative. When he hears the good news, he says, "Great! I'm tired of taking this medicine." What will be the nurse's response?

9. The health care provider is planning intravenous amphotericin B (Fungizone) therapy for a patient.

   a. What guidelines does the nurse follow in diluting the drug?

   b. What adverse effects can the nurse expect the patient to experience? Explain your answer.

   c. Should the nurse stop the infusion if those effects occur? Explain your answer.

10. Lewis has a severe fungal infection for which the health care provider has prescribed ketoconazole. During the nursing assessment, Lewis tells the nurse that he hopes the infection will clear up soon because he is going on a cruise ship in a week and plans to "party every night." What patient teaching issues should the nurse discuss with Lewis?

11. Chrissie has a prescription for nystatin oral troches to treat thrush. After a few days, she calls the nurse practitioner to report that her mouth is not better. "I've been chewing them slowly every time I take one. I don't understand why it's not working." How should the nurse respond to Chrissie's concern?

Match each definition with its corresponding term.

12. _____ Single-celled fungi that reproduce by budding

13. _____ One of the major chemical groups of antifungal drugs; includes amphotericin B and nystatin

14. _____ A very large, diverse group of eukaryotic, thallus-forming micro-organisms that require an external carbon source

15. _____ Another of the major groups of antifungal drugs; includes ketoconazole

16. _____ A term for a fungal infection of the mouth

17. _____ One of the older antifungal drugs that acts by preventing susceptible fungi from reproducing

18. _____ The drug of choice for many severe, systemic fungal infections; also the oldest antifungal drug

a. Thrush

b. Moulds

c. griseofulvin

d. Mycosis

e. Polyenes

f. Fungi

g. Imidazoles

h. amphotericin B (Fungizone)

i. nystatin

j. Yeast

19. _____ An antifungal drug commonly used to treat candidal diaper rash

20. _____ An infection caused by fungi

21. _____ Multicellular fungi characterized by long, branching filaments called hyphae, which entwine to form a mycelium

Case Study

Read the scenario and answer the following questions on a separate document.

Sally is a 68-year-old retiree with pneumonia secondary to invasive aspergillosis. She has been treated for 2 weeks without much improvement, and the health care provider is considering starting voriconazole (Vfend) therapy. Sally is also receiving a drug for treatment of a cardiac dysrhythmia.

1. What is the reason for starting voriconazole therapy now rather than earlier?

2. What consideration may arise depending on the cardiac drug she is taking?

3. What should be monitored while she is taking voriconazole?

CHAPTER 48

Antimalarial, Antiprotozoal, and Anthelmintic Drugs

Chapter Review and Examination Preparation

Choose the best answer for each of the following:

1. Before beginning antiprotozoal therapy, the nurse should assess the patient for which priority contraindications?
   a. Pregnancy and underlying renal, cardiac, thyroid, or hepatic disease
   b. Porphyria and glucose-6-phosphate dehydrogenase deficiency
   c. Glaucoma, cataracts, anemia, and petechiae
   d. Constipation, gastritis, and lactose intolerance

2. A patient was prescribed quinine sulphate. What possible adverse effect should the nurse teach the patient to monitor when on this drug?
   a. Constipation
   b. Irritation to the gastro-intestinal mucosa
   c. A metallic taste in the mouth
   d. Severe halitosis

3. A patient is taking quinine therapy for a mild case of malaria. The health care provider has decided to add a sulphonamide or tetracycline drug along with the quinine. When the nurse gives the patient the prescription for this new drug, the patient is upset about having to take "another pill." What is the nurse's best word-for-word explanation for the second drug?
   a. "The antibiotic treats bacterial infections that accompany malaria."
   b. "The antibiotic reduces the severe adverse effects of quinine."
   c. "The antibiotic will help the quinine to work more effectively against the malaria."
   d. "The antibiotic therapy is also needed to kill the parasite that causes malaria."

4. What are the possible adverse effects of taking metronidazole? (Select all that apply.)
   a. Reddish-orange urine
   b. Anorexia
   c. Cough
   d. Weakness
   e. Headache
   f. A metallic taste in the mouth

5. Which of the following drugs is used mainly for the management of *Pneumocystis jiroveci* (formerly called *Pneumocystis carinii*) pneumonia? (Select all that apply.)
   a. metronidazole (Flagyl)
   b. pentamidine
   c. primaquine
   d. pyrantel (Combantrin)
   e. atovaquone (Mepron)

6. Which of the following is true regarding anthelmintic therapy?
   a. The drug can be stopped once symptoms disappear and can be restarted if the symptoms re-appear.
   b. Anthelmintics are more effective in their parenteral forms.
   c. Anthelmintics are broad in their actions and can be substituted easily if one drug is not well tolerated.
   d. The drug is used to target specific organisms and must be taken exactly as prescribed.

7. The nurse is reviewing the drug list of a patient with a new prescription for mefloquine (Lariam). Which of the following drugs may interact with the mefloquine? (Select all that apply.)
   a. β-blockers
   b. Antidiabetic drugs
   c. Calcium channel blockers
   d. Proton pump inhibitors
   e. Thiazide diuretics

8. A patient with *Pneumocystis jiroveci* pneumonia will be receiving pentamidine intravenously; the order reads, "Give 4 mg/kg/day once daily." The drug comes in a 300 mg vial and is to be reconstituted with 5 mL of sterile water, for a resulting concentration of 60 mg/mL. The dose will then be added to a 100 mL bag of 5% dextrose in water for the infusion. The patient weighs 69.3 kg. What is the dose for this patient and how many millilitres of drug will the nurse add to the infusion bag? (Record answer using one decimal place.) _____

9. A patient is to receive mefloquine 1,250 mg in a single dose for treatment of malaria. The drug is available in 250 mg tablets. How many tablets will the patient receive? _____

Critical Thinking and Application

Answer the following questions on a separate document.

10. Bryant is a humanitarian aid worker in Africa, where he did not adequately protect himself from mosquito exposure; thus, he has contracted malaria. What kind of parasite causes malaria? Which drug is recommended if the parasite is in the exoerythrocytic phase of development?

11. Bryant's partner, who accompanied him on his trip to Africa, has begun to develop signs of malaria. She is given chloroquine, a 4-aminoquinoline derivative. Unlike Bryant, however, she sees no diminishing of her symptoms. Her strain of malaria appears to be chloroquine resistant. What alternative(s) will the nurse practitioner suggest for Bryant's partner?

12. The heath care clinic has a full waiting room this morning. Patient A is being seen for an intestinal disorder that was acquired after swimming in a local lake. Patient B has acquired immune deficiency syndrome and is showing early signs of pneumonia. Patient C is being treated and evaluated on a regular basis for a sexually transmitted infection. The nurse is challenged with finding a commonality between all three patients.
   a. Describe what the commonality could be.
   b. Based on that commonality, predict what disorder, of those discussed in this chapter, each patient might have. (Hint: One patient has giardiasis.)
   c. What drug does the nurse think the health care provider is likely to prescribe for each patient?

Case Study

Read the scenario and answer the following questions on a separate document.

Sandra, aged 15 years, has been diagnosed with an intestinal roundworm infestation, specifically ascariasis, after a visit to another country. The nurse is preparing to medicate her with pyrantel (Combantrin).

1. How is this infestation diagnosed?

2. What are the contraindications to therapy with pyrantel?

3. The recommended dosage for pyrantel is 11 mg/kg, up to a maximum of 1 g, in a one-time dose. If Sandra weighs 57 kg, what dose should she receive?

4. What are the expected adverse effects of this drug?

CHAPTER 49

Anti-Inflammatory and Antigout Drugs

Chapter Review and Examination Preparation

Choose the best answer for each of the following:

1. When teaching a patient about nonsteroidal anti-inflammatory drugs (NSAIDs), for what possible adverse effect should the nurse tell the patient to monitor?
   a. Dizziness
   b. Heartburn
   c. Palpitations
   d. Diarrhea

2. A 13-year-old patient presents at the family health clinic with a fever of 39.4°C secondary to the flu. What drug will the health care provider recommend to treat the fever?
   a. acetylsalicylic acid (Aspirin)
   b. acetaminophen (Tylenol)
   c. indomethacin
   d. naproxen (Naprosyn)

3. A patient is receiving treatment with allopurinol (Zyloprim) for an acute flare-up of gout. Which of the following should the nurse say to this patient when giving instructions? (Select all that apply.)
   a. "Be sure to avoid alcohol and caffeine."
   b. "Take the drug with meals to prevent stomach problems."
   c. "You need to take this drug on an empty stomach to improve absorption."
   d. "You need to increase fluid intake to 3 litres per day."
   e. "Call your provider immediately if you note any skin rashes or abnormalities."

4. When reviewing the health history of a patient who is to receive NSAID therapy, the nurse should keep in mind that contraindications for the use of these drugs include which condition?
   a. Pericarditis
   b. Osteoarthritis
   c. Bleeding disorders
   d. Juvenile rheumatoid arthritis

5. The nurse is reviewing use of celecoxib (Celebrex). For which of the following is celecoxib indicated? (Select all that apply.)
   a. Osteoarthritis
   b. Prevention of thrombotic events
   c. Rheumatoid arthritis
   d. Primary dysmenorrhea
   e. Fever reduction

6. The nurse is reviewing a patient's drugs and sees an order for ketorolac (Toradol). This drug is ordered for which condition?
   a. Fever
   b. Mild pain
   c. Moderate to severe acute pain
   d. Long-term persistent pain conditions

7. A child is to receive celecoxib as part of treatment for juvenile rheumatoid arthritis. The dose ordered is 100 mg twice daily orally (PO). The child weighs 14.9 kg. According to the text, the dosing chart for the pediatric administration of celecoxib is as appears below:

<25 kg	50 mg twice daily PO
>25 kg	100 mg twice daily PO

Is the ordered dose appropriate for this child? Explain your answer.

8. The order reads, "Give ketorolac (Toradol) 20 mg IV every 6 hours as needed for pain." The drug is available in a concentration of 15 mg/mL. How much will the nurse draw up for each dose? Mark the syringe to indicate your answer. (Record answer using one decimal place.)

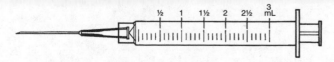

Critical Thinking and Application

Answer the following questions on a separate document.

9. Layla is brought into the emergency department with severe tinnitus, hearing loss, and some confusion. On examination, the nurse discovers that the patient's blood glucose level is 2.89 mmol/L. Layla's husband tells you that she has been experiencing back pain and has been using "a lot of Aspirin" over the past few weeks. What do her symptoms and history suggest? Explain your answer.

10. Sergio comes to the emergency department with symptoms that are similar to Layla's but not as extensive. He is experiencing drowsiness, lethargy, and disorientation, and had a seizure while en route to the hospital. His girlfriend tells the nurse that she noticed an empty bottle of ibuprofen (Advil) by his bed when she found him. What do his symptoms and history suggest? What would the nurse expect if the situation were allowed to progress?

11. Sammy has come to the clinic complaining of a severe flare-up of his gout. He tells the nurse that he does not take his medicine on a regular basis because it "kills" his stomach. He also says that he hates to take medicine but hates the gout more. He has a prescription for allopurinol (Zyloprim) and a follow-up appointment for next month. What patient teaching does Sammy need?

12. Eileen has had arthritic joint pain for months, and her current pain management regimen has been less than success-ful. During a checkup today, she tells the nurse that she has heard of a drug, Toradol, that "works wonders." She wants to try it for "a couple of months" to see if it can help her.

    a. What will the nurse tell her?

    b. What could happen if Eileen takes Toradol on a long-term basis?

Case Study

Read the scenario and answer the following questions on a separate document.

Sadie has been taking indomethacin as part of therapy for osteoarthritis but lately has noticed that it has been less effective. Her health care provider has decided to try celecoxib (Celebrex). Sadie has a history of hepatitis (15 years ago).

1. What advantages might there be to treatment with celecoxib rather than indomethacin?

2. What potential adverse effects should the nurse warn Sadie about before she takes this drug? What should the nurse report to the health care provider?

3. Sadie asks the nurse if she can drink her usual glass of wine each evening while on this drug. What does the nurse tell her?

CHAPTER **50**

Immunosuppressant Drugs

Chapter Review and Examination Preparation

Choose the best answer for each of the following:

1. When monitoring patients on immunosuppressant therapy, the nurse must keep in mind that the major risk factor for patients taking these drugs is which condition?
   a. Severe hypotension with potential kidney failure
   b. Increased susceptibility to opportunistic infections
   c. Decreased platelet aggregation
   d. Increased bleeding tendencies

2. A patient is experiencing rejection of a transplanted organ. The nurse expects which drug to manage this?
   a. azathioprine (Imuran)
   b. cyclosporine (Neoral)
   c. muromonab-CD3
   d. tacrolimus (Advagraf)

3. The nurse is discussing drug therapy with cyclosporine (Sandimmune). Which food product inhibits metabolism enzymes and possibly increases the activity of cyclosporine?
   a. Dairy products
   b. Orange juice
   c. Grapefruit juice
   d. Red wines

4. When teaching patients who are taking oral doses of immunosuppressants, what priority instructions should the patient receive from the nurse when taking this drug?
   a. Take with food to minimize gastro-intestinal upset.
   b. Take on an empty stomach to increase absorption rates.
   c. Take only when adverse effects are tolerable.
   d. Take with antacids.

5. Which of the following information will the nurse include when educating patients who are taking immunosuppressants? (Select all that apply.)
   a. The mouth and tongue should be inspected carefully for white patches.
   b. Allergic reactions to these drugs are rare.
   c. Patients should avoid crowds to minimize the risk of infection.
   d. Patients should report any fever, sore throat, chills, or joint pain.
   e. Patients should take oral forms with food to avoid gastro-intestinal upset.

6. Which drugs are indicated for the treatment of multiple sclerosis? (Select all that apply.)
   a. glatiramer acetate (Copaxone)
   b. azathioprine (Imuran)
   c. basiliximab (Simulect)
   d. fingolimod (Gilenya)

7. A patient will be taking cyclosporine (Sandimmune) after transplant surgery. Which of the following are potential adverse effects of cyclosporine therapy? (Select all that apply.)
   a. Hypertension
   b. Fever
   c. Nephrotoxicity
   d. Fluid retention
   e. Hypotension
   f. Post-transplant diabetes mellitus

8. The order reads, "Give mycophenolate mofetil (CellCept) 1 g PO [orally] twice daily." The capsules are available in 250 mg strength. How many capsules will the patient receive per dose?

   _____

9. A patient is about to undergo transplant surgery and will be receiving a preoperative dose of cyclosporine (Sandimmune) 8 hours before the surgery. The order is "cyclosporine, 6 mg/kg/dose, IV [intravenous], give 8 hours preoperatively." The patient weighs 124 kg. The drug is available in a 50 mg/mL formulation.

a. The dose for this patient is how many milligrams? _____

b. How many millilitres will the nurse administer for this dose? _____

Critical Thinking and Application

Answer the following questions on a separate document.

10. A patient on cyclosporine (Neoral) therapy is convinced that the cyclosporine is causing stomach upset. What can the patient be encouraged to take to alleviate this problem?

11. John has relapsing remitting multiple sclerosis and is in hospital because of an acute exacerbation. The health care provider talks to him about a "different type" of therapy with an immunosuppressant drug. What drug will be used, and how can it help John?

Case Study

Read the scenario and answer the following questions on a separate document.

Kellum had kidney transplant surgery 6 months ago and so far has had no problems with organ rejection. He is taking cyclosporine (Neoral) in a maintenance dose. He wants to return to work and is in for a checkup before approval is given for a return to his job.

1. He asks if he will have to continue the cyclosporine. What is the nurse's response?

2. He complains of difficulty swallowing. As his mouth is examined, the nurse looks for signs of oral candidiasis. What findings would indicate that Kellum has this condition?

3. After 2 weeks at work, Kellum calls to report that he has the flu; he has a sore throat, chills, and aching joints, and he feels tired. What is the nurse's best response with respect to his symptoms?

4. Kellum tells the nurse that his job sometimes requires him to travel to remote areas of the world. What concerns are there with vaccinations, if any?

CHAPTER 51

Immunizing Drugs and Pandemic Preparedness

Chapter Review and Examination Preparation

Choose the best answer for each of the following:

1. The immunity that is passed from a mother to her nursing infant through antibodies in breast milk is known as what type of immunity?
   a. Artificially acquired passive immunity
   b. Naturally acquired passive immunity
   c. Active immunity
   d. Immunoglobulins

2. Which of the following contain substances that trigger the formation of antibodies against specific pathogens?
   a. Antivenins
   b. Serums
   c. Toxoids
   d. Vaccines

3. When reviewing various immunizing drugs, the nurse recalls that some products provide long-lasting immunity against a particular pathogen. Which of the following is an example of this type of product?
   a. Live oral poliovirus vaccine
   b. Tetanus immunoglobulin
   c. $Rh_0(D)$ immunoglobulin
   d. Black widow spider antivenin

4. The nurse is preparing to give a second dose of diphtheria and tetanus toxoids and acellular pertussis (DTaP) vaccine to a 6-month-old infant. The infant's mother tells the nurse that the last time he received this vaccination, the injection site on his leg became warm, slightly swollen, and red. Which of the following is the nurse's best response?
   a. Explain that these effects can be expected, and administer the drug.
   b. Give half the prescribed dose this week and the other half next week if tolerated well.
   c. Skip the dose, and notify the health care provider.
   d. Wait 6 months, then administer the dose.

5. A nurse has been stuck by a used needle while starting an intravenous line. Which preparation is used as prophylaxis against disease after exposure to blood and body fluids?
   a. *Haemophilus influenzae* type B (Hib) vaccine
   b. $Rh_0(D)$ immunoglobulin
   c. Hepatitis B immunoglobulin
   d. Hepatitis antitoxin

6. The nurse is teaching a 24-year-old woman about the human papillomavirus vaccine. Which statement by the woman indicates that more teaching is needed? (Select all that apply.)
   a. "This vaccine only takes one injection."
   b. "I need to have this vaccine before I turn 26."
   c. "It is safe to take this vaccine if I am pregnant."
   d. "This vaccination prevents the virus that commonly causes genital warts."

7. A newborn will be receiving a first dose of hepatitis B vaccine (inactivated). The dose is 5 mcg IM (intramuscular) at birth, then again at 1 month and 6 months. Five micrograms is equivalent to how

   many milligrams? _____

Critical Thinking and Application

Answer the following questions on a separate document.

8. Emily, aged 25 years, has stepped on a rusty piece of metal and will be receiving a tetanus booster after the wound is cleansed and stitched. Her last tetanus booster, a tetanus and diphtheria (Td) booster, was administered 10 years ago. Which booster is she likely to receive today? Explain your answer.

9. Jim, a cabinetmaker, is cut by a woodworking tool and comes to the clinic for stitches. When the nurse asks him about his tetanus vaccination history, he says, "I have no idea when my last tetanus shot was. I thought that once I had all the shots for school, I was set for life! I don't need any more." How should the nurse respond to Jim?

10. Betty, an 82-year-old widow, is in the office for a follow-up appointment to evaluate her emphysema. The health care provider recommends that she have an influenza virus vaccine. As the nurse prepares the injection, Betty says, "I had a flu shot last year. Why do I need another one this year?" What is the nurse's explanation to her?

11. Paul has received several immunizations in preparation for an overseas trip. He expects to feel some soreness at the injection sites, but the next morning, he wakes up with swelling of the face and tongue, difficulty breathing, shortness of breath, nausea and vomiting, and a fever of 38.9°C. What is happening, and what should he do?

12. **Complete the following chart by filling in all missing information:**

Drug or Vaccine	Active or Passive?	Purpose
a.	b.	chicken pox
Hib	c.	d.
e.	active	hepatitis B virus prophylaxis
f.	g.	postpartum antibody suppression
bacillus Calmette-Guérin (BCG)	h.	i.
DTaP	j.	k.
tetanus immunoglobulin	l.	m.
Td	n.	o.

Case Study

Read the scenario and answer the following questions on a separate document.

The nurse is volunteering at a local animal shelter and helping to care for a sick dog that has just been admitted. During the examination, the dog nips both the nurse and the veterinarian. A while later, the veterinarian tells the nurse that the dog is feared to have rabies and thinks that both of them have been exposed. The veterinarian has had a rabies vaccine but says the nurse will need to be vaccinated immediately.

1. Is rabies a virus or a bacterium?

2. Did the vaccine the veterinarian received previously provide active or passive immunization? Explain.

3. Will the vaccine the nurse receives provide active or passive immunization? Explain why this particular type of vaccine is preferred in his situation.

CHAPTER 52

Antineoplastic Drugs Part 1: Cancer Overview and Cell Cycle–Specific Drugs

---

Chapter Review and Examination Preparation

Choose the best answer for each of the following:

1. Which of the following conditions are general adverse effects of antineoplastic drugs? (Select all that apply.)
   a. Bone marrow suppression
   b. Infertility
   c. Diarrhea
   d. Urinary retention
   e. Nausea and vomiting
   f. Stomatitis

2. A patient will be receiving chemotherapy with paclitaxel. What priority actions must the nurse prepare to do when administering this drug?
   a. Administer platelet infusions.
   b. Provide acetaminophen as needed.
   c. Keep the patient on "nothing-by-mouth" status.
   d. Premedicate with a steroid, an H_2 receptor antagonist, and an antihistamine.

3. As the nurse is preparing to administer chemotherapy to a patient, the patient asks why more than one drug is used. The nurse should explain to the patient that the purpose of having a combination of chemotherapeutic drugs is to do which of the following?
   a. Prevent drug resistance
   b. Reduce the incidence of adverse effects
   c. Decrease the cost of treatment
   d. Reduce treatment time

4. If extravasation of a neoplastic drug occurs, what should the nurse do first?
   a. Remove the intravenous catheter immediately.
   b. Stop the drug infusion without removing the intravenous catheter.
   c. Aspirate residual drug or blood from the tube if possible.
   d. Administer the appropriate antidote.

5. A patient is on chemotherapy drugs. What symptoms of stomatitis should the nurse monitor for?
   a. Indigestion and heartburn
   b. Ulceration of the mouth
   c. Severe vomiting and anorexia
   d. Diarrhea and perianal irritation

6. A patient is receiving leucovorin as part of a chemotherapy regimen. Which antineoplastic drug can the nurse expect this patient to be receiving?
   a. cladribine
   b. fluorouracil
   c. vincristine
   d. methotrexate

7. The nurse is monitoring a patient who developed thrombocytopenia after two rounds of chemotherapy. Which symptoms will the nurse look for in this patient? (Select all that apply.)
   a. Bruising
   b. Increased fatigue
   c. Ulcerations on mucous membranes inside the mouth
   d. Temperature above 38.1°C
   e. Increased bleeding from venipunctures

8. A patient will be receiving daily doses of asparaginase. The order is for 200 units/kg per day up to 40,000 units per dose intravenously. The patient weighs 124 kg. How many units will the patient receive per dose? Is this dose within the safe limit?

   _____

9. A patient will be receiving chemotherapy with IV (intravenous) cladribine. The order reads, "Give 0.09 mg/kg each day for 7 days." The drug is to be added to 500 mL of normal saline and is available in a 1 mg/mL solution. The patient weighs 90 kg.
   a. How many milligrams constitute each daily dose? (Record answer using one decimal place.)

      _____

   b. How many millilitres of drug will be added to each infusion? _____

Critical Thinking Crossword

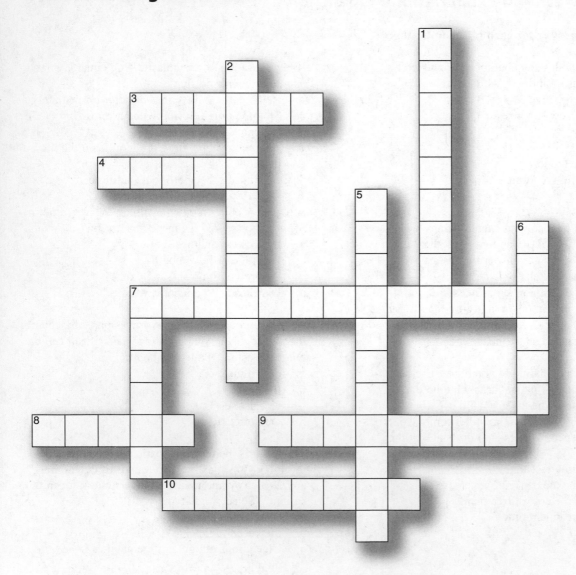

Across

3. A patient is told that his cancer has metastasized. His health care practitioner explains to him that this means it has _____ to other areas of his body.
4. Your patient is receiving methotrexate. Your instructor asks for a full description of its mechanism of action, so you explain that it will inhibit dihydrofolic reductase from converting _____ acid to a reduced folate and thus ultimately prevent the synthesis of deoxyribonucleic acid (DNA) and cell reproduction. The result, you explain, is that the cell will die.
7. A patient has just undergone a series of chemotherapeutic treatments when it is discovered that the antineoplastic drug has leaked into surrounding tissues; in other words, _____ of the drug has occurred.
8. A patient is very interested in his chemotherapy process. As you are discussing a drug's action, the patient hears you use the term _____ and asks what it means. You explain that this is the point at which the lowest neutrophil count occurs after administration of a chemotherapy agent that causes bone marrow suppression.
9. A patient has been given her first chemotherapy treatment. However, it soon becomes apparent that the adverse effects she is experiencing prevent her from being given dosages that will be high enough to be effective. These are dose _____ adverse effects.
10. A patient has a hematologic malignancy; the bone marrow is being rapidly replaced with leukemic blasts, there are abnormal numbers (and forms) of immature white blood cells in the circulation, and even the patient's lymph nodes, spleen, and liver are being infiltrated. This type of cancer is known as _____.

Down

1. A patient had a biopsy performed on the same day as the patient in 6 Down. When this first patient's biopsy specimen is analyzed, however, the results are the opposite of those of the patient in 6 Down, so the first patient's lump is considered _____.
2. A patient has been treated with methotrexate for its folate-antagonistic properties. Now, however, he seems to be experiencing a toxicity reaction. The treatment he will receive will be _____ rescue.
5. A patient is receiving chemotherapy with a drug that is considered cytotoxic during any phase of the cellular growth cycle. This drug is known as cell cycle _____.
6. A patient recently underwent a biopsy of a lump near her breast. Several days later, her health care practitioner calls and tells her that the lump is noncancerous and therefore not an immediate threat to life. She is relieved to hear, then, that it is _____.
7. A patient's health care practitioner is not surprised to find that this patient is experiencing nausea and vomiting; the methotrexate therapy is displaying a strong _____ potential in this patient.

Case Study

Read the scenario and answer the following questions on a separate document.

Allen, a 40-year-old health care practitioner, has been diagnosed with acute lymphocytic anemia and will be receiving chemotherapy with methotrexate. He is scheduled to receive his first treatment today.

1. What is methotrexate's classification, and how does methotrexate work?

2. What laboratory test results should be checked before Allen receives this drug?

3. Allen tells the nurse that he often has problems with ankle pain from an old injury and that he takes ibuprofen for relief. Is this a concern? Explain your answer.

4. What other drugs may be given along with the methotrexate chemotherapy, and why?

CHAPTER 53

Antineoplastic Drugs Part 2: Cell Cycle–Nonspecific and Miscellaneous Drugs

Chapter Review and Examination Preparation

Choose the best answer for each of the following:

1. While hanging a new infusion of a chemotherapy drug, the nurse accidentally spills a small amount of solution onto the floor. What is the nurse's best course of action to address the spillage?
   a. Let it dry; then wipe up the floor.
   b. Wipe the area with a paper towel.
   c. Use a spill kit to clean the area.
   d. Ask the housekeeping staff to wipe the floor.

2. The nurse is reviewing the drug list for a patient who will be receiving mitotane (Lysodren) treatments. What type of drug would cause the most concern if administered along with the mitotane?
   a. A benzodiazepine
   b. A thyroid replacement hormone
   c. Insulin
   d. A beta-blocker

3. A patient receiving chemotherapy for a testicular tumour complains of hearing a "loud ringing sound" in his ears. What can the nurse expect to happen next regarding chemotherapy?
   a. The therapy will continue as ordered.
   b. The therapy will be stopped until the patient's hearing is evaluated.
   c. The therapy will be withheld for a day and then resumed.
   d. The therapy will be stopped until renal studies are performed.

4. When a patient who is receiving outpatient chemotherapy is being taught about potential problems, what signs and symptoms that are considered to constitute an oncologic emergency must the nurse instruct the patient to watch for? (Select all that apply.)
   a. Swollen tongue
   b. Alopecia
   c. Blood in the urine
   d. Nausea and vomiting
   e. Temperature of 37.8°C
   f. Chills

5. Which drug requires the nurse to closely monitor the patient for liver and renal toxicity? (Select all that apply.)
   a. doxorubicin (Caelyx)
   b. mitomycin hydrochloride
   c. idarubicin hydrochloride
   d. hydroxyurea (Hydrea)

6. A patient who has cancer is to receive a course of chemotherapy with doxorubicin (Adriamycin). Which coexisting condition will require very close monitoring while the patient is taking this drug?
   a. Hypertension
   b. Diabetes mellitus
   c. Gout
   d. Cardiomyopathy

7. A patient will be receiving mitotane (Lysodren), and the nurse is reviewing the patient's drug list for potential interactions. Which drugs may interact with mitotane? (Select all that apply.)
   a. digoxin
   b. warfarin
   c. phenytoin
   d. spironolactone

8. The orders read, "Administer normal saline, 2 L, over 24 hours, beginning 12 hours before the cisplatin chemotherapy begins." At what rate will the nurse program the infusion pump to deliver

   the normal saline? _____

9. A patient will be receiving cisplatin chemotherapy. The order reads, "Give 75 mg/m^2 in 1000 mL D$_5$W [5% dextrose in water] over 20 hours." At what rate will the nurse program the infusion pump to deliver

   the infusion? _____

Critical Thinking and Application

Answer the following questions on a separate document.

10. Selena has been receiving bleomycin to treat a lung tumour, and lately she has been experiencing increased difficulty breathing. She tells the nurse, "I guess this cancer is getting worse. The medicine is not working." What priority action must the nurse take next? What possible health condition is occurring?

11. During a busy evening shift, a health care provider tells the nurse to mix Amal's chemotherapy drugs "as soon as possible." The health care provider wants to start Amal's chemotherapy immediately. What should the nurse do next? Explain your answer.

12. Describe the concept of cytoprotection, and provide at least two examples of how cytoprotection may be accomplished during chemotherapy.

Case Study

Read the scenario and answer the following questions on a separate document.

Gabby, aged 63 years, has been diagnosed with mid-stage ovarian cancer and will be receiving chemotherapy with cisplatin after surgery. She is very anxious about the therapy but says she wants to "beat the cancer."

1. Cisplatin is associated with three main toxicities. Describe each one.

2. Before Gabby receives the therapy, what priority assessment must be completed?

3. During therapy, Gabby complains of an "odd tingling" in her toes. Is this a concern? Explain.

4. Gabby tells the nurse that she would rather "drink nothing" when she is feeling nauseated. Is this a concern? Explain what the nurse needs to teach her about fluid intake.

CHAPTER 54

Biological Response–Modifying Drugs and Antirheumatic Drugs

Chapter Review and Examination Preparation

Choose the best answer for each of the following:

1. A patient with a critically low hemoglobulin level and hematocrit is to receive a drug that will stimulate the production of red blood cells. Which drug should the nurse begin to prepare?
   a. filgrastim (Neupogen)
   b. epoetin alfa
   c. pegfilgrastim (Neulasta)
   d. ferrous gluconate

2. What are the adverse effects of interferon drug? (Select all that apply.)
   a. Myalgia
   b. Fever
   c. Diarrhea
   d. Fatigue
   e. Chills
   f. Dizziness

3. A patient is starting therapy with adalimumab (Humira) after a course of methotrexate failed to improve the patient's condition. What health condition is this patient being treated for?
   a. Advanced-stage cancer
   b. Multiple sclerosis
   c. Severe rheumatoid arthritis
   d. Systemic lupus erythematosus

4. A patient will be starting etanercept (Enbrel) therapy to treat severe rheumatoid arthritis. Which of the following health conditions are contraindications for this drug? (Select all that apply.)
   a. Latex allergy
   b. Active bacterial infection
   c. Diabetes mellitus
   d. Latent tuberculosis
   e. Acute hepatitis B
   f. Peanut allergy

5. A patient is to receive 400 mcg of filgrastim subcut daily for 1 week. The vial contains 480 mcg/1.6 mL. How many millilitres will the nurse draw up into the syringe for the dose? _____

Critical Thinking and Application

Answer the following questions on a separate document.

6. Pedro is to receive interferon as part of the treatment for cancer. Pedro is athletic and participates in sports activities on a regular basis. The health care provider explains that a dose-limiting adverse effect of this type of drug may have undesired effects on his daily activities. What is this adverse effect, and how will it concern Pedro?

7. Takashi is receiving chemotherapy as part of his treatment for Hodgkin's disease. As he begins therapy, he tells the nurse, "I've seen those commercials about the drugs that increase your white blood cell count. Can't I start taking one of them now to keep my counts from getting so low?" What are the drugs that Takashi is referring to? How can the nurse best address Takashi's concerns?

8. Dustin will be receiving treatments with methotrexate for severe rheumatoid arthritis. The nurse is reviewing the drug administration record and sees the following transcribed order: "methotrexate, 7.5 mg per day PO." What is the most appropriate action for the nurse to take?

Match each definition below with its corresponding term. (Not all terms are used.)

9. _____ A type of cytokine that promotes resistance to viral infection in uninfected cells

10. _____ Cytokines that regulate the growth, differentiation, and function of bone marrow stem cells

11. _____ Cytokines that are produced by sensitized T lymphocytes upon contact with antigen particles

12. _____ An immunoglobulin that binds to antigens to form a special complex

13. _____ A substance that is considered foreign by the body's immune system

14. _____ Leukocytes functional cells of the cell-mediated immune system

15. _____ Leukocytes of the humoral immune system

a. Colony-stimulating factors

b. Antibody

c. B lymphocytes (B cells)

d. T lymphocytes (T cells)

e. Interferons

f. Lymphokine-activated killer cells

g. Lymphokines

h. Antigen

i. Memory cells

Case Study

Read the scenario and answer the following questions on a separate document.

Connie, a 58-year-old woman, presents in the emergency department with extreme weakness. She has a pre-existing condition of chronic renal failure that was diagnosed 3 years ago. She receives hemodialysis treatment three times a week. Laboratory results reveal a critically low hemoglobin and hematocrit level, and the health care provider has ordered a transfusion of 2 units of packed red blood cells. However, Connie states that she cannot accept the blood transfusion because of her beliefs. As a result, there are orders to begin therapy with epoetin alfa.

1. What is the rationale for epoetin therapy?

2. What laboratory test results should be monitored while Connie is taking this drug, and why?

3. Connie is concerned about the source of this drug. What can the nurse tell her about this?

4. Connie will be taking this drug at home. By what route will the epoetin be taken?

5. When Connie realizes that she will be giving herself injections up to three times a week, she complains, "Isn't there something else that I can take? I don't want that many shots." Is there an alternative?

CHAPTER 55

Anemia Drugs

Chapter Review and Examination Preparation

Choose the best answer for each of the following:

1. Three days after beginning therapy with oral iron tablets, a patient calls the office. "I'm worried because my bowel movements are black!" What should the nurse do?
   a. Instruct the patient to stop the iron tablets.
   b. Instruct the patient to take the tablets every other day instead of daily.
   c. Ask the patient to come into the office for a checkup.
   d. Explain to the patient that this is an expected effect of the drug.

2. A patient is prescribed oral iron supplements. What should the nurse tell the patient to monitor with respect to possible adverse effects? (Select all that apply.)
   a. Dizziness
   b. Nausea
   c. Vomiting
   d. Drowsiness
   e. Orthostatic hypotension
   f. Stomach cramps

3. The nurse is preparing to administer folic acid. What occurs if folic acid is given to treat anemia without the underlying cause of the anemia having been determined?
   a. Erythropoiesis is inhibited.
   b. Excessive levels of folic acid may accumulate, causing toxicity.
   c. Symptoms of pernicious anemia may be masked, delaying treatment.
   d. Intestinal intrinsic factor is destroyed.

4. A patient is about to receive folic acid supplementation. The nurse knows that indications for folic acid supplementation include which condition? (Select all that apply.)
   a. Iron deficiency anemia
   b. Tropical sprue
   c. Prophylaxis of fetal neural tube defects
   d. Hemolytic anemia

5. When teaching patients about oral iron preparations, what priority instructions should the nurse provide? (Select all that apply.)
   a. Mix the liquid iron preparations with antacids to reduce gastro-intestinal distress.
   b. Take the iron with meals if gastro-intestinal distress occurs.
   c. Take liquid forms through a straw to avoid discolouration of tooth enamel.
   d. Take oral forms with juice or water, not milk.
   e. Iron products will turn the stools black.

6. A patient asks the nurse, "What foods are good sources of iron? I know meat contains iron, but what other choices are there?" Which of the following should the nurse suggest?
   a. Apples
   b. Citrus fruits
   c. Wheat crackers
   d. Raisins

7. The nurse is preparing to give iron sucrose (Venofer) to a 58-year-old patient. For which common adverse effect will the nurse monitor?
   a. Hypotension
   b. Dyspnea
   c. Itching
   d. Cramps

8. A 5-year-old child who is receiving hemodialysis is to receive 8 doses of sodium ferric gluconate (Ferrlecit) 1.5 mg/kg intravenously, with future dialysis sessions. The child weighs 17 kg. How many milligrams is each dose? (Record answer using a whole number.) _____

Critical Thinking and Application

Answer the following questions on a separate document.

9. Jack is prescribed an intramuscular iron dextran. However, before the nurse can give him his first injection, the health care provider suggests administering a smaller dose of 25 mg first. What is the rationale for the smaller dose?

10. Selma will be taking iron for treatment of anemia, and her health care provider instructed her to take it with orange juice. She asks the nurse for an explanation of this. What will the nurse tell her?

11. A child accidentally ingests large doses of iron, resulting in intoxication. Outline the treatment response for this situation.

Case Study

Read the scenario and answer the following questions on a separate document.

Maureen has been given ferrous fumarate capsules with instructions to take two capsules twice a day as part of her treatment for iron deficiency anemia.

1. She asks the nurse if she can take ferrous fumarate with meals. What is an appropriate answer?

2. What else should the nurse warn her to expect with this drug?

3. After a week, Maureen calls the nurse because she does not like to swallow capsules. She says that her mother has iron tablets that are labelled ferrous sulphate. She wants to know if she can take those tablets instead. What does the nurse tell her?

4. Because Maureen does not like the capsules, her iron preparation has been switched to an oral liquid suspension. While the nurse is teaching Maureen how to give herself the correct dosage, what else is important to tell her about liquid iron preparations?

CHAPTER 56

Dermatological Drugs

Chapter Review and Examination Preparation

Choose the best answer for each of the following:

1. Which statement accurately describes antifungal therapy for topical infections?
   a. The treatment required to eradicate the organism may last from several weeks to as long as a year.
   b. Antifungal therapy works best when the affected area is exposed to sunlight.
   c. Oral drugs are the preferred drugs for treating topical fungal infections.
   d. Antifungal therapy is palliative only; fungi are rarely eradicated from topical areas.

2. When instructing a patient on how to use miconazole (Monistat) vaginal cream for vaginal yeast infections, what should the nurse tell the patient as to when to insert this drug?
   a. Insert once every other day at bedtime for 1 week.
   b. Insert once daily at bedtime for 7 consecutive days.
   c. Administer a one-time dose in the morning.
   d. Insert every night at bedtime until symptoms stop.

3. A patient with a sunburn affecting a large area on her back requests the nurse for "something to help make it feel better." Which of the following forms of topical drugs will be easiest to use to cover such a large area and should thus be recommended to the patient?
   a. Aerosol spray
   b. Gel
   c. Oil
   d. Cream

4. A patient needs a drug that has excellent emollient properties. Because she works as a swimming coach, the drug prescribed should not wash off when it comes in contact with water. If each has the same healing properties, which drug is the most appropriate for this patient?
   a. Aerosol spray
   b. Gel
   c. Oil
   d. Cream

5. A nurse is educating a patient on topical antiviral drugs. Which of the following information should the nurse include for the patient? (Select all that apply.)
   a. Common adverse effects include stinging, itching, and rash.
   b. Topically applied acyclovir (Zovirax) does not cure viral skin infections but does seem to decrease the healing time and pain.
   c. Topically applied acyclovir can cure viral skin infections if applied as soon as symptoms appear.
   d. Antiviral drugs are applied topically for the treatment of both initial and recurrent herpes simplex infections.
   e. Topical antiviral drugs are used more often than systemic antiviral drugs for the treatment of viral skin conditions.

6. A patient is taking isotretinoin (Accutane) as part of her treatment for severe cystic acne. Which statement about her isotretinoin therapy is correct?
   a. This drug reduces acne by causing skin peeling.
   b. Its use is contraindicated if the patient is allergic to erythromycin.
   c. The patient will need to apply it twice a day to her face, after washing her face thoroughly.
   d. The patient will need to use two forms of birth control while taking this drug.

7. Before using povidone-iodine (Betadine) solution to prepare skin for surgery, the nurse will ask the patient about allergies to which substance?
   a. Shellfish
   b. Penicillin
   c. Mercury
   d. Milk

8. A patient will be given fluorouracil (Efudex) cream as part of treatment for basal cell carcinoma of the skin on her nose. Which possible adverse effects will the nurse teach the patient about? (Select all that apply.)
   a. Swelling
   b. Scaling
   c. Pallor
   d. Burning
   e. Tenderness

9. The order for a patient who has a severely infected skin wound reads, "Administer clindamycin 300 mg diluted in 50 mL 0.9% NS [normal saline] IVPB every 6 hours. Infuse over 30 minutes." What rate for this IVPB (intravenous piggyback) will the nurse set the infusion pump to? _____

10. A patient will be receiving intravenous amphotericin B (Fungizone) for a severe fungal infection that has not responded to other drugs. The order reads, "75 mg in 1,000 mL D_5W [5% dextrose in water] to infuse over 6 hours." The nurse will set the infusion pump to what rate? _____

Critical Thinking and Application

Answer the following questions on a separate document.

11. Lester has a topical skin infection. He is prescribed clindamycin. He has never used this drug before. What priority assessments must the nurse consider prior to administering this drug?

12. The nurse is getting ready to apply erythromycin to a patient's skin. The affected area of the skin is not oozing or even moist. Why must the nurse wear gloves?

Case Study

Read the scenario and answer the following questions on a separate document.

Judy is in the clinic today because she burned her arm last evening while frying chicken. She has a second-degree burn over a 12.7 cm area of her forearm. She did not apply anything to it overnight, and the wound is reddened and peeling.

1. The health care provider tells the nurse to apply silver sulphadiazine cream to the site. What will the nurse need to do before applying this cream?

2. The nurse tells Judy that the area will need to be kept covered. Why is this necessary?

3. What is the rationale for wearing gloves when applying silver sulphadiazine?

4. Are there any adverse effects associated with this drug?

CHAPTER **57**

Ophthalmic Drugs

Chapter Review and Examination Preparation

Choose the best answer for each of the following:

1. When reviewing the medical record of a patient with a new order for a carbonic anhydrase inhibitor, the nurse recognizes that which of the following conditions is a potential problem for a patient taking this drug?
   a. Glaucoma
   b. Ocular hypertension
   c. Allergy to sulpha drugs
   d. Allergy to penicillin

2. During an ophthalmic procedure, the patient receives ophthalmic acetylcholine. What is the purpose of administering this drug?
   a. To produce mydriasis for ophthalmic examinations
   b. To produce immediate miosis during ophthalmic surgery
   c. To cause cycloplegia to allow for measurement of intraocular pressure
   d. To provide topical anaesthetic during ophthalmic surgery

3. The nurse is preparing to administer latanoprost (Xalatan) eyedrops to a patient. What possible adverse effects must the nurse monitor the patient for?
   a. Temporary eye colour changes, from light colours to brown
   b. Permanent eye colour changes, from light colours to brown
   c. Photosensitivity
   d. Bradycardia and hypotension

4. Willis has come to the emergency room with an eye injury. After the application of fluorescein (AK Fluor), the health care provider sees an area with a green halo. What does this clinical finding indicate?
   a. A corneal defect
   b. A conjunctival lesion
   c. The presence of a hard contact lens
   d. A foreign object

5. What instructions must the nurse adhere to when administering ophthalmic drugs to a patient? (Select all that apply.)
   a. Apply drops directly onto the cornea.
   b. Apply drops into the conjunctival sac.
   c. Apply pressure to the inner canthus for 1 minute after drug administration.
   d. Apply ointments in a thin layer.
   e. Avoid touching the eye with the tip of the drug dropper.

6. A newborn infant is about to be given erythromycin (Ak-Mycin) ointment, when the mother asks, "Why are you giving my baby this drug?" What is the most appropriate response by the nurse?
   a. "This will prevent urinary tract infections for your baby."
   b. "It ensures that the baby has the proper immunity."
   c. "This prevents gonorrheal eye infections from occurring."
   d. "It determines the type of infection the baby is exposed to."

7. A patient has an order for an IV (intravenous) line to infuse at 75 mL per hour. The IV line will infuse by gravity drip; the administration set delivers 15 gtt/mL. How many drops per minute will the nurse need to use for this infusion? (Round to a whole number without any decimals.) _____

Critical Thinking and Application

Answer the following questions on a separate document.

8. Jonathan has blue eyes; Julie has brown eyes. Why would the effects of miotics on the iris be less pronounced in Julie?

9. Jin, 60 years old, has open-angle glaucoma. The health care provider prescribes dipivefrin.

   a. Why might this drug be chosen over epinephrine (Epifrin)?

   b. What effects should the nurse advise Jin to report when first taking this drug?

   c. Considering Jin's overall uncomplicated health, would the nurse expect any serious reactions to the drug? Explain your answer.

10. The health care provider prescribes a β-adrenergic blocker for Ned, who has ocular hypertension. Ned experiences what he calls "an allergic reaction" to the drug. Consequently, the health care provider changes Ned's drug to another beta-blocking drug, timolol (Tim-AK). Because both of these drugs are β-adrenergic blockers and Ned had a reaction to the first drug, what is the rationale for switching Ned to another drug in the same category?

11. Louisa has an inflammatory disorder of the eye for which the nurse practitioner has prescribed a topical ophthalmic nonsteroidal anti-inflammatory drug (NSAID). Why was an NSAID chosen over a corticosteroid?

12. Luna has been prescribed ophthalmic corticosteroid drops for an inflammation of her eyes. The next day, she calls the clinic and tells the nurse, "These drops sting so much when I use them that I can't even put in my contacts." What would the nurse explain to Luna?

13. The nurse is administering drugs to a patient. The patient is due to receive both latanoprost (Xalatan) eyedrops and pilocarpine eye gel at the same time. Which drug should the nurse administer first? Explain your answer.

Match each definition with its corresponding term. (Not all terms will be used.)

14. _____ Adjustment of the lens to variation in distance

15. _____ Inflammation of the eyelids

16. _____ The clear, watery fluid that circulates in the anterior and posterior chambers of the eye

17. _____ An abnormal condition of the lens of the eye, characterized by loss of transparency

18. _____ Paralysis of the ciliary muscles, which prevents accommodation of the lens to variations in distance

19. _____ Excessive intraocular pressure caused by elevated levels of aqueous humor

20. _____ The mucous membrane that lines the eyelids and the exposed anterior surface of the eye

21. _____ Drugs that constrict the pupil

22. _____ The vascular middle layer of the eye, containing the iris, ciliary body, and the choroid

23. _____ Drugs that dilate the pupils

a. Cycloplegia

b. Conjunctiva

c. Accommodation

d. Glaucoma

e. Mydriatics

f. Miotics

g. Uvea

h. Blepharitis

i. Vitreous humor

j. Aqueous humor

k. Cataract

Case Study

Read the scenario and answer the following questions on a separate document.

Wey, aged 72 years, has developed a bacterial ocular infection and has a prescription for erythromycin ocular ointment. You are teaching him how to self-administer the drug.

1. How will this drug be administered?

2. You will educate Wey about what safety precautions to take after he receives a dose of this drug?

3. After receiving the first dose, Wey complains that the drug "burns and stings." What will you say to Wey about this?

4. Wey tells you, "I have some eyedrops from a few months ago when I had some allergy problems. I am sure they will help me now. Can I take them with this ointment?" What is your best response?

CHAPTER 58

Otic Drugs

Chapter Review and Examination Preparation

Choose the best answer for each of the following:

1. When assessing for otitis media, the nurse recalls that common symptoms of this condition include which of the following? (Select all that apply.)
   a. Pain
   b. Malaise
   c. Ear drainage
   d. Hearing loss
   e. Fever

2. A patient with a middle-ear infection will generally require treatment with which type of drug?
   a. Topical steroids
   b. Systemic steroids
   c. Topical antibiotics
   d. Systemic antibiotics

3. An older adult has a buildup of cerumen in his left ear. The nurse expects that this patient will receive which type of drug for this problem?
   a. Antifungal
   b. Wax emulsifier
   c. Steroid
   d. Local analgesic

4. The nurse is preparing to administer ear drops for a patient. What contraindication must the nurse assess for prior to giving the drug?
   a. Eardrum perforation
   b. Infection
   c. The presence of cerumen
   d. Mastoiditis

5. A child has a case of otitis media. The nurse knows that otitis media in children is usually preceded by which of the following?
   a. Participation on a swim team
   b. Injury with a foreign object
   c. Upper respiratory tract infection
   d. Mastoiditis

6. A child with an ear infection will be receiving amoxicillin (Amoxil) suspension by mouth (PO). The order reads, "Give 125 mg (5 mL) three times a day PO." The child weighs 11 kg.
   a. How many milligrams of drug will this child receive in 24 hours? _____
   b. The safe dosage range of the drug is 20 to 40 mg/kg/day. What is the safe range (in milligrams) for this child? _____
   c. Is the ordered dose within the safe range?

   _____

Critical Thinking and Application

Answer the following questions on a separate document.

7. A patient calls the health care provider's office complaining of severe pain in his left ear and drainage from it. He also says he "had a little mishap" on his motorcycle yesterday. What does the nurse tell him?

8. Why are anti-infective otic drugs frequently combined with steroids?

9. André, a 30-year-old teacher, has an ear infection and a new prescription for eardrops.

    a. What might be done before he takes the eardrops?

    b. What safety measures are important to tell André about regarding his self-administration of the eardrops?

10. Frannie, a 52-year-old office manager, has come to the clinic today complaining of a painful, "itchy" left ear. The health care provider diagnoses an infection of the external auditory canal and prescribes eardrop drug that contains a combination of polymyxin B and hydrocortisone.

    a. What is the advantage of using a product containing hydrocortisone?

    b. What would be a contraindication to Frannie's use of this type of drug?

11. Why do so many otic combination products contain local anaesthetic drugs?

12. Ben is a 2-year-old who attends day care, and his brother Drew is a 6-year-old in kindergarten. They both require otic drugs for ear infections.

    a. What instructions does the nurse give the boys' parents regarding instillation of the drops?

    b. A few days after they are first seen, the boys' mother brings them back for a follow-up visit. Ben and Drew do not seem to be in pain, and there is no redness or swelling in either child's ears. What does this mean?

13. During a home visit, the nurse observes Esther's husband preparing her eardrops. The husband puts a glass of water in the microwave oven, saying that he will soak the bottle of eardrops in hot water to warm them up.

    a. Is this a good way to warm the eardrops?

    b. Immediately after her husband instills the drops, Esther sits up and asks whether they are now doing everything right. What will the nurse tell her?

Case Study

Read the scenario and answer the following questions on a separate document.

Mark, who is 45 years old, is in the office complaining of a "heavy" feeling in his left ear, along with slight pain and decreased hearing. When the nurse walks into the examination room, she finds Mark inserting a cotton-tipped applicator into his ear "to scratch it."

1. What is the possible source of Mark's symptoms?

2. What can be done to address this problem?

3. The nurse gives Mark a container of urea hydrogen peroxide (Murine Ear Drops). He asks her how many times a day he needs to take this drug and whether he can take it with meals. In what form is this drug given, and how should Mark administer the drug?

Overview of Dosage Calculations

Disclaimer: *Please note that the drugs and dosages mentioned in this chapter are examples for educational purposes only. Please refer to appropriate drug resources for dosage information.*

Accurate drug calculation skills are important, as a mistake in calculating can result in a medication error that causes unwanted consequences for the patient. There are many important aspects to consider when doing calculations, but the most important one may be common sense. If a drug dose calculation does not seem right, then most likely it is not. The administration of drug to patients is a shared responsibility among the patient, physician, pharmacist, and nurse. All those involved have moral, ethical, and legal responsibilities to ensure that the administration of drugs takes place in a safe and effective way. The nurse has both a legal and a professional responsibility to ensure that patients receive the right dose of the right drug at the right time and by the right route. There are many checks and balances in the system to ensure that this happens. The necessary basic calculations involved in the safe and accurate administration of medications to patients are described in this section.

Calculating drug doses is one part of the overall process of pharmacological therapy. Before actually calculating a drug dose, the nurse must follow several steps. The nurse should assess the patient and the prescribed medication according to the traditional "five rights": right patient, right drug, right dose, right time, and right route. Other principles to follow to decrease the likelihood of mistakes are to calculate doses systematically and to do the calculations consistently time after time so that the process becomes easier with each calculation. It also helps to have a peer check the calculations, especially if the dose seems unusual or the math is difficult. Remember, common sense should prevail. If a calculation shows that you should give 25 mg of digoxin and the strongest strength is 0.25 mg, common sense should tell you that the patient should not be given 100 pills, especially since drug dosage forms are usually manufactured with the most commonly prescribed dosages in mind.

You must have basic arithmetic skills before beginning. The following basic principles may need to be reviewed:

- Basic multiplication
- Basic division
- Roman numerals
- Fractions (addition, subtraction, multiplication, division, mixed numbers, reducing to lowest terms)
- Decimals (addition, subtraction, multiplication, division)
- Ratios and percentages (changing a fraction to a percentage; changing a ratio to a percentage)
- Solving for "*x*" in a simple equation

RULES TO REMEMBER

- Before calculating a drug dose for a particular patient, you must first convert all units of measure to a single system. The best approach is to convert to the system used on the drug label. Although metric is the preferred system in Canada, it may still be necessary to convert the patient's weight from pounds to kilograms if the medication is ordered to be given per kilogram of weight.

Rounding

- Always round your answers to the nearest dose that is measurable, after verifying that the dose is correct for that patient.
  - If a tablet is scored, you may round to the nearest half tablet.
    - **Example:** 1.8 tablets, give 2 tablets
      1.2 tablets, give 1 tablet

- If a tablet is unscored, call the pharmacy to check if there is a lower dosage tablet available or if a pill cutter is suitable to use to split the pill. It is difficult to cut an unscored tablet into fourths accurately. Remember that enteric-coated, sustained-release, or extended-release pills cannot be cut or crushed!
- Recheck your calculations if the dose is more than one or two tablets.
- To round liquids, look at the equipment you plan to use. Some syringes are marked in tenths or hundredths of a millilitre. Larger syringes are marked in 0.2 mL increments. Tuberculin syringes are marked in one-hundredths. For liquid medications, never round up to the nearest whole number. If the answer is 1.8 mL, do not round up to 2 mL. Rounding up in these situations may lead to overdosing. However, if you are using an electronic infusion pump, you will probably need to round to the nearest whole number.
- To round to the nearest tenth, look at the hundredths column. If it is 0.5 or more, round up to the next tenth.
  Example: To round to the nearest tenth,
  1.78 or 1.75, round to 1.8
  1.32 or 1.34, round to 1.3
- A syringe calibrated in hundredths permits more exact measurement of small dosages. To round to the nearest hundredth, look at the thousandth column. If it is 0.005 or more, round up to the next hundredth.
  Example: To round to the nearest hundredth,
  1.847, round to 1.85
  1.653, round to 1.65
- NOTE: Never round up liquid medications to the nearest whole number. If the answer is 1.6 mL, do not round up to 2 mL! Such increases may lead to overdoses.
- Children's doses are rounded to the tenths place, not whole numbers. Rounding to whole numbers may lead to overdoses.

Leading Zeros

■ Always insert a zero in front of decimals when the number is less than a whole number. This draws attention to the decimal and avoids potential errors.
  Example: 0.05 is correct.
  .05 is not correct.

Trailing Zeroes

■ Never place a lone zero after a decimal point. If the decimal is not noticed, a dangerous dosage error may occur.
  Example: 3 is correct.
  3.0 is not correct and may be mistaken for 30.

Labelling

■ Always label your answers with the appropriate unit. If the problems asked for a number of tablets, write "tablets." If you are to give an injection, use "mL." For heparin and insulin, however, use "units" instead of "mg" or "mcg." Intravenous drips will be written in terms of "mL/hr." Problems using an intravenous infusion pump are always asking for mL/hr. Think about what the question is asking, and label your answer appropriately.

Common Sense

■ Use common sense! Drug companies typically formulate medications that are close to the usual doses and medications that can provide the ordered dose with one or two tablets. If your answer indicates that you should give 60 mL intramuscularly, check it again! Remember, you can give only 2 to 3 mL intramuscularly, depending on institution policies, so a dosage of 60 mL would be inappropriate.

INTERPRETING MEDICATION LABELS

Medication labels contain a tremendous amount of information, much of it in small print. Some labels are printed by the manufacturer; others are prepared by pharmacy technicians or pharmacists for institutional use. The most important information is as follows:

- Generic name: the first letter is lowercased. This is the name used by all companies that produce the drug.
- Trade, brand, or proprietary name: the first letter is usually capitalized. This name is used only by the manufacturer of the drug and may be followed by the "®" symbol.
- Drug Identification Number (DIN): a "computer-generated 8-digit number assigned by Health Canada to a drug product prior to being marketed in Canada. It uniquely identifies all drug products sold in a dosage form in Canada and is located on the label of prescription and over-the-counter drugs that have been evaluated and authorized for sale in Canada" (Health Canada, 2009).
- Unit dose per millilitre, per tablet, per capsule, and so on
- Total amount in the container
- Route
- Directions for preparation, if needed
- Directions for storage
- Expiration date

Other information, such as a specification for adult or child use, may be noted on the label.

Example:

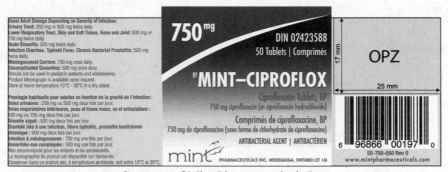

Courtesy of Mint Pharmaceuticals Inc.

Generic name:	ciprofloxacin hydrochloride
Trade name:	Mint-Ciproflox
Unit dose:	750 mg per tablet
Total amount in container:	50 tablets
Route:	(It is assumed that tablets are for oral route.)

For the following labels, identify the information requested:

1.

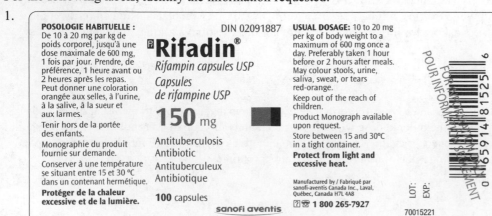

Courtesy of Sanofi Canada

Generic name: _____

Trade name: _____

Unit dose: _____

Total amount in container: _____

Route: _____

2.

DEPO-PROVERA ®/MD

DIN 00030848

MEDROXYPROGESTERONE ACETATE
INJECTABLE SUSPENSION USP
SUSPENSION INJECTABLE D'ACÉTATE
DE MÉDROXYPROGESTÉRONE, USP

50 mg/mL medroxyprogesterone acetate / d'acétate de médroxyprogestérone

250 mg/5 mL

Sterile Aqueous Suspension /
Suspension aqueuse stérile

Progestogen / Progestatif

**For intramuscular use only
Pour usage intramusculaire
seulement**

1 x 5 mL Single dose vial / Fiole unidose
Discard unused portion /
Jeter toute portion inutilisée

Pfizer

PROGESTOGEN
Each mL contains:
Medroxyprogesterone acetate . . . . 50 mg
Methylparaben & . . . . 1.3 mg
Propylparaben (as preservatives) . . . . 0.14 mg
Polyethylene glycol 3350 . . . . 28.8 mg
Polysorbate 80 . . . . 1.9 mg
Sodium chloride . . . . 8.6 mg
Water for Injection . . . . q.s.
When necessary, pH adjusted with sodium
hydroxide and/or hydrochloric acid.

PROGESTATIF
Un mL contient:
Acétate de médroxyprogestérone . . . . . 50 mg
Méthylparaben et . . . . 1,3 mg
Propylparaben (comme agents
de conservation) . . . . 0,14 mg
Polyéthylèneglycol 3350 . . . . 28,8 mg
Polysorbate 80 . . . . 1,9 mg
Chlorure de sodium . . . . 8,6 mg
Eau pour injection . . . . q.s.
Le pH est ajusté, au besoin, avec de l'hydroxyde de
sodium et/ou de l'acide chlorhydrique.

**FOR INTRAMUSCULAR USE ONLY.
SHAKE WELL BEFORE USING.**
Usual Adult Dose:
Contraception: 150 mg every 3 months within the
first 5 days of onset of normal menstrual period or of
post-partum if not breast feeding.
Endometriosis: 50 mg weekly or 100 mg every
2 weeks for at least 6 months.
See enclosed package insert for complete dosage,
administration and direction for use. Store **upright** at
controlled room temperature (between 15 and 30°C).
Protect from freezing.
Keep out of reach of children.
Pharmacist: Dispense with enclosed Patient Infor-
mation leaflet and instruct patient to read it before use.
Product Monograph available on request.

6 21745 02518 1

Pfizer

Courtesy of Pfizer Inc.

Generic name: _____

Trade name: _____

Unit dose: _____

Total amount in container: _____

Route: _____

SECTION I: BASIC CONVERSIONS USING RATIO AND PROPORTION

A proportion is a way of stating a relationship of equality between two ratios. The first ratio listed is equal to the second ratio listed. The double colon (::) that separates the two ratios means "as." The numbers at each end of the ratio equation can be called the "outside," and the two numbers in the middle of the ratio (around the "::") can be called the "inside." Ratio and proportion problems can be used to calculate one of the numbers in the equation if it is not known. The simple rule to use is this:

The product of the outside terms equals the product of the inside terms.

If one of the terms is not known, it is designated as "x." The problem is then set up to solve for "x."

Example:

1 : 100 :: 4 : x means:
"The relationship of 1 to 100 is the same as the relationship of 4 to x." ("x" is unknown.)

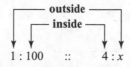

outside

inside

1 : 100   ::   4 : x

1 and x are the "outsides;" 100 and 4 are the "insides." To solve for x, multiply the outsides (1 × x), multiply the insides (100 × 4), and form an equation:

$(1 \times x) = (100 \times 4)$
$1x = 400$
$x = 400$

Proof: You may prove your equation as follows: Insert the answer for x in the original equation, then solve.

$1 \times 400 = 400$ (outsides)
$100 \times 4 = 400$ (insides)
$400 = 400$; the answer for x is correct.

Example:

$5 : 25 :: 15 : x$
Multiply the outsides and the insides and form an equation; then solve for x.
$(5 \times x) = (25 \times 15)$
$5x = 375$
$x = 375/5$
$x = 75$

Proof:

$5 \times 75 = 375$
$25 \times 15 = 375$
$375 = 375$

Calculating ratios is one of the major foundations of dosage calculations. When calculating a dosage, the nurse will use the medication on hand to calculate how much of it to give for a desired dosage. The nurse uses the principle of proportion to calculate accurately how much medication to give. The following chart provides a few common equivalents used in pharmacology. These equivalents are then used in ratio and proportion problems to calculate appropriate dosages.

BASIC EQUIVALENTS

Metric Equivalent	Approximate Equivalent
Weight 1 mg = 1000 mg or mcg (micrograms) 1 g = 1000 mg (milligrams) 1 kg = 1000 g (grams)	
Volume 1000 mL = 1 L	1 tsp = 5 mL 1 tbsp = 15 mL 2 tbsp = 30 mL 1 oz = 30 mL 1 kg = 2.2 lb 1 mL (weighs approximately 1 g)

To find basic equivalents from one unit of measure to another, use the ratio-and-proportion approach.

Example 1: The drug dosage is 500 mg. You have scored tablets that are 1 g each. How many tablets will you give?

You have grams on hand. You need to change the milligrams needed to the equivalent grams on hand.
Find the proper equivalents:
    Equivalent: 1 g = 1000 mg

Next, set up the ratio and proportion equation.

On the left side, put the ratio that you know: 1 g is 1000 mg

On the right side, put the ratio that you want to know: how many g ("x") is 500 mg?

Know   ***Want to Know***

1 g : 1000 mg :: x g : 500 mg

Solve for x: $(1 \times 500) = (1000 \times x)$; $500 = 1000x$; $x = 500/1000$; $x = 0.5$

You will give 0.5 (half) of the 1 g tablet.

To double-check your answer, substitute your answer for the x and solve. The outsides should equal the insides.

$1 \times 500 = 500$; $1000 \times 0.5 = 500$; $500 = 500$

Example 2: Mabel weighs 122 lb. How many kilograms does she weigh?

Equivalent: 1 kg = 2.2 lb

Know   ***Want to Know***

1 kg : 2.2 lb :: x kg : 122 lb

$(1 \times 122) = (2.2 \times x)$; $122 = 2.2x$; $122/2.2 = x$; $x = 55.45$ kg. Round off to tenths: 55.5 kg

Proof: $1 \times 122 = 122$; $2.2 \times 55.45 = 121.99$ (rounds to 122)

Example 3: You have an injectable solution that is 50 mg strength. How many micrograms are in 50 mg?

Equivalent: 1 mg = 1000 mcg

Know   ***Want to Know***

1 mg : 1000 mcg :: 50 mg : x mcg

$(1 \times x) = (1000 \times 50)$; $1x = 50,000$; $x = 50,000$; therefore, 50 mg = 50,000 mcg

Proof: $1 \times 50,000 = 50,000$; $1000 \times 50 = 50,000$

Example 4: An elixir is ordered as follows: "Give 2 tsp twice a day." How many millilitres would you give?

Equivalent: 1 tsp = 5 mL

Know   ***Want to Know***

1 tsp : 5 mL :: 2 tsp : x mL

$(1 \times x) = (5 \times 2)$; $1x = 10$; $x = 10$ mL

Proof: $1 \times 10 = 10$; $5 \times 2 = 10$; $10 = 10$

Thus, to equal 2 tsp, give 10 mL.

Example 5: You have an injection that delivers 75 mcg. How many milligrams does it deliver?

Equivalent: 1 mg = 1000 mcg

Know   ***Want to Know***

1 mg : 1000 mcg :: x mg : 75 mcg

$(1 \times 75) = (1000 \times x)$; $75 = 1000x$; $x = 75/1000$; $x = 0.075$

So, 75 mcg = 0.075 mg. (Do not forget the leading zero!)

Proof: $1 \times 75 = 75$; $1000 \times 0.075 = 75$; $75 = 75$

PRACTICE PROBLEMS

Calculate the following conversions:

1. 600 mg = _____ mcg
2. 1500 mg = _____ mcg
3. 5000 mcg = _____ mg
4. 5 g = _____ mg
5. 2.5 g = _____ mg
6. 900 mg = _____ g
7. 8 kg = _____ g
8. 750 mL = _____ L
9. 975 L = _____ mL
10. 500 mL = _____ L
11. 90 g = _____ g
12. 4 tsp = _____ mL
13. 60 mL = _____ tsp
14. 90 mL = _____ tbsp
15. 90 kg = _____ lb
16. 150 lb = _____ kg
17. 11 kg = _____ lb

SECTION II: CALCULATING ORAL DOSES

To calculate oral dosages of medications, use the same ratio and proportion procedures described in Section I. Label all terms, and check your answers by proving them.

The first step in doing medication dosage calculation problems is examining the order and the medication on hand. The units for both the order and the medicine on hand must be the same units (e.g., milligrams, millilitres). If they are not the same, a conversion must first be done to change the ordered dose to the same units as the medication on hand.

Remember these rules:

■ Never substitute one form of a medication for another, even if the dosage amount is the same. Parenteral forms of oral drugs are much stronger, and the resulting effects might be dangerous.
■ Do not forget to place a zero in front of a decimal point (e.g., 0.75 mg). It reminds you that the number is a decimal, not a whole number.
■ Are the medication ordered and the medication on hand in the same units? If not, convert the drug ordered to the units of the drug on hand.
■ Place what you have on hand (what you know)—information from the label—on the left side of the equation.
■ Place what is ordered (what you want to know) on the right side of the equation.
■ Solve the equation as described in Section I.
■ Always label the units of your answer (tablets, capsules, millilitres, etc.).

Example 1: The prescription reads, "Give 500 mg PO." The unit dose is 250 mg per tablet. How many tablets will you give?

Ordered: 500 mg   Unit dose: 250 mg per tablet
NOTE: Units match (milligrams).

Know   *Want to Know*
250 mg : 1 tablet :: 500 mg : x tablet
$(250 \times x) = (1 \times 500); 250x = 500; x = 500/250 = 2$
Answer: Give 2 tablets.
Proof: $250 \times 2 = 500; 1 \times 500 = 500; 500 = 500$

Example 2: The order is to give 175 mg. The tablets on hand are 350 mg scored tablets. How many tablets will you give?

Ordered: 175 mg   Unit dose: 350 mg per tablet
NOTE: Units match (milligrams).

Know   *Want to Know*
350 mg : 1 tablet :: 175 mg : x tablet
$(350 \times x) = (1 \times 175); 350x = 175; x = 175/350 = 0.5$
Answer: Give 0.5 tablet (one half of the scored tablet).
Proof: $350 \times 0.5 = 175; 1 \times 175 = 175; 175 = 175$

Example 3: You are asked to administer 100 mg of a drug. You have 0.05 g tablets on hand. How many tablets will you give?

Ordered: 100 mg   Unit dose: 0.05 g per tablet
NOTE: Units do not match (milligrams and grams).

First: Calculate: 100 mg = x g (equivalent: 1 g = 1000 mg)

Know   *Want to Know*
1 g : 1000 mg :: x g : 100 mg
$(1 \times 100) = (1000 \times x); 100 - 1000x; x = 100/1000 = 0.1$
100 mg = 0.1 g
Now that you have the ordered dose and the dose on hand in the same units, you can complete the problem.

Ordered: 0.1 g (100 mg)   Unit dose: 0.05 g per tablet

Know   *Want to Know*
0.05 g : 1 tablet :: 0.1 g : x tablet
$(0.05 \times x) = (1 \times 0.1); 0.05x = 0.1; x = 0.1/0.05 = 2$
Answer: Give 2 tablets.
Proof: $0.05 \times 2 = 0.1; 1 \times 0.1 = 0.1; 0.1 = 0.1$

Example 4: You are instructed to give 0.5 g of a drug. You have 250 mg tablets on hand. How many tablets will you give?

Ordered: 0.5 g   Unit dose: 250 mg per tablet
NOTE: Units do not match (grams and milligrams).

First: Calculate: 0.5 g = x mg (equivalent: 1 g = 1000 mg)

Know   *Want to Know*
1 g : 1000 mg :: 0.5 g : x mg
$(1 \times x) = (1000 \times 0.5); 1x = 500; x = 500$
0.5 g = 500 mg
Now that you have the ordered dose and the dose on hand in the same units, you can complete the problem.
Ordered: 500 mg (0.5 g)   Unit dose: 250 mg per tablet

Know   *Want to Know*
250 mg : 1 tablet :: 500 mg : x tablet
$(250 \times x) = (1 \times 500); 250x = 500; x = 500/250 = 2$
Answer: Give 2 tablets.
Proof: $250 \times 2 = 500; 1 \times 500 = 500; 500 = 500$

Example 5: You are to administer 200 mg of guaifenesin syrup. You have a bottle labelled 100 mg/5 mL. How many millilitres will you give?

Ordered: 200 mg   Unit dose: 100 mg/5 mL
NOTE: Units match (milligrams).

Know   ***Want to Know***
100 mg : 5 mL :: 200 mg : x mL
$(100 \times x) = (5 \times 200); 100x = 1000; x = 1000/100 = 10$
Answer: Give 10 mL.
Proof: $100 \times 10 = 1000; 5 \times 200 = 1000; 1000 = 1000$

PRACTICE PROBLEMS

1. Dose ordered: ascorbic acid 0.5 g PO (orally)
   Dose on hand: 500 mg tablets
   How many tablets will you give? _____

2. Dose ordered: digoxin 0.5 mg PO
   Dose on hand: 250 mcg tablets
   How many tablets will you give? _____

3. Dose ordered: sulphisoxazole 0.25 g PO
   Dose on hand: 500 mg tablets
   How many tablets will you give? _____

4. Dose ordered: diphenhydramine elixir 50 mg PO
   Dose on hand: elixir 12.5 mg/5 mL
   How many millilitres will you give? _____

5. Dose ordered: cefaclor 0.1 g PO
   Dose on hand: liquid 125 mg/5 mL
   How many millilitres will you give? _____

6. Dose ordered: zidovudine 0.3 g PO
   Dose on hand: 100 mg tablets
   How many tablets will you give? _____

7. Dose ordered: potassium chloride elixir 30 mmol PO
   Dose on hand: 20 mmol/15 mL
   How many millilitres will you give? _____

8. Dose ordered: pentobarbital 0.15 g PO
   Dose on hand: 50 mg capsules
   How many capsules will you give? _____

9. Dose ordered: levodopa 2 g PO
   Dose on hand: 500 mg tablets
   How many tablets will you give? _____

SECTION III: RECONSTITUTING MEDICATIONS

Many medications come in powder or crystal form and must be reconstituted by the addition of a diluent to create a liquid form. Many parenteral medications must be reconstituted before administration. Instructions for dissolving medications can be found in the literature that accompanies the medication or on the medication label. Most of the time, medications that need to be reconstituted are in delivery systems that match 50 or 100 mL intravenous (IV) bags, and reconstitution occurs as the nurse prepares the medication for use. However, there are still instances where the nurse may be required to reconstitute a drug and then draw up the proper dose for parenteral use. These examples are for those instances.

For example, the instructions may read:

Add 1.2 mL normal saline to make 2 mL of reconstituted solution that yields 100 mg/mL.

This tells the user that the medication takes up 0.8 mL of space: 1.2 mL + 0.8 mL = 2 mL of medication solution. The label of the medication container will tell the user how many units, grams, milligrams, or micrograms are in each millilitre of the reconstituted medication. In this example, the dose on hand after reconstitution is 100 mg/mL.

Remember these rules:

- Read all instructions for reconstitution before doing anything! Be sure to ask a pharmacist if you have any questions.
- When reconstituting medications, be certain to use the exact type of diluent, and add the exact amount of diluent as directed. Substitutions or inaccurate amounts of diluent can inactivate the medication or alter the concentration, thus altering the dose received by the patient.
- If the vial is a multiple-dose vial, the nurse who reconstitutes the medication must put the date, time, amount of diluent used, and the nurse's initials on the label.
- Many solutions are unstable after being reconstituted. Be sure to follow the directions on the label for proper storage of reconstituted medications.
- Make note of the time limit or expiration date of the reconstituted medication. Do not use the medication after it has expired.
- Ratio solutions indicate the number of grams of the medication per total millilitres of solution. For example, a medication that is designated 1:1000 has 1 g of medication per 1000 mL of solution.

In order to avoid overdosing, it is essential that the nurse chooses the correct ratio solution!

- Percentage solutions indicate the number of grams of the medication per 100 mL of solution. For example, a medication that is designated 10% has 10 g of drug per 100 mL of solution.
- Compare: "1:1000" indicates 1 g per 1000 mL
                    "10%" indicates 10 g per 100 mL

As you calculate parenteral dosages, observe the following:

- If the amount is greater than 1 mL, round x (the amount to be given) to tenths, and use a 3 mL syringe to measure it.
- Small (less than 0.5 mL, or child) dosages should be rounded to hundredths and measured in a tuberculin syringe. The tuberculin syringe is calibrated in 0.01 mL increments.
- Think! For adults, the maximum volume of an intramuscular (IM) injection is usually 3 mL. Sometimes the dose might have to be given in two divided doses; for example, a dose of 4 mL IM would usually be divided into two 2 mL doses. However, if your calculations yield an unusual number, such as 10 mL IM, look over your calculation and repeat your math! Double-check your calculations with a peer.

Always remember to note the route ordered. Intramuscular doses and IV doses are not always the same amount, and the drug formulations may differ. Confusing the route can have fatal results.

Example 1: You receive an order for morphine 12 mg IM. The medication vial reads 10 mg/mL.

How much morphine would you give?
Does this medication require reconstitution?
Would you use a 3 mL or a tuberculin syringe to measure this drug?

Ordered: 12 mg   Unit dose: 10 mg/mL

Know   *Want to Know*
10 mg : 1 mL :: 12 mg : x mL
$(10 \times x) = (1 \times 12)$; $10x = 12$; $x = 12/10 = 1.2$
Answer: 1.2 mL measured in a 3 mL syringe. This medication does not require reconstitution.
Proof: $10 \times 1.2 = 12$; $1 \times 12 = 12$

Example 2: The ordered dose is cloxacillin sodium 500 mg IV. The medication label reads as shown below:

500 mg CLOXACILLIN SODIUM FOR INJECTION
For IM or IV use
Add 2.7 mL sterile water for injection.
Each 1.5 mL contains 250 mg cloxacillin.

How much cloxacillin would you give?
Does this drug require reconstitution?
Would you use a 3 mL or a tuberculin syringe to measure this drug?

Ordered: 500 mg   Unit dose: 250 mg/1.5 mL

Know   **_Want to Know_**
250 mg : 1.5 mL :: 500 mg : x mL
$(250 \times x) = (1.5 \times 500); 250x = 750; x = 750/250 = 3$
Answer: 3 mL measured in a 3 mL syringe. Reconstitute by adding 2.7 mL of sterile water to the vial.
Proof: $250 \times 3 = 750; 1.5 \times 500 = 750; 750 = 750$

Example 3: You receive an order for penicillin G potassium 400,000 units IM. The medication label reads as shown below:

ONE MILLION UNITS
Penicillin G potassium
Use sterile saline as diluent as follows:

Add	Units per mL reconstituted solution
18.2 mL	250,000
8.2 mL	500,000
3.2 mL	1,000,000

Which dilution would you choose for the ordered dose?
How much penicillin G potassium would you give?
Would you use a 3 mL or a tuberculin syringe to measure this drug?

Ordered: 400,000 units   Unit dose: Choosing the 8.2 diluent amount, the unit dose is 500,000/mL.

Know   **_Want to Know_**
500,000 units : 1/mL :: 400,000 : x mL
$(500,000 \times x) = (1 \times 400,000); 500,000x = 400,000; x = 400,000/500,000 = 0.8$
Answer: 0.8 mL measured in either a 3 mL or tuberculin syringe
Proof: $500,000 \times 0.8 = 400,000; 1 \times 400,000 = 400,000; 400,000 = 400,000$

NOTE: Choose the concentration that is close to the ordered dose. Choosing the 8.2 diluent amount allows for the injection amount to be small yet easily measured. If you had chosen the 18.2 diluent amount, the injection would have been 1.6/mL; choosing the 3.2 diluent would have made the injection amount very small (0.04/mL).

Example 4: You receive an order for epinephrine 0.6/mg SC. The medication label reads as shown below:

1/mL ampule
Epinephrine 1:1000
For SC or IM use

What is the dose on hand?
How much epinephrine would you give?
Would you use a 3 mL or a tuberculin syringe to measure the drug?
First: Figure the dose on hand.
1:1000 = 1/g in 1000/mL = 1000/mg in 1000/mL = 1/mg in 1/mL

Then complete the problem:

Ordered: 0.6/mg   Unit dose: 1/mg/mL

Know   *Want to Know*

1 mg : 1 mL :: 0.6 mg : x mL
$(1 \times x) = (1 \times 0.6)$; $1x = 0.6$; $x = 0.6$
Answer: 0.6 mL measured in either a 3 mL or tuberculin syringe.
Proof: $1 \times 0.6 = 0.6$; $1 \times 0.6 = 0.6$; $0.6 = 0.6$

Example 5: Magnesium sulphate 5/g IV over 3 hours is the dosage ordered. The medication label reads as shown below:

> 10/mL vial
> Magnesium sulphate 10%
> For IM or IV use

What is the dose on hand?
How much magnesium sulphate would you give?
First: Figure the dose on hand.
10% = 10 g in 100 mL = 0.1 g per 1 mL

Then complete the problem:

Ordered: 5 g   Unit dose: 0.1 g/mL

Know   *Want to Know*

0.1 g : 1 mL :: 5 g : x mL
$(0.1 \times x) = (1 \times 5)$; $0.1x = 5$; $x = 5/0.1$; $x = 50$
Answer: 50 mL
Proof: $0.1 \times 50 = 5$; $1 \times 5 = 5$; $5 = 5$

PRACTICE PROBLEMS

1. Dose ordered: thiamine 200 mg
   On hand: 10 mL vial, 100 mg/mL

   How much will you give? _____

2. Dose ordered: gentamicin 60 mg IM
   On hand: 40 mg/mL

   How much will you give? _____

3. Dose ordered: heparin 8000 units SC (subcut)
   On hand: 1 mL vial, 10,000 units/mL

   How much will you give? _____

4. Dose ordered: methicillin 750 mg IV
   On hand: 1 g vial
   Instructions for reconstitution: Add 1.5 mL sterile water. Reconstituted solution will contain approximately 500 mg methicillin solution per mL.

   How much will you give? _____

5. Dose ordered: ampicillin 500 mg IV
   On hand: 1 g vial
   Instructions for reconstitution: Add 66 mL sterile water. Reconstituted solution will contain 125 mg/5 mL.

   How much will you give? _____

6. Dose ordered: penicillin G potassium 300,000 units IM
   On hand: 1,000,000-unit vial
   Instructions for reconstitution: Using only sterile water, add 9.6 mL to provide 100,000 units/mL, or 4.6 mL to provide 200,000 units/mL.
   Which concentration would you choose for this dose? _____

   How much will you give? _____

7. Dose ordered: epinephrine 750 mcg SC
   On hand: 1:1000

   How much will you give? _____

8. Dose ordered: isoproterol hydrochloride 0.2 mg
   On hand: 1:5000

   How much will you give? _____

9. Dose ordered: calcium gluconate 900 mg
   On hand: calcium gluconate 10%, 100 mg/mL vial

   How much will you give? _____

10. Dose ordered: magnesium sulphate 4 g
    On hand: magnesium sulphate 50%, 10 mL vial

    How much will you give? _____

SECTION IV: CHILD CALCULATIONS

Doses used in children must differ from those used in adults. The most common method for calculating doses for children is weight based (i.e., mg/kg). In some cases, dosages may be calculated using body surface area calculations.

Body Surface Area–Based Calculations

The body surface area (BSA) is a common method of calculating therapeutic children's dosages. It requires the use of a chart, called a West nomogram (see Figure 4-1 in the text), that converts weight to square metres (m^2) of BSA. The average adult is assumed to weigh 63.5 kg (140 lb) and have a BSA of $1.73/m^2$. The BSA may be used to calculate the child dose of certain medications.

- For a child of normal height and weight, find the BSA in square metres for that weight on the shaded area of the nomogram chart.
  Example: Using Figure 4-1 in your text, find the BSA for a child who weighs 18.1 kg (25 lb) and is 95 cm (38 inches) tall (normal weight for her height). According to the nomogram, the BSA for 40 lb is 0.74 m^2.

- For a child who is underweight or overweight, the BSA is indicated at the point where a straight line connecting the height and weight intersects the unshaded surface area (SA) column.
  Example: Using Figure 4-1, find the BSA for a child who weighs 11.4 kg (25 lb) and has a height of 75 cm (30 inches) (underweight). According to the nomogram, the BSA for this child is 0.51 m^2.

There are two types of BSA problems:

1. The first type involves medications for which the literature provides recommended dosages in square metres.

   Step 1: Check the order, and look up the recommended dose.
   The order is for 15 mg PO.
   The literature states that 40 mg/m^2 is safe for children.

   Step 2: Determine the child's height and weight. Then consult the appropriate nomogram to obtain the BSA in square metres. This child weighs 10 kg (22 lb) and has a normal height of 70 cm. The BSA is approximately 0.46 m^2.

   Step 3: Calculate the recommended mg/m^2 dose (from the literature), using ratio and proportion. Then for a safety check, compare it with the dose ordered.
   For this calculation, what you know is the literature's recommendation (40 mg/m^2). What you *want to know* is the milligrams per the child's BSA (which is 0.46 m^2).

   Know   *Want to Know*
   40 mg : 1 m^2 :: x mg : 0.46 m^2
   $(40 \times 0.46) = (1 \times x)$; $18.4 = 1x$; $x = 18.4$ (Child doses are rounded to tenths place; do not round to whole numbers.)
   Answer: 18.4 mg is the safe dose limit.
   Decision: The order for 15 mg is safe.

   Practice:
   The medication ordered is 100 mg.

   Step 1: The literature recommends 50 mg/m^2 for children.

   Step 2: The child weighs 4.5 kg (10 lb) and has a normal height for his weight. The BSA is 0.27 m^2.

   Step 3: Calculate the dose for this child's BSA:

Know   *Want to Know*

50 mg : 1 m² :: *x* mg : 0.27 m²

$(50 \times 0.27) = (1 \times x)$; $13.5 = 1x$; $x = 13.5$ (Child doses are rounded to tenths place; do not round to whole numbers.)

Answer: 13.5 mg is the safe dose limit.

Decision: The order for 15 mg exceeds the safe dose limit and therefore is *not* safe. Notify the physician.

2. The second type of BSA involves situations when a recommended dose is cited in the literature for adults but not for children.

   Step 1: Determine the BSA (in square metres) of the child by dividing the adult dose by 1.73 m² (the average adult's BSA).

   Step 2: Multiply the result by the average adult dose.

   $$\frac{\text{child's BSA (m}^2)}{\text{average adult's BSA (m}^2)} \times \text{average adult dose of drug} = \text{estimated child dose}$$

   Example: A 2.7 kg (6-lb) child has a BSA of 0.20 m², and the average adult dose of a drug is 300 mg. What would be the estimated safe dose for a child?

   $$\frac{0.20 \text{ m2}}{1.73 \text{ m2}} \times 300 \text{ mg} = 34.68 \text{ mg}$$

   Answer: 34.7 mg is the estimated safe dose for this child. (Round to tenths place for child doses.)

   Practice:

   The average adult dose for a medication is 20 mg. The child has a BSA of 0.6 m².

   What would be the estimated safe dose for a child?

   $$\frac{0.6 \text{ m}^2}{1.73 \text{ m}^2} \times 20 \text{ mg} = 6.94 \text{ mg}$$

   Answer: 6.9 mg is the estimated safe dose for this child. (Round to tenths place for child doses.)

Weight-Based Calculations

Step 1 involves changing the weight from pounds to kilograms (if necessary) when calculating the proper dose according to weight.

■ Be careful when converting ounces and pounds to kilograms. First, ounces must be converted to part of a pound (by dividing the ounces by 16). Remember, 16 ounces = 1 pound. Therefore, 8 oz does not convert to 0.8 lb! Convert 8 ounces to pounds by dividing by 16: 8/16 = 0.5; 8 oz = 0.5 lb.

■ Once you have converted ounces to pounds, add the ounces to the pounds. For example, 10 lb 8 oz would equal 10.5 lb. You are now ready to convert pounds to kilograms.

■ Remember, 1 kg = 2.2 lb. To convert 10.5 lb to kilograms, divide the pounds by 2.2. 1 kg : 2.2 lb :: *x* kg : 10.5 lb; $(1 \times 10.5) = (2.2 \times x)$; $10.5 = 2.2x$; $x = 10.5/2.2 = 4.8$ kg (rounded to tenths)

■ Do not round child weights to whole numbers!

Once you have converted the child's weight to kilograms, you are ready for Step 2.

Step 2 involves calculating the therapeutic dosage ranges for a child, based on his or her weight. The nurse uses the child's weight (in kilograms) to calculate the low and high acceptable doses for that medication. This will give a range of dosages that this child could receive for this medication.

Step 3 involves thinking and comparing the ordered dose with the therapeutic dosage range that was calculated for that child. If the ordered dose is under or over the calculated therapeutic dosage range, then do not give the medication, and notify the physician.

- **Step 1:** Convert the child's weight from pounds to kilograms.

- **Step 2:** Calculate the therapeutic dose range (low and high).

- **Step 3:** (1) Is the ordered dose safe (i.e., does not exceed the dosage range)?
  (2) Is the ordered dose therapeutic (i.e., falling within the recommended dosage range, not too low)?

Example 1: The ordered dose is 50 mg of acetaminophen. The infant weighs 15 lb. The therapeutic dosage range for acetaminophen is 10 to 15 mg/kg/dose.

Step 1: Convert pounds to kilograms by dividing 15 by 2.2.
15/2.2 = 6.82; 15 lb = 6.8 kg (Round child weights to tenths, not to whole numbers.)

Step 2: Calculate the therapeutic dosage range for this infant based on his weight.
Low dose: 10 mg/kg/dose × 6.8 kg = 68 mg/dose (Note that the "kg" cancels out.)
High dose: 15 mg/kg/dose × 6.8 kg = 102 mg/dose (Note that the "kg" cancels out.)
The therapeutic dosage range for this infant is 68 to 102 mg per dose for acetaminophen.

Step 3: Compare the ordered dose with the therapeutic dosage range calculated in Step 2.
Answer: The ordered dose of 50 mg is not therapeutic, because it falls under the low recommended dose.

If the doctor orders 110 mg of acetaminophen for this infant, would that be a safe and therapeutic dose?

Answer: No, it would be neither safe nor therapeutic, because it is higher than 102 mg.

Example 2: The ordered dose is amoxicillin 275 mg q8h PO. The child weighs 35 lb. The therapeutic dosage range for amoxicillin is 20 to 40 mg/kg per 24 hours.

Step 1: Convert pounds to kilograms by dividing 35 by 2.2.
35/2.2 = 15.9; 35 lb = 15.9 kg

Step 2: Calculate the therapeutic dosage range for this child based on his weight.
Low dose: 20 mg/kg per 24 hours × 15.9 kg = 318 mg per 24 hours
High dose: 40 mg/kg per 24 hours × 15.9 kg = 636 mg per 24 hours

NOTE: These ranges are for 24 hours! The dosage is every 8 hours, so dividing 24 hours by 8 tells us that there will be 3 doses within 24 hours. To figure out the single dosage for the low and high ranges, divide each 24-hour dose by 3:
318 mg per 24 hours divided by 3 doses = 106 mg per dose
636 mg per 24 hours divided by 3 doses = 212 mg per dose
Answer: The safe range for a single dose of amoxicillin for this child is 106 to 212 mg per dose.

(An alternative way to figure a single dose is to calculate the amount of medication the ordered dose would provide in 24 hours. In this example, knowing there are three doses given every 8 hours in a 24-hour period, multiplying the dose ordered by 3 would yield the ordered dose for 24 hours: 275 mg × 3 doses = 825 mg per 24 hours.)

Step 3: Is the ordered dose of 275 mg therapeutic for this child?
Answer: No, the ordered dose of 275 mg exceeds the therapeutic dosage range for this child. Consult the physician. (Note also that the calculated 24-hour dose of 825 mg per 24 hours exceeds the high range of 636 mg per 24 hours calculated for this child.)

Many pediatric medications come in several concentrations. It is essential to use the correct concentration of medication to ensure accurate dosage and prevent accidental underdosage or overdosage.

Example: Acetaminophen comes in many forms, including the following:
    Drops, 80 mg/mL
    Syrup, 80 or 120 or 160 mg/5 mL
    Liquid oral solution, 32 or 80 or 160 mg/mL
    Liquid suspension, 160 mg/5 mL
    Chewable tablets, 80 or 160 mg
    Tablets, 80 or 325 or 500 mg
    Tablets, extended-release, 650 mg
    Suppositories, 120 mg, 160 mg, 125 mg, 325 mg, or 650 mg

A 4-month-old infant weighs 13 lb and has a fever of 38.6°C. What would be the therapeutic dosage range of acetaminophen this infant could receive?

Step 1: 13 lb = 5.9 kg

Step 2: Low dose: 10 mg/kg per dose × 5.9 = 59 mg per dose
    High dose: 15 mg/kg per dose × 5.9 = 88.5 mg per dose
Answer: The therapeutic dosage range for this infant is 59.0 to 88.5 mg per dose.
Referring to the forms of acetaminophen listed above, which form would you choose if this infant was to receive an 80 mg dose?
Answer: Choose the drops or suspension, 80 mg/mL, and administer 1 mL with a calibrated oral syringe or dropper.

Step 3: Is the ordered dose of 60 mg therapeutic for this infant?
Answer: Yes, the 60 mg dose falls within the 59 to 88.5 mg per dose range for this infant.

Why choose the drops? Remember, you are giving medication to an infant. The infant cannot take tablets; suppositories are not the first choice unless the infant cannot take oral medications, and rectal doses may be a little higher than oral doses. You should choose the medication form that is manufactured for infants and the form that will deliver the dose in an amount that is easily measured yet not too much for the infant to swallow. For example, if you chose the elixir or liquid suspension, 160 mg/5 mL, then you would need to give 2.5 mL. The 0.6 mL would be easier to administer to an infant. Note: Most liquid medication packages for infants and children have specific instructions for dosing and include the specific dropper to use for measuring liquids.

PRACTICE PROBLEMS

1. Your 6-year-old patient weighs 40 lb. Morphine sulphate via continuous infusion is ordered at 1 mg/hr. The therapeutic dosage range for continuous IV infusion is 0.025 to 2.6 mg/kg/hr.
    a. What are the low and high doses for this child?

    _____

    b. Is the ordered dose within a safe and therapeutic range? _____

2. A 5-year-old weighs 33 lb. Ibuprofen is ordered at 120 mg PO every 8 hours (q8h). The therapeutic dosage range is 5 to 10 mg/kg per dose q6h to q8h, and the maximum dose is 40 mg/kg per 24 hours.
    a. What are the low and high doses for this child?

    _____

    b. What is the maximum amount this child can receive in 24 hours? _____
    c. Is the ordered dose within a safe and therapeutic range? _____

3. A 10-year-old patient weighs 70 lb. Ceftazidine is ordered at 1.7 g q8h IV. The therapeutic dosage range is 100 to 150 mg/kg per 24 hours (divided q8h IV).
    a. What are the low and high doses for this child in 24 hours? _____
    b. What are the low and high doses for this child per individual dose? _____
    c. Is the ordered dose within a safe and therapeutic range? _____

4. Your patient weighs 15 lb. The medication ordered is 150 mcg twice a day (bid). The therapeutic dosage range of the medication is 0.02 to 0.05 mg/kg/d.
   a. What are the low and high doses for this child in 24 hours? _____
   b. What are the low and high doses for this child per individual dose? _____
   c. Is the ordered dose within a safe and therapeutic range? _____

5. A child weighs 34 lb. The medication ordered is 30 mg IM preoperatively. The therapeutic dosage range is 1 to 2.2 mg/kg.
   a. What are the low and high doses for this child per individual dose? _____
   b. Is the ordered dose within a safe and therapeutic range? _____

6. For a child weighing 50 lb, medication is ordered at 0.2 mg daily IV. The therapeutic dosage range is 4 to 5 mcg/kg/d.
   a. What are the low and high doses for this child per individual dose? _____
   b. Is the ordered dose within a safe and therapeutic range? _____

SECTION V: BASIC INTRAVENOUS CALCULATIONS

Intravenous fluids and medications are given over a designated period of time. For instance, the order may read as follows:

Give 1000 mL normal saline over 8 hours IV.

For IVs that infuse with an infusion pump, the rate in millilitres per hour is calculated.

For IVs that infuse by gravity, the rate at which an IV is given is measured in terms of drops per minute (gtt/min).

To calculate millilitres per hour and drops per minute, consider what the order contains and what equipment is used. In order to calculate drops per minute, it is important to know the drop factor of the IV tubing. The size of the drops delivered per millilitre can vary with different types of tubing. The drop factor of a certain tubing set is printed on the packaging label.

Adding to the above order,

The drop factor for the IV tubing is 15 gtt/mL.

The order now reads as follows:

Give 1000 mL normal saline over 8 hours IV. The drop factor is 15 gtt/mL.

Step 1: Calculate millilitres per hour.
We know that 1000 mL is to infuse over 8 hours. We want to know how much is to infuse over 1 hour. Set up the equation as follows:

Know   *Want to Know*
1000 mL : 8 hours :: x mL : 1 hour
$(1000 \times 1) = (8 \times x)$; $1000 = 8x$; $x = 8/1000$; $x = 125$ mL/hr
Rate: To give 1000 mL normal saline over 8 hours, give 125 mL/hr for 8 hours.
A quick way to determine the hourly rate is to divide the total volume by the total time (if the time is in hours):
1000 mL $\times$ 8 hours = 125 mL/hr.

Step 2: Calculate the drops per minute.

To set up a gravity IV drip, further calculations are needed. To ensure the proper rate, one must count the drops per minute.

We know the rate is 125 mL/hr and the drop factor is 15 gtt/mL. Since we need to change from hours to minutes, another equivalent we will need is 60 minutes = 1 hour.

When the millilitres per hour are known, the formula for calculating the drops per minute is as follows:

$$\frac{\text{drop factor}}{\text{time (min)}} \times \text{hourly rate (mL/hr)} = \text{gtt/min}$$

Plugging in what we know:

$$\frac{15 \text{ gtt/mL*}}{60 \text{ min/hr}} \times 125 \text{ mL/hr} = \text{x gtt/min}$$

*To make it easier to calculate, reduce the 15/60 fraction to 1/4 before multiplying by 125.

1/4 × 125 = 125/4 = 31.25 (Round millilitres per hour to whole numbers.)
Answer: 31 gtt/min for a gravity drip

Points to remember:
- The drop factor varies according to the manufacturer of the IV tubing set. It can range from 10 to 60 gtt/min.
- Infusion sets that deliver 60 gtt/min are called microdrips.
- Step 1: To calculate millilitres per hour, divide the total volume by the total time (in hours).
- Step 2: To calculate drops per minute when the hourly rate is known, use the following formula:

$$\frac{\text{drop factor (gtt/mL)}}{\text{time (min)}} \times \text{hourly rate (mL/hr)} = \text{gtt/min}$$

- Think! If you are using an infusion pump, you need to calculate millilitres per hour.
- Think! Round off your answer to the nearest whole number. You cannot count a partial drop! Also, IV electronic infusion pumps will usually use the nearest whole number in millilitres. (Exceptions to this may occur in pediatric settings.)

Example 1: The order reads "200 mL to be infused for 1 hour." If the drop factor is 15 gtt/mL, how many drops per minute will be given?
Start at Step 1 or Step 2?
Start at
Step 1: Calculate millilitres per hour.
Step 1: Divide the total volume by the total time (in hours).
200 mL over 1 hour = 200 mL/hr
Step 2: Calculate the drops per minute, using the formula given above.

$$\frac{\text{drop factor}}{\text{time (min)}} \times \text{hourly rate} = 15/60 \times 200 = 1/4 \times 200 = 50$$

Answer: 50 gtt/min

Example 2: The order is for 1000 mL to infuse at 150 mL/hr. The drop factor is 20 gtt/mL. How many drops per minute will be given?
Start at Step 1 or Step 2?
Start at Step 2. The hourly rate, 150 mL/hr, has been given.
Step 2: Calculate the drops per minute:

$$\frac{\text{drop factor}}{\text{time (min)}} \times \text{hourly rate} = 20/60 \times 150 = 1/3 \times 150 = 50$$

Answer: 50 gtt/min

Example 3: You receive an order for 200 mL to be infused for 90 minutes. You have a microdrip set (60 gtt/mL). How many drops per minute will be given?

Start at Step 1 or Step 2?

Start at Step 1. Calculate the hourly rate. Remember, 60 minutes = 1 hour.

Step 1:

Know	Want to Know

200 mL : 90 min :: x mL : 60 min

$(200 \times 60) = (90 \times x)$; $12{,}000 = 90x$; $x = 12{,}000/90$ $x = 133.33$

Rate: 133 mL/hr (Round to nearest whole number.)

Step 2: Calculate the drops per minute:

$$\frac{\text{drop factor}}{\text{time (min)}} \times \text{hourly rate} = 60/60 \times 133 = 1 \times 133 = 133$$

Answer: 133 gtt/min

Shortcut: For microdrips, when the drip factor is 60 and the time is 60 minutes, the "60s" cancel out to "1," and the result is that the ordered millilitres per hour equal the drops per minute.

PRACTICE PROBLEMS

Calculate the following, and prove your answers.

1. Give 1000 mL lactated Ringer's solution over 6 hours. The drop factor is 15 gtt/mL.
   Start at Step 1 or Step 2?

   a. mL/hr: _____

   b. gtt/min: _____

2. Infuse 600 mL blood over 3 hours. The blood administration set has a drop factor of 10 gtt/mL.
   Start at Step 1 or Step 2?

   a. mL/hr: _____

   b. gtt/min: _____

3. Infuse 1000 mL normal saline over 12 hours, using tubing with a drop factor of 15 gtt/mL.
   Start at Step 1 or Step 2?

   a. mL/hr: _____

   b. gtt/min: _____

4. Infuse 200 mL 5% dextrose in normal saline (D$_5$NS) over 2 hours, using a microdrip set.
   Start at Step 1 or Step 2?

   a. mL/hr: _____

   b. gtt/min: _____

   c. What is the drop factor? _____

5. Infuse D$_5$W at 75 mL/hr. The drop factor is 10 gtt/mL.
   Start at Step 1 or Step 2?

   gtt/min: _____

6. Infuse D$_5$W at 75 mL/hr. The drop factor is 15 gtt/mL.
   Start at Step 1 or Step 2?

   gtt/min: _____

7. Infuse D$_5$W at 75 mL/hr. The drop factor is 20 gtt/mL.
   Start at Step 1 or Step 2?

   gtt/min: _____

8. After looking at your answers for questions 5, 6, and 7, what observation can you make about the relationship between the drop factor and the resulting drops per minute?

9. Give 50 mL of an antibiotic over 30 minutes. You will be using an infusion pump.
   Start at Step 1 or Step 2?

   a. mL/hr: _____

   b. gtt/min: _____

   c. Do you need to calculate both millilitres per hour and drops per minute for this situation?

10. Infuse 500 mL normal saline over 4 hours, using tubing with a drop factor of 60 gtt/mL.
    Start at Step 1 or Step 2?

    a. mL/hr: _____

    b. gtt/min: _____

REFERENCE

Health Canada (2009). Drug identification number (DIN). Retrieved December 15, 2009, from http://www.hc-sc. gc.ca/dhp-mps/prodpharma/activit/fs-fi/dinfs_fd-eng.php

PRACTICE QUIZ

Convert the following.

1. 750 mcg   = _____ mg
2. 8 g   = _____ mg
3. 250 lb   = _____ kg
4. 75 kg   = _____ lb
5. 3 tsp g   = _____ mL

Calculate the following, and prove your answers.

6. Dose ordered: indomethacin (oral suspension) 50 mg four times a day (qid)
   Dose on hand: oral suspension 25 mg/5 mL

   How much would you give per dose? _____

7. Dose ordered: procainamide 0.5 g q4h
   Dose on hand: 500 mg tablets

   How much would you give per dose? _____

8. Dose ordered: phenytoin 100 mg IV now
   Dose on hand: 5 mL ampules labelled "0 mg/mL"

   How much would you give per dose? _____

9. Dose ordered: lidocaine 50 mg IV now
   Dose on hand: lidocaine 1% in 5 mL ampules

   How much would you give? _____

10. Dose ordered: epinephrine 0.25 mg SC now
    Dose on hand: epinephrine 1:1000 ampules

    How much would you give? _____

11. Dose ordered: heparin 15,000 units IV bolus
    Dose on hand: heparin 10,000 units/mL (5 mL vial)

    How much would you give? _____

12. Dose ordered: hydrochlorathiazide 1 mg/kg PO daily
    Child's weight: 22 lb
    Therapeutic dosage range: 2 mg/kg divided bid
    a. What is the safe and therapeutic range for this child? _____
    b. Is the ordered dose safe and therapeutic?

    _____

13. Ordered: Infuse normal saline 500 mL over 8 hours. The tubing drop factor is 15.

    a. What is the rate of the IV? _____
    b. What is the number of drops per minute?

    _____

14. Ordered: D5 1/2NS to infuse at 50 mL/hr via an infusion pump.
    a. How will this be administered? As millilitres

       per hour or as drops per minute? _____

    b. What is the rate? _____

15. Ordered: 1000 mL D$_5$W to infuse over 24 hours. The tubing drop factor is 60.

    a. What is the rate of the IV? _____
    b. What is the number of drops per minute?

    _____

16. Ordered: cefuroxime 500 mg IVPB [intravenous piggyback] q6h
    Dose on hand: cefuroxime powder for injection (see label)

    > 750 mg vial
    > CEFUROXIME
    > Add 8 mL sterile water for injection.
    > Solution will contain 90mg/mL

    a. How much does this vial contain? _____
    b. How much will you give for each dose?

    _____

17. Ordered: penicillin G 200,000 units IM qid
    Dose on hand: penicillin G 5,000,000 units
    The medication label reads as shown below:

FIVE MILLION UNITS multidose vial
Penicillin G
Use sterile saline as diluent as follows:

Add	Units per mL reconstituted solution
23 mL	200,000
18 mL	250,000
8 mL	500,000
3 mL	1,000,000

a.   What concentration should you choose?

_____

b.   How much sterile saline should you add to the

vial to obtain this concentration? _____

c.   How much medication will you give?

_____

d.   How do you label the vial? _____

18. A child weighs 31 lb.
Dose ordered: ceftriaxone sodium 600 mg IV q12h
Dose on hand: See label.
Maximum safe dose: up to 100 mg/kg/d in two
divided doses

1 g
ceftriaxone sodium
DIRECTIONS: Add 9.6 mL sterile water for injection to equal 100 mg/mL.

a.   How much would you give for this dose?

_____

b.   What is the maximum safe dose for this child

(in 24 hours)? _____

c.   What is the maximum safe dose for this child

(per dose)? _____

d.   Is the ordered dose within a safe and therapeu-

tic range? _____

19. Dose ordered: digoxin 125 mcg daily
Dose on hand: pediatric elixir 0.05 mg/mL

How much would you give? _____

20.

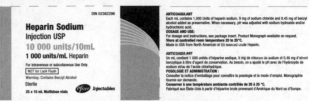

Courtesy of Pfizer Inc.

Dose ordered: heparin 15,000 IV push now
Dose on hand: See label.
How much would you give for this dose?

_____

21.

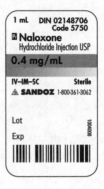

Dose ordered: ranitidine 75 mg IM now
Dose on hand: See label.

How much would you give for this dose? _____

Answers

CHAPTER 1
Nursing Practice in Canada and Drug Therapy

Chapter Review

1. a
2. d
3. c
4. b
5. a, e, f
6. b
7. d
8. 1 = c; 2 − b; 3 = d; 4 = e; 5 = a

Critical Thinking and Application

9. S, O, O, O, S, S
10. Answers may vary slightly with each one but should include the following:
    - ***Right drug (or right medication):*** Compare drug orders and drug labels. Consider whether the drug is appropriate for that patient. Obtain information about the patient regarding past and present medical history, and obtain a thorough updated medication history, including over-the-counter (OTC) medications.
    - ***Right dose:*** Check the order and the label on the medication, and check for all of the ten "rights" at least three times before administering the medication. Recheck the math calculations for dosages, and contact the health care provider when clarification is needed.
    - ***Right time:*** Assess for a conflict between the pharmacokinetic and pharmacodynamic properties of the drugs prescribed and the patient's lifestyle and likelihood of adherence.
    - ***Right route:*** Never assume the route for administration or change it; always check with the health care provider.
    - ✓ ***Right patient:*** Check the patient's identity before administering a medication. Ask for the patient's name, and check the identification band or bracelet to confirm the patient's name, identification number, age, and allergies.
    - ***Right reason:*** Ensure that the drug ordered is being given for the right reason. This necessitates a prior knowledge of the drug's actions and adverse effects.
    - ***Right documentation:*** Ensure that documentation of the administration is done after the drug has been administered, not before; moreover, ensure that any unusual variance in time, dose, and adverse reactions is properly recorded, as well as any refusal of the drug, if applicable.
    - ✓ ***Right evaluation (or right assessment):*** Ensure that any special assessment requirements have been made prior to the drug administration, such as specific pulse rate and blood pressure readings, and laboratory results. Moreover, ensure that appropriate monitoring of the patient has been done following medication administration and that follow-up measures are taken if the drug has not achieved its desired effect.
    - ✓ ***Right patient education:*** Ensure that the patient has been given a proper explanation of the drug being given and told the reason for its administration and what to expect in terms of the drug's effects and possible adverse effects.
    - ***Right to refuse:*** Ensure that patients know they have a right to refuse the drug being administered, and inform them properly of the potential consequences of refusal.
11. a. Assessment
    b. Objective
    c. Subjective
    d. Analyze
    e. Goals
    f. Outcome criteria
    g. Implementation
    h. Evaluation
12. The nurse must be sure to question the patient for any allergies, especially drug allergies, before giving this medication. If an allergy is present, question the patient about the type of reaction that occurs, and do not give the medication until the order is clarified with the prescriber.

Case Study

1. See the discussion in Chapter 1, under Assessment. Important points include the following:
   - Use of prescription and OTC medications
   - Use of natural health products, including home remedies and vitamins
   - Intake of alcohol, tobacco, and caffeine
   - Current or prior use of illicit drugs
   - Personal health history
   - Family history
   - Allergies
2. The medication order is missing the route of delivery and the dose amount. The nurse should contact the health care provider to clarify the incomplete order.
3. Again, the nurse should contact the health care provider and should never change the medication route without an order.
4. After administering a drug, the nurse should evaluate the patient's response to the drug therapy. In this case, monitoring intake and output, monitoring vital signs, and observing for postural hypotension would be important.

CHAPTER 2
Pharmacological Principles

Chapter Review

1. 1= e; 2 = c; 3 = d; 4 = a; 5 = b
2. c
3. b
4. d
5. a
6. c
7. b
8. c
9. d
10. b
11. h
12. i
13. f
14. g
15. a
16. d
17. e
18. c

Critical Thinking and Application

19. Because muscles have a greater blood supply than the skin, drugs injected intramuscularly are typically absorbed more quickly than those injected subcutaneously. Absorption can be increased by applying heat to the injection site or by massaging it, which increases the blood flow to the area and thus enhances absorption.
20. This is an example of maintenance therapy—drug therapy that does not eradicate the patient's medical condition but rather prevents the progression of the condition.
21. Extended-release oral dosage forms must not be crushed, as this could cause the accelerated release of drug from the dosage form and cause possible toxicity. Enteric-coated tablets also are not recommended for crushing, as this would cause disruption of the tablet coating that is designed to protect the stomach lining from the local effects of the drug and protect the drug from being prematurely disrupted by stomach acid.

Case Study

1. Half-life is the time it takes for one-half of the original amount of a drug in the body to be eliminated and is a measure of the rate at which drugs are excreted by the body. If the half-life is 2 hours, then in this example, the drug level would be reduced as follows:
   1600 = 200 mg/L
   1800 = 100 mg/L
   2000 = 50 mg/L
   2200 = 25 mg/L
2. a. He has nausea and vomiting and cannot take medications by mouth. His medications will need to be given parenterally.
   b. Because of his decreased serum albumin level, a lesser amount of drugs that are usually protein bound will be bound to protein, and as a result, more free drug will be circulating and the duration of drug action may be increased. In addition, the patient has heart failure that may result in decreased cardiac output and thus decreased distribution.
   c. The patient has liver failure that will result in decreased metabolism of drugs.
   d. Because the patient's liver may not be able to effectively metabolize drugs and convert them to water-soluble compounds, excretion through the kidneys may be decreased.
3. This situation illustrates therapy to prevent illness or other undesirable outcomes. Prophylactic intravenous antibiotic therapy may be used to prevent infection during a high-risk surgery or procedure, such as the placement of a peripherally inserted central catheter.
4. Therapeutic index is the ratio between the toxic and therapeutic concentrations of a drug. A low therapeutic index means that the range between a therapeutically active dose and a toxic dose is small. As a result, the drug has a greater

likelihood of causing an adverse reaction. The nurse should monitor the patient's response carefully when a drug has a narrow therapeutic index.

CHAPTER 3
Legal and Ethical Considerations

Chapter Review

1. b
2. a
3. d
4. b
5. b
6. c, e
7. d
8. b
9. c
10. b
11. c
12. a
13. d
14. b

Critical Thinking and Application

15. Answers will vary depending on the group identified.
    a. Barriers may include language, poverty, access, pride, freedom, and beliefs regarding medical practices.
    b. Attitudes will vary depending on the group identified.
    c. Questions may include the following topics: health beliefs and practices, past use of medicine, folk remedies, home remedies, use of over-the-counter drugs and treatments, usual responses to illness, responsiveness to medical treatments, religious practices and beliefs, and dietary habits.

Case Study

1. You should not give the drugs until it is established that the study has been reviewed by an institutional review board and that the patient has given informed consent. As a professional, the nurse has the responsibility to provide safe nursing care, and it is within the nurse's realm of practice to provide information and assist the patient facing decisions regarding health care. The nurse also has the right to refuse to participate in any treatment or aspect of a patient's care that violates personal ethical principles.

2. These principles include the following:
   • Autonomy—the patient's right to self-determination. The nurse supports this by ensuring informed consent.
   • Beneficence—the duty to do good. Will the patient be best served by this course of action?
   • Nonmaleficence—the duty to do no harm.
   • Veracity—the duty to tell the truth, especially with regard to investigational drugs and informed consent.
3. Some patients believe strongly in using home remedies instead of medications. Sometimes these remedies can be integrated into the treatment of human immunodeficiency virus infection. You should assess and consider health beliefs and practices at the beginning of the therapeutic relationship. Because the patient believes drugs are not needed, the nurse has a duty to provide education so that the patient has the knowledge needed in order to make a sound judgment.
4. The issue of confidentiality should be discussed. The researchers have a duty to respect privileged information about a patient. Measures that the researchers will use to ensure the confidentiality of participants should be discussed.

CHAPTER 4
Patient-Focused Considerations

Chapter Review

1. b
2. a, c, e
3. d
4. c
5. a, b, d
6. d
7. b
8. e
9. a
10. c

Critical Thinking and Application

11. Keep in mind that older patients take a greater proportion of both prescription and over-the-counter (OTC) medications, and they commonly take multiple medications on a daily basis. In addition, older adults also have more chronic diseases than younger people. They may see several different specialists, each of whom may prescribe a different set of medications. In addition, some patients self-administer OTC products to ease the discomfort of even more

ailments. This use of multiple medications is called *polypharmacy*.

12. Drawing on the information in Table 4-3: Physiological Changes in the Older Patient, a variety of physiological changes affecting the cardiovascular, gastro-intestinal, hepatic, and renal systems may be described.

Case Study

1. Children and teenagers should not take acetylsalicylic acid (Aspirin) to treat chicken pox or influenza-like symptoms because Reye's syndrome, a rare but serious illness, has been associated with Aspirin use at these ages. It is important to check for precautions when giving any medication to children.

2. If the toddler does not like or cannot take pills, have the parent ask the pharmacist for a liquid form of the medication, which may be flavoured and may be better accepted than a pill.

3. The most common dosage calculation for children is the milligrams per kilogram formula. However, for OTC medications, the manufacturer will convert kilograms to pounds in order to make dosing by the parents an easier process.

4. The 5-year-old child received 240 mg (at 160 mg per teaspoon, 1.5 teaspoons = 240 mg).

5. The parents should monitor the children's fever; the expected response is that the fever will go down. In addition, because the medication also has analgesic effects, signs of discomfort may decrease. The parents should also monitor for any adverse effects of the medication or worsening of the child's illness.

CHAPTER 5
Gene Therapy and Pharmacogenomics

Chapter Review

1. a, c, d
2. a, e
3. a
4. b
5. c
6. d

Case Study

1. This information about Riley's cousin may be significant. An unusual or other-than-expected reaction to a drug in family members may point to a difference in the patient's ability to metabolize certain drugs. Genetic factors may alter a patient's metabolism of a particular drug, resulting in either increased or decreased drug action.

2. The nurse will ask about the type of medication Riley's cousin received, the type of surgery, and the reaction that occurred, as well as the treatment. The nurse will also ask if any other family members have had unusual reactions to drugs and whether Riley himself has had any problems.

3. The family history needs to cover at least three generations and include the current and past health status of each family member.

4. The surgeon and anaesthesiologist will work to adjust the planned drug therapy for Riley's surgery according to the genetic variation that has been identified. In addition, during surgery, the patient will be monitored closely for any unusual responses.

CHAPTER 6
Medication Errors: Preventing and Responding

Chapter Review

1. Medication error
2. Idiosyncratic
3. Allergic reaction
4. Adverse drug reaction (ADR)
5. Adverse drug event (ADE)
6. False. High-alert medications are not necessarily involved in more errors than other drug. However, the potential for patient harm is higher with these medications.
7. False. ADEs include medication errors and ADRs.
8. To avoid medication errors, follow the "10 rights" of medication administration. Carefully read all drug labels and confirm that the drug, dose, time and frequency of administration, patient, and route of administration are correct. Verbal orders should be minimized, but if a verbal order must be taken, repeat the order to confirm it with the prescriber, and spell the drug name aloud, speaking slowly and clearly. Never assume a route of administration; if an order is unclear or incomplete, clarify the order with the prescriber. Always read the label three times, and check the medication order before administering the medication. See the text for other possible answers.
9. Refer to Box 6-1 (p. 95 in the textbook). Chemotherapeutic drugs; neuromuscular blocking drugs; adrenergic agonists, adrenergic antagonists; opiates; thrombolytics; and local anaesthetics in large containers
10. digoxin 250 micrograms PO now
furosemide 40 mg IV daily
Discontinue all medications
NPH insulin 8 units subcutaneously with breakfast daily
garamycin otic drops, 2 drops right ear bid

11. a. One-half of a 50 mg tablet
    b. A 50 mg dose, which is a double dose
    c. Because this medication can have an effect on the patient's blood pressure and heart rate, the nurse will immediately check and record the patient's vital signs and caution the patient about getting out of bed without help. The patient's prescriber will be notified, and the patient must be monitored frequently throughout the day. In addition to telling the patient about the double dose, the nurse will need to follow facility protocol for reporting a medication error.
12. b
13. 5 mL

Case Study

1. The nursing student should immediately inform her instructor of the error. Together they should then monitor the patient's response and follow the institution's procedure for reporting a medication error. Reporting medication errors is a professional and ethical responsibility.
2. By checking the "rights" of medication administration before giving this medication; in this situation, the student missed the right dose. In addition, if the student had understood the rationale for the medication (i.e., the low dose needed for antiplatelet therapy), she might have avoided this error. One must be knowledgeable about medications and the rationale for their use in a particular patient before administering them.
3. According to Chapter 3, the recommendation is that the patient be told of the error, both as ethical practice and because of the legal implications.
4. Yes. A medication error is defined as any "preventable ADE involving inappropriate medication use by a patient or health care provider." It may or may not cause harm to the patient.
5. The Canadian Medication Incident Reporting and Prevention System (CMIRPS) exists to gather and disseminate safety information regarding medications. By reporting this error, CMIRPS is able to add to the database of medication errors and their causes and thus help identify to all health care providers the potential errors. This service is confidential.

CHAPTER 7
Patient Education and Drug Therapy

Chapter Review

1. c
2. d
3. a

4. a, b
5. 10 mL for each dose
6.

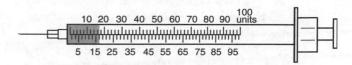

Critical Thinking and Application

7. Refer to the information in Chapter 23 for specific information about antihypertensive drug therapy. In addition, Table 7-1 provides information relevant to the development of teaching strategies for the 72-year-old patient.
8. Refer to Box 7-1. Ideally, a health care provider who speaks the mother's language should do the teaching. It is essential that an interpreter be found so that questions from the mother can be answered adequately. Other strategies include using pictures and illustrations and demonstrating by example. In addition, the parent needs to be provided with detailed written instructions in her native language.
9. a. Answers will vary, but the nursing diagnosis addresses deficient knowledge.
   b. Answers will vary, but the nursing diagnosis addresses noncompliance or ineffective health maintenance.
10. Teaching plans will vary somewhat in format, but each should contain the following information:
    a. Some of the assessment items listed in the text in the section Assessment of Learning Needs Related to drug Therapy
    b. Deficient knowledge
    c. A measurable goal with outcome criteria related to the nursing diagnosis
    d. Specific educational strategies for providing the information needed
    e. Specific questions designed to determine whether learning has occurred

Case Study

1. Both "deficient knowledge" and "noncompliance" are possible answers. In this case, "deficient knowledge" is probably the most correct, because this nursing diagnosis exists when the patient has a lack of or limited understanding about his or her medications. For example, as you will read in Chapter 24, nitroglycerin tablets should not be stored in one's pants pockets, because the body's heat may destroy the active compounds in the tablets. In addition, the patient is not aware of the importance of not missing doses of antihypertensive medication. Noncompliance exists when the patient

does not take the medication as directed or at all, and the data collected indicate that the patient's condition has recurred or has not resolved. In this case, his blood pressure has improved from previous readings, despite what he has said about taking his medications.

2. Answers may vary. A goal for the nursing diagnosis of "deficient knowledge" in this case may be the following: "The patient self-administers his prescribed medications on schedule without missing doses." Outcome criteria may include the following: "The patient is able to describe the schedule of medications ordered"; "The patient is able to state the rationale for consistent dosing of antihypertensive medications"; "The patient is able to state the proper storage and administration of sublingual nitroglycerin tablets"; and "The patient is able to identify potential adverse effects of the prescribed medications and knows when to report them."

3. Answers may vary. Refer to Box 7-1.
   Suggestions include the following:
   - Conduct a teaching session regarding medication administration with both the patient and his wife in attendance. If necessary, find out whether they have any children or neighbours nearby who may be able to assist with medications as needed.
   - Assist the patient in developing a daily time calendar for taking the medications prescribed.
   - Suggest the use of a daily or weekly pill container that can assist in reminding when doses are due. If necessary, a neighbour or the patient's son or daughter can come over periodically to fill this container.
   - Discuss and provide written literature on the purposes and adverse effects of each medication ordered and on other important issues regarding these medications.

4. Confirm whether learning has occurred by asking the patient and his wife questions related to the teaching session. Assess their understanding of the time calendar and the concept of using pill containers. Follow-up can be accomplished via telephone as needed, and a return visit to review medications can be scheduled. In addition, the patient must keep return appointments to the office so that the therapeutic outcomes of the drug therapy (i.e., blood pressure readings) can be measured.

CHAPTER 8
Over-the-Counter Drugs and Natural Health Products

Double Puzzle

Valerian
Garlic

Feverfew
St. John's wort
Ginkgo
Saw palmetto
Ginseng
Echinacea
Aloe
Goldenseal
Herbal therapy

Chapter Review

1. a, b, d, f
2. d
3. a
4. b
5. c
6. 8000 mg total per day
7. YES, there is a concern! Acetaminophen doses must not exceed a total of 4000 mg per day; hepatic toxicity may occur with excessive doses.
8. a, c, d, e
9. See the "Natural Health Products" Box, p. 123. These natural health products interfere with the therapeutic ability of the anticoagulant. For example, chamomile increases the risk of bleeding with an anticoagulant.

Case Study

1. The Aspirin and the garlic tablets may interfere with platelet and clotting functions. If the wine is taken with the kava or the valerian or both, central nervous system depression may occur.
2. Health Canada has issued a warning about the use of kava and possible liver toxicity. Also, tachyphylaxis may develop in patients who use *Echinacea* for more than 8 weeks.
3. Because she is trying to conceive, this patient needs to consider the fact that the herbal agents have not been tested or been proved safe for use in pregnancy. Also, acetylsalicylic acid (Aspirin) is contraindicated in pregnancy because of its antiplatelet effects.
4. Assuming the natural health products are all purchased from reputable sources in Canada and not through a foreign website, then the products are considered safe, because Health Canada regulations enforce standards of quality and safety assessment for all natural health products sold in Canada.
5. Many patients believe that if a product is "natural," then it is safe. The nurse should discuss each product with the patient and instruct the patient about possible contraindications, safe use, frequency of dosing, specifics about how to take the product, and the way to monitor for both therapeutic effects and complications or toxic effects.

CHAPTER 9
Vitamins and Minerals

Chapter Review

1. c
2. g
3. b
4. h
5. e
6. k
7. i
8. d
9. j
10. a
11. l
12. f
13. a, d, e
14. b
15. d
16. d
17. 0.5 mL

Critical Thinking and Application

18. By "endogenous," the health care provider was referring to the endogenous synthesis of a form of vitamin D synthesized in the skin by ultraviolet irradiation. Dietary sources of vitamin D include fish oils, salmon, sardines, and herring; fortified milk, bread, and cereals; and animal livers, tuna, eggs, and butter.

19. a. Pernicious anemia
    b. The oral absorption of cyanocobalamin (vitamin B_{12} or extrinsic factor) requires the presence of intrinsic factor, which is a glycoprotein secreted by the gastric parietal cells. Damage to the gastro-intestinal tract may reduce the amount of available intrinsic factor.
    c. The patient education card for this patient should focus on foods containing cyanocobalamin; these include foods of animal origin, such as liver, kidney, fish, shellfish, meat, and dairy foods.

20. When given intravenously, calcium should be given via an intravenous infusion pump to avoid venous irritation. It should be given slowly (less than 1 mL/min for adults) to avoid cardiac dysrhythmias and cardiac arrest. The health care provider is correct in ordering infusion with 1% procaine. This will reduce vasospasm and dilute the effects of calcium on surrounding tissues. In either case, monitor for extravasation; if it occurs, the nurse should discontinue administration immediately. The nurse should also watch for signs of hypercalcemia.

21. The orange juice contains ascorbic acid (vitamin C), which enhances the absorption of iron.

Case Study

1. At 0.067 mmol/L, the patient's magnesium level is critically low. The patient should receive intravenous magnesium to raise the serum magnesium to therapeutic levels of 0.65 to 1.05 mmol/L.

2. During intravenous magnesium infusion, monitor the patient's electrocardiogram and vital signs, and rate patellar or knee-jerk reflexes. Impaired reflexes are an indication of drug-related central nervous system (CNS) depressant effects. CNS depression may quickly lead to respiratory or cardiac depression; thus, perform frequent monitoring. Document the infusion and infusion site, and record each set of vital-sign measurements and ratings of reflexes appropriately. Other signs that require immediate attention are confusion, irregular heart rhythm, cramping, unusual fatigue, lightheadedness, and dizziness.

3. Contact the prescriber immediately, stop the infusion, and monitor the patient.

4. Calcium gluconate must be readily accessible for use as an antidote to magnesium toxicity.

CHAPTER 10
Principles of Drug Administration

Chapter Review

1. b
2. c
3. a
4. b
5. c
6. c
7. b
8. a
9. c
10. a
11. b
12. d
13. b
14. a
15. a, b, c, e

Critical Thinking and Application

16. a. Palpate sites for masses or tenderness, and assess the amount of subcutaneous tissue.
    b. Note the integrity and size of the muscle, and palpate for tenderness.
    c. Note any lesions or discolouration of the forearm.

17. a. Use a 25-gauge, 12 to 16 mm needle. (For insulin, a 6 mm or 8 mm needle is recommended.) A 90-degree angle is used for a

patient of average size; a 45-degree angle may be used for patients who are thin, emaciated, or cachectic and for children. To ensure the correct needle length, grasp the skinfold with the thumb and forefinger, and choose a needle that is approximately one-half the length of the skinfold from top to bottom.

b. Locate the proper site for the injection, and cleanse the site with an alcohol or antiseptic swab. Apply the swab at the centre of the site, and cleanse outward in a circular direction for about 5 cm (see Figure 10-47); then let the skin dry. Keep a sterile gauze pad nearby for use after the injection. With your nondominant hand, pull the skin taut. Follow the instructions for the Z-track method (see later), if appropriate. Grasp the syringe with your dominant hand, as if holding a dart, and hold the needle at a 90-degree angle to the skin. Tell the patient to expect a "stick" feeling as you insert the needle. Insert the needle quickly and firmly into the muscle. Grasp the lower end of the syringe with the nondominant hand while still holding the skin back, to stabilize the syringe. With the dominant hand, pull back on the plunger for 5 to 10 seconds to check for blood return. If no blood appears in the syringe, inject the medication slowly, at the rate of 1 mL every 10 seconds. After injecting the drug, wait 10 seconds, and then withdraw the needle smoothly while releasing the skin.

c. Use a tuberculin or 1-mL syringe with a 26- or 27-gauge needle that is 10 to 16 mm long. Be sure to choose an appropriate site for the injection. Avoid areas of bruising, rashes, inflammation, edema, or skin discolouration. Help the patient to a comfortable position. Extend and support the elbow and forearm on a flat surface. In general, three to four finger-widths below the antecubital space and one hand-width above the wrist are the preferred locations on the forearm. Areas on the back that are also suitable for subcutaneous injections may be used if the forearm is not appropriate for the intradermal injection. Cleanse the site with an alcohol or antiseptic swab. Apply the swab at the centre of the site, and cleanse outward in a circular direction for about 5 cm; then let the skin dry. After cleansing the site, stretch the skin over the site with your nondominant hand. With the needle almost against the patient's skin, insert the needle, bevel up, at a 5- to 15-degree angle until resistance is felt, and then advance the needle approximately 3 mm through the epidermis (Figures 10-44 and 10-45). The needle tip should still be visible

under the skin. Do not aspirate. This area under the skin contains few blood vessels. Slowly inject the medication. It is normal to feel resistance, and a bleb that resembles a mosquito bite (about 6 mm in diameter) will form at the site if accurate technique is used. Withdraw the needle slowly while gently applying a gauze pad at the site, but do not massage the site.

18. Remove the needle, and ensure that the site is not bleeding. Discard the medication and syringe, draw up new medication, and repeat the procedure in a different location.
19. Rather than pouring it into a medication cup, draw small volumes of liquid medication into a calibrated oral syringe.
20. Two-hundred fifty divided by four (4 puffs/day) comes to 62.5 days before the inhaler is empty.

Case Study

1. For the adult, the ventro-gluteal site is the preferred injection site. If the woman is of average size, choose a needle that is 4 cm long and 21 to 25 gauge, and insert the needle at a 90-degree angle. For an infant, the preferred site is the vastus lateralis site. The needle should be of the correct length to ensure that it reaches muscle tissue, not the subcutaneous layer.
2. For an infant or child younger than 3 years, the pinna of the ear should be pulled down and back before the drops are administered. The drops should be directed along the sides of the ear rather than directly onto the eardrum. The drops should be taken out of refrigeration about 30 minutes before giving them. The mother should stay with her child and should ensure that she lies on her side for 5 to 10 minutes. Gentle massage of the tragus area of the ear with her finger will help distribute the medication down the ear canal.
3. Liquid medication doses under 5 mL should be drawn up in a calibrated oral syringe.
4. Liquids are usually ordered because infants cannot swallow pills or capsules. A plastic disposable oral dosing syringe is recommended for measuring small doses of liquid medications. Position the infant so that the head is slightly elevated. Place the plastic dropper or syringe inside the infant's mouth, beside the tongue, and administer the liquid in small amounts while allowing the infant to swallow each time. Take great care to prevent aspiration. A crying infant can easily aspirate medication. Do not add the medication to a bottle of formula. The infant may refuse the feeding or may not drink all of it and, as a result, would not receive the entire dosage of medication.

CHAPTER 11
Analgesic Drugs

Chapter Review

1. b
2. d
3. c
4. d
5. b, c, e
6. 3 mL
7. 1.2 mL
8.

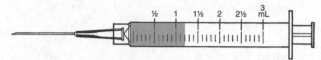

9. g
10. f
11. i
12. h
13. d
14. b
15. j
16. c
17. e

Critical Thinking Crossword

Across
3. Agonist
5. Acute
11. Superficial
13. Visceral

Down
1. Antagonist
2. Adjuvant
4. Tolerance
6. Threshold
7. Somatic
8. Chronic
9. Opioid
10. Opiate
12. Partial

Case Study

1. Superficial pain, which originates from the skin or mucous membranes.
2. A back rub. Massage to the affected area often decreases the pain. When an area is rubbed or liniment is applied to an area, large sensory fibres from peripheral receptors carry impulses to the spinal cord. This causes impulse transmission to be inhibited and the gate to be closed. This in turn reduces the recognition of the pain impulses arriving by means of the small fibres. This is the same pathway that the opioid analgesics use to alleviate pain.
3. All opioids cause some histamine release. It is thought that this histamine release is responsible for many of the unwanted adverse effects, such as itching.
4. The most serious adverse effect of opioids is central nervous depression, which may lead to respiratory depression. Naloxone, an opioid reversal agent, may need to be administered to reverse severe respiratory depression.
5. The use of a non-opioid analgesic with an opioid is known as adjuvant analgesic therapy. This allows the use of smaller doses of opioids, which accomplishes two important functions. First, it diminishes some of the adverse effects that are seen with higher doses of opioids, such as respiratory depression, constipation, and urinary retention. Second, adjuvant therapy approaches the pain stimulus from another mechanism and has a resulting synergistic beneficial effect in reducing the pain.

CHAPTER 12
General and Local Anaesthetics

Chapter Review

1. d
2. b
3. a
4. b
5. b, c, e
6. c
7. d
8. 1 = c; 2 = a; 3 = b

Critical Thinking and Application

9. Children are more susceptible to problems such as central nervous depression, toxicity, atelectasis, pneumonia, and cardiac abnormalities because their hepatic, cardiac, respiratory, and renal systems are not fully developed or fully functional.
10. These drugs cause paralysis of the respiratory muscles. The nurse will need to monitor the mechanical ventilation closely because if the ventilator does not work, this patient will not be able to breathe on his own. Emergency resuscitation equipment must be kept nearby. In addition, these drugs do not cause sedation, and the patient is still able to hear and feel. Most facilities have protocols for sedation during the use of these drugs. However, it is important to remain professional at all times and to take the

time to reassure the patient and orient him to his surroundings, to what noises mean, and to what procedures are going to be done to him. Remind the family that he is still able to hear what is said.

11. She will be given a combination of intravenous medications that will produce analgesia and also amnesia in regard to the procedure, but she will still be alert enough to breathe on her own and follow verbal directions as needed. In some cases, local anaesthesia will be used to enhance patient comfort. This type of sedation is called moderate (or procedural, or conscious) sedation; it is associated with fewer complications and a shorter recovery time than is general anaesthesia.

12. Lidocaine with epinephrine is used when the vasoconstriction effects of epinephrine are needed. The vasoconstriction confines the anaesthetic (lidocaine) to the local area of injection, and also acts to reduce bleeding. The two types of lidocaine are not interchangeable.

Critical Thinking Crossword

Across
3. Pancuronium
6. General
7. Topical
8. Adjunctive
9. Local

Down
1. Atropine
2. Anaesthetics
3. Parenteral
4. Balanced
5. Regional

Case Study

1. In balanced anaesthesia, minimal doses of a combination of anaesthetic drugs (both intravenous and inhaled) are used to achieve the desired level of anaesthesia for the surgical procedure. Adjunctive drugs may also be used and commonly include sedative–hypnotics, narcotics, and neuromuscular blocking drugs (NMBDs) (depolarizing drugs such as succinylcholine and the nondepolarizing or competitive drugs such as atracurium and pancuronium). Combining several different drugs makes it possible for general anaesthesia to be accomplished with smaller amounts of anaesthetic gases and thus reduces the adverse effects.

2. The main therapeutic use of the NMBD succinylcholine is to maintain controlled ventilation during surgical procedures. When respiratory muscles are paralyzed by NMBDs, mechanical ventilation is easier because the body's drive to control respirations is eliminated by the drug; this allows the ventilator to have total control of the respirations.

3. Multiple medical conditions (listed in Box 12-4 on p. 227 of the textbook) can predispose an individual to toxicity. These conditions increase the sensitivity of an individual to NMBDs and prolong their effects. Because the patient's temperature has decreased, hypothermia may lead to an increased sensitivity to the medication.

4. Anticholinesterase drugs such as neostigmine are antidotes and are used to reverse the muscle paralysis.

5. Local anaesthesia is most commonly used in settings in which loss of consciousness, whole-body relaxation, and loss of unresponsiveness are either unnecessary or not wanted. A lower incidence of toxic effects is associated with the use of local anaesthetics because little is systemically absorbed.

6. Regardless of the type of anaesthesia a patient is receiving, one of the most important nursing considerations during this time is close and frequent observation of the patient and all body systems, with specific attention to the ABCs of nursing care (*a*irway, *b*reathing, and *c*irculation) and vital signs. Resuscitative equipment, as well as any antidote, should be kept nearby in case of cardiorespiratory distress or arrest. Other nursing actions include monitoring all aspects of body functions (including the ABCs of care), instituting safety measures, and implementing the health care provider's orders.

CHAPTER 13
Central Nervous System Depressants and Muscle Relaxants

Chapter Review

1. a
2. b
3. a
4. d
5. b
6. c
7. a, c, d, e
8. a. 7.5 mg
   b. 3.75 mL
9. 10 mL

10.

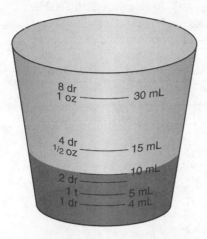

8 dr
1 oz ——— 30 mL

4 dr
1/2 oz ——— 15 mL

——— 10 mL
2 dr ———
1 t ——— 5 mL
1 dr ——— 4 mL

Critical Thinking and Application

11. Answers should reflect the discussion under Toxicity and Management of Overdose in the textbook. The priority of care would be to maintain the ABCs (*a*irway, *b*reathing, *c*irculation), particularly respirations, because respiratory depression is likely. Overdose of barbiturates produces central nervous system (CNS) depression ranging from sleep to profound coma and death. Respiratory depression progresses to Cheyne-Stokes respiration, hypoventilation, and cyanosis. Patients often have cold, clammy skin or are hypothermic, and later they can exhibit fever, areflexia, tachycardia, and hypotension. The priority of care would be to maintain the ABCs (airway, breathing, and circulation), especially respirations, because respiratory depression is likely. There is no antidote for barbiturate overdose.

12. Benzodiazepines can be used for insomnia only if they are limited to short-term use (i.e., less than 2–4 weeks). With long-term use, rebound insomnia and severe withdrawal can develop. If Jackie needs to take something to help her sleep while she is on her trip, the nonbenzodiazepine hypnotics may be an option, and of course, the nurse can provide patient teaching on nonpharmacological methods to aid sleep.

13. Older adults should be started on lower doses because they generally experience a more pronounced effect from benzodiazepines. Benzodiazepines can create a significant fall hazard in older adults, and the lowest effective dose must be used in this patient population.

14. a. Ask about allergies, CNS disorders, sleep disorders, diabetes, addictive disorders, personality disorders, thyroid conditions, and kidney and liver function status
     b. Other measures should include alcohol and CNS depressants but also all prescribed or over-the-counter medications.

c. The patient's age matters because these drugs cause increased effects in older adults and small children.

15. a. Patient teaching should include information about potential adverse effects and potential drug interactions. In addition, safety measures to prevent injury stemming from decreased sensorium must be emphasized.
     b. These medications are most effective when used in conjunction with rest and physical therapy.

Case Study

1. Barbiturates are considered controlled substances because of the potential for misuse and the severe effects that result if they are not used appropriately. Other hypnotic drugs are now used more frequently than barbiturates because they have fewer adverse effects and are safer than the older barbiturates. They also do not suppress rapid eye movement (REM) sleep to the same extent as do barbiturates.

2. Barbiturates deprive people of REM sleep (dreaming sleep), and long-term use can result in agitation and the inability to deal with normal stress. In addition, when the barbiturate is stopped, the returning REM sleep may be more intense than before and lead to nightmares (a rebound effect). Barbiturates are habit forming, they have a low therapeutic index, and severe withdrawal effects may occur when the medication is stopped. Other drugs have been shown to be safer to use for treatment of insomnia.

3. Other CNS depressants, particularly alcohol, should be avoided. There may also be an additive effect with the intake of the natural health product valerian.

4. Zopiclone (Imovane) is indicated for the short-term treatment of insomnia and has been shown to be effective for up to 5 weeks. Zopiclone has a short half-life; thus, the patient should be taught that if sleep difficulties include early awakening, a dose can be taken as long as there is at least 4 hours before the patient must arise. In addition, the patient should explore other nonpharmacological options to use for the treatment of insomnia and try to find the cause of the sleep problems. See Box 13-1 for information on nonpharmacological measures to promote sleep.

CHAPTER 14
Central Nervous System Stimulants and Related Drugs

Chapter Review

1. c
2. a

3. c
4. d
5. b
6. b, c, e
7. b, c, d
8. 100 mg
9. 37.5 mg

Critical Thinking and Application

10. a.   Riley has narcolepsy.
    b.   Methylphenidate, an amphetamine, may be ordered. Amphetamines increase mental alertness, increase motor activity, and diminish the patient's sense of fatigue by stimulating the cerebral cortex and possibly the reticular activating system.
    c.   (i) Riley should take her medication exactly as her health care provider prescribes, without skipping, omitting, or doubling up on the doses.
         (ii) Riley should avoid other sources of central nervous system stimulants, particularly caffeine-containing products (e.g., coffee, tea, colas, and chocolate). She should check with her doctor before taking any over-the-counter drug, and she should not consume any substance that contains alcohol.

11. Specialists sometimes recommend periodic "medication holidays" (e.g., 1 day per week without medication) to diminish the addictive tendencies of the stimulant drugs. School-aged children often do not take these drugs on weekends and school vacations.

Case Study

1. Serotonin agonists work by stimulating 5-hydroxy-tryptamine (5-HT$_1$) receptors in the brain. This stimulation results in constriction of dilated blood vessels in the brain and decreased release of inflammatory neuropeptides.
2. Orally administered medications often may not be tolerated because of the nausea and vomiting that often accompany the headaches. Alternative formulations such as subcutaneous self-injections and nasal sprays are advantageous. They also have a more rapid onset of action, producing relief in some patients in 10 to 15 minutes compared with 1 to 2 hours with tablets.
3. The use of sumatriptan succinate (Imitrex DF) is contraindicated in patients with ischemic heart disease, signs and symptoms consistent with ischemic heart disease, Prinzmetal's angina, and uncontrolled hypertension.
4. Foods containing tyramine should be avoided because tyramine is known to precipitate severe headaches.

Tyramine-containing foods include beer, wine, aged cheese, food additives, preservatives, artificial sweeteners, chocolate, and caffeine.

5. Keeping a journal of the occurrence of headaches, precipitating factors, and response to drug therapy is also encouraged in order to follow the patient's progress and response to drug therapy.

CHAPTER 15
Antiepileptic Drugs

Chapter Review

1. d
2. a
3. c
4. c
5. b
6. c
7. a, b, c
8. a. 450 mg per day; 150 mg per dose
   b. 3 mL per dose
9.

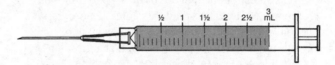

Critical Thinking and Application

10. Autoinduction is the process by which the metabolism of a medication increases over time, which leads to lower-than-expected drug concentrations. Carbamazepine is one antiepileptic drug that undergoes this process.
11. Jay's mother should be told that topiramate should be taken whole and should not be crushed, broken in half, or chewed. It does have a bitter taste and seems to be better tolerated when taken with food. She can still give it with gelatin, as long as the dosage form remains whole.

Critical Thinking Crossword

Across
2. Emergency
6. Primary
10. Hepatotoxicity
11. Seizure
12. Slowly

Down
1. Secondary
3. Convulsion

4. Benzodiazepines
5. Idiopathic
6. Phenobarbital
7. Autoinduction
8. Epilepsy
9. Phenytoin

Case Study

1. The signs and symptoms that Mattie is experiencing are typical of absence seizures. These are most often seen in children.
2. She needs to be sure to measure the dose carefully with an exact graduated device or oral syringe rather than by using a household teaspoon, and to give the medication at the same time daily. She needs to report excessive sedation, confusion, lethargy, or decreased movement. See the Patient Teaching Tips in your textbook for more information.
3. Encourage her to keep a journal to record Mattie's signs and symptoms before, during, and after any seizure activity, to measure the therapeutic effectiveness of the medication.
4. A therapeutic response to antiepileptic drugs does not mean that the patient has been cured of the seizures but only that seizure activity is decreased or absent. Further evaluation will be needed before a decision is made to stop the medication. Treatment may need to last for years or may be lifelong.

CHAPTER 16
Antiparkinsonian Drugs

Chapter Review

1. b
2. a
3. c
4. c
5. b
6. b
7. a, c, e
8. 2.5 tablets

Critical Thinking and Application

9. a. Dopamine must be given in this form because exogenously administered dopamine cannot pass through the blood–brain barrier; levodopa can.
   b. The addition of carbidopa avoids the high peripheral levels of dopamine and the unwanted adverse effects induced by the large doses of levodopa necessary when the drug is given alone.
   c. Carbidopa does not cross the blood–brain barrier and thus prevents levodopa breakdown in the periphery. This in turn allows levodopa to reach and cross the blood–brain barrier without carbidopa doing so. Once in the brain, the levodopa is then broken down to dopamine, which can be used directly.

10. The nurse must ask whether Hayley is lactating; if so, amantadine is contraindicated.
11. Older adults, particularly men who have a diagnosis of benign prostatic hypertrophy, are at risk for urinary retention. Jane's neighbour may or may not have that condition, but his age is a major factor. Jane's age is not a concern at this time. This drug may also cause palpitations.

Case Study

1. The primary cause of Parkinson's disease is an imbalance in the two neurotransmitters dopamine and acetylcholine (ACh) in the basal ganglia of the brain. This imbalance is caused by a failure of the nerve terminals in the substantia nigra to produce dopamine, which acts in the basal ganglia to control body movements. A correct balance between dopamine and ACh is needed for the proper regulation of posture, muscle tone, and voluntary movement. The deficiency of dopamine can also lead to excessive ACh activity due to the lack of dopamine's normal balancing effect. Symptoms of Parkinson's disease do not appear until approximately 80% of the dopamine store in the substantia nigra of the basal ganglia has been depleted.
2. Drug therapy is aimed at increasing the levels of dopamine at the remaining functioning nerve terminals. It is also aimed at blocking the effects of ACh and slowing the progression of the disease.
3. Amantadine facilitates the release of dopamine from nerve endings that are still intact. The result is higher levels of dopamine in the central nervous system.
4. Amantadine is most effective in the early stages of Parkinson's disease, but as the disease progresses and the number of functioning nerves diminishes, amantadine's effect is also reduced. It is usually effective for only 6 to 12 months.
5. The patient with Parkinson's disease often experiences rapid swings in response to levodopa; this fluctuating response is known as the "on-off phenomenon." This phenomenon is seen in patients taking levodopa for a long time. Such patients may experience periods when they have good control ("on" time) and periods when they have bad control or breakthrough Parkinson's disease ("off" time). Carbidopa is a peripheral decarboxylase inhibitor that does not cross the blood–brain barrier. As a result, carbidopa prevents levodopa from breaking down in the periphery and allows

more levodopa to reach and cross the blood–brain barrier. Levodopa and carbidopa combinations, such as Sinemet CR, may help reduce the "off" periods.

CHAPTER 17
Psychotherapeutic Drugs

Chapter Review

1. b
2. b, c
3. c
4. c
5. a, c, d
6. c
7. 3 tablets
8. 900 mg of lithium; three capsules per dose
9. l
10. f
11. g
12. o
13. b
14. i
15. j
16. k
17. c
18. n
19. a
20. d
21. h
22. e
23. m

Critical Thinking and Application

24. a. Carl may have taken an overdose of the benzodiazepine.
    b. If an overdose of benzodiazepine is suspected, flumazenil may be given to reverse the effect of the benzodiazepine overdose. The treatment for benzodiazepine overdose is generally supportive.
25. a. David needs to be aware of the foods and drinks, including red wine, that he can no longer have because they contain tyramine.
    b. It appears that David may have inadvertently ingested something containing tyramine, which has caused a hypertensive crisis.
26. Second-generation antidepressants offer an advantage over other antidepressants because they have fewer and less severe adverse effects.
27. If the antidepressant taken is a first-generation (tricyclic) antidepressant, excessive dosages could result in lethal cardiac dysrhythmias as well as seizures. These dysrhythmias are responsible for

most of the deaths due to tricyclic antidepressant overdoses.

Case Study

1. See Table 17-3 (p. XXX of the textbook) for potential adverse effects of benzodiazepines. Most are related to the effects on the central nervous system. Patient teaching includes warning George to avoid driving or operating heavy equipment or machinery until he becomes accustomed to the adverse effects of the medication. In addition, measures should be taken to avoid orthostatic hypotension. Finally, he should avoid alcohol and other central nervous system depressants while taking this medication.
2. If George is experiencing life-altering anxiety, he should also consider undergoing psychotherapy.
3. Benzodiazepines are potentially habit forming and addictive and may cause withdrawal symptoms such as anxiety, panic attacks, convulsions, nausea, and vomiting. The medication should not be withdrawn abruptly. Patients should always be advised to take the medication as directed and never to stop taking the medication abruptly.
4. There is a potential for benzodiazepines to cause serious life-threatening toxicities, but when taken alone in normal doses in otherwise healthy patients, they are safe and effective anxiolytics. When taken with other sedating medications or with alcohol, however, life-threatening respiratory depression or arrest can occur. An overdose of benzodiazepines may result in one or more of the following symptoms: somnolence, confusion, coma, and respiratory depression. Overdose may be treated with administration of activated charcoal and a cathartic. The benzodiazepine-specific antidote flumazenil may be used in severe cases.
5. Buspirone has the advantage of being both nonsedating and non–habit forming (lacks dependency) compared with benzodiazepines.

CHAPTER 18
Substance Misuse

Chapter Review

1. a, c, f
2. d
3. b, c, e
4. c
5. b
6. 2 mL
7. h
8. i
9. f

10. e
11. g
12. d
13. j
14. a
15. c
16. b

Critical Thinking and Application

17. The nicotine transdermal (patch) system and nicotine polacrilex (gum) can be used to provide nicotine without the carcinogens in tobacco. The patches provide a stepwise reduction in delivery and work by gradually reducing the nicotine dose over time. Rapid chewing of the gum releases an immediate dose of nicotine, but this dose is approximately one-half of what the average smoker receives from one cigarette, and the onset of action is longer than with smoking. Therefore, the re-inforcement and self-reward effects of smoking are minimized. Zyban is a sustained-release form of the antidepressant bupropion and is the first nicotine-free prescription medicine used to treat nicotine dependence.

18. For all three levels of ethanol withdrawal, benzodiazepines such as diazepam (Valium, Vivol), lorazepam (Ativan), and chlordiazepoxide (Librax) are used in various doses and frequencies. The doses are lower for mild withdrawal; for moderate ethanol withdrawal, higher doses of the benzodiazepines are used, and dosage is tapered over 5 days as needed. For severe withdrawal, also known as delirium tremens, the dosages of diazepam, lorazepam, or chlordiazepine are at their highest until the patient's agitation has subsided. In addition, thiamine injections may be given.

19. Dextromethorphan is an ingredient in several over-the-counter products, including Robitussin DM cough syrup and Mucinex DM tablets. Some adolescents have discovered that taking dextromethorphan in large amounts leads to a "high" that is accompanied by hallucinations. The hallucinations have been documented to be similar to those associated with the "street drug" phencyclidine (PCP). In addition, it has been found that teens who abuse dextromethorphan may also abuse other medications such as lysergic acid diethylamide (LSD), PCP, ecstasy, and inhalants. The hazardous short- or long-term effects that may occur with these drugs include nausea, hot flashes, reduced mental status, dizziness, seizures, loss of coordination and balance, brain damage, and death.

Case Study

1. Ethanol causes central nervous system depression and is thus a depressant.

2. Acute severe alcoholic intoxication may cause cardiovascular depression, and long-term excessive use has largely irreversible effects on the heart. Moderate amounts may either stimulate or depress respirations, but large amounts produce lethal respiratory depression.

3. The nurse should monitor the patient's respiratory and cardiovascular status and prevent (1) injury from falling and (2) aspiration from vomiting. In addition, the nurse should be alert to the patient's behaviour and mental status to identify changes in his condition. Withdrawal from alcohol can lead to serious conditions such as delirium tremens (see Question 4). Careful assessment of vital signs and mental status is imperative at this time; early withdrawal symptoms may be an increase in blood pressure and pulse with an altered mental status.

4. Fahim should stay in the hospital for observation and possible treatment of delirium tremens, which may begin with tremors and agitation and progress to hallucinations and sometimes death. See Box 18-6 in the textbook for information on treatment of ethanol withdrawal.

5. Chronic excessive ingestion of ethanol is directly associated with several serious mental and neurological disorders. Nutritional and vitamin B deficiencies that result in conditions such as Wernicke's encephalopathy, Korsakoff's psychosis, polyneuritis, and nicotinic acid deficiency encephalopathy can occur. Seizures may also occur. In addition, long-term ingestion of ethanol may result in alcoholic hepatitis or liver cirrhosis.

CHAPTER 19
Adrenergic Drugs

Chapter Review

1. d
2. b, d
3. a, b, d
4. a
5. c
6. a, b, e
7. 50 mcg per dose (see Overview of Dosage Calculations, Section IV)
8. 0.5 mL (see Overview of Dosage Calculations, Section III)

Critical Thinking and Application

9. a. The α-adrenergic activity of this drug causes vasoconstriction in the nasal mucosa. This produces shrinkage of the mucosa and promotes easier nasal breathing.

b. Perhaps the spray was administered too often. Excessive use of nasal decongestants can lead to greater congestion because of a rebound phenomenon.

10. Use of the drug is contraindicated in patients who have a tumour that secretes catecholamines, such as a pheochromocytoma.

11. The action of dopamine depends on the dosage. At low dosages, it can dilate blood vessels in the brain, heart, kidneys, and mesentery, increasing blood flow to these areas. Increased renal flow may help remove excess fluid volume. At higher infusion rates, dopamine can improve contractility and cardiac output.

12. The toxic effects of adrenergic drugs are mainly an extension of their common adverse effects, such as seizures, hypotension or hypertension, dysrhythmias, and other effects, but the two most life-threatening toxic effects involve the central nervous system and the cardiovascular system. Seizures can be managed effectively with diazepam. An extreme elevation in blood pressure poses the risk of hemorrhage in the brain and elsewhere in the body. To lower the blood pressure quickly, a rapid-acting β-adrenergic blocking drug can be used to reverse the adrenergic effects. Most of the adrenergic drugs have very short half-lives; therefore, their effects are relatively short-lived. Stopping the drug should quickly cause the toxic symptoms to subside. The treatment of overdoses often focuses on treating the symptoms and supporting the patient's respiratory and cardiac functions.

13. a. He is probably having an anaphylactic reaction to the penicillin.

b. First, the nurse must stop the medication! Then she will have someone else notify the health care provider while she stays with the patient to monitor and support the airway, breathing, and circulation (the "ABCs").

c. Epinephrine is the drug of choice for anaphylactic reactions.

Case Study

1. Before giving this medication, the nurse should assess for hypersensitivity to salbutamol and assess breath sounds and vital signs (blood pressure, pulse rate, respiratory rate) to obtain a baseline for comparative purposes. Because this medication may cause tachycardia and cardiac dysrhythmias, Maureen's pulse rate and rhythm should be monitored during the treatment. Afterward, Maureen's vital signs and breath sounds should be assessed again, as well as her therapeutic response to the medication.

2. Salbutamol given orally has an onset of action of 30 minutes and peaks in 2.5 hours. Inhaled salbutamol has an onset of action of 5 to 15 minutes and peaks in 1 to 1.5 hours. Therefore, the inhaled form will take effect faster than the oral form.

3. These are expected adverse effects of the salbutamol and will soon wear off.

4. Salmeterol is indicated for asthma and the prevention of bronchospasms in patients who may need long-term maintenance of their asthma. Patients should be taught that salmeterol is not to be used for relief of acute symptoms, and education about its dosing is important. Dosing of salmeterol is usually at two puffs twice daily 12 hours apart for maintenance. For prevention of exercise-induced asthma, the recommendation is two puffs 30 minutes to 1 hour before exercise and no additional dosing for 12 hours. If Maureen is still taking the inhaled steroid, then the bronchodilator should be taken first; then she should wait approximately 5 minutes before taking the steroid inhaler. All equipment should be rinsed, and the patient should be encouraged to perform mouth care after the use of any inhaled forms of medication.

CHAPTER 20
Adrenergic-Blocking Drugs

Chapter Review

1. a, b, d
2. a
3. d
4. b
5. d
6. c
7. 83 mL per hour (see Overview of Dosage Calculations, Section V.)
8. 4 mL

Critical Thinking and Application

9. Extravasation can cause vasoconstriction and ultimately tissue death (necrosis). If the vasoconstriction is not reversed quickly, the whole limb can be lost. Phentolamine, an α-adrenergic, can reverse this potent vasoconstriction and restore blood flow to the ischemic, vasoconstricted area. When phentolamine is injected subcutaneously in a circular fashion around the extravasation site, it causes α-adrenergic receptor blockade and vasodilation. This in turn increases blood flow to the ischemic tissue, thus preventing permanent damage.

10. Some beta-blockers are considered cardioprotective because they inhibit stimulation by the circulating catecholamines released during muscle damage, such as that caused by a myocardial infarction. When a beta-blocker occupies their receptors,

the circulating catecholamines cannot bind to their receptors. Thus the beta-blockers protect the heart from being stimulated by these catecholamines, which would only further increase the heart rate and the contractile force, thereby increasing myocardial oxygen demand.

11. Anna should take her apical pulse for 1 full minute and monitor her blood pressure because cardiac depression can occur with these drugs. If her systolic blood pressure decreases to less than 100 mm Hg or her pulse decreases to less than 60 beats per minute, she should contact her health care provider. She should also report any weight gain, especially a gain of more than 1 kg in 24 hours or 2 kg in a week, as well as any weakness, shortness of breath, or edema.

12. A common problem with the alpha-blockers such as tamsulosin is that when patients first start taking these drugs, they may experience lightheadedness and orthostatic hypotension. Patients usually quickly develop a tolerance to this effect. Trevor should be taught to take care when standing up to prevent falling if he gets lightheaded; taking the first dose at bedtime may help. In addition, other adverse effects of blurred vision, dizziness, and drowsiness may lead to injuries if he should fall. Special care must be taken for safety until he knows how he responds to the medication.

Case Study

1. Nonselective ß-blockers (which block both ß$_1$ and ß$_2$ receptors) may precipitate bradycardia and hypotension; their use is contraindicated in asthma. Therefore, if the patient has heart disease as well as respiratory disease, then a ß1-blocker, or a "cardioselective" drug, would be beneficial because it would not produce constriction or increased airway resistance, as would a ß2-blocker.

2. When a ß-blocker is given, it occupies receptors and prevents circulating catecholamines (which are released when a myocardial infarction occurs) from binding to these receptors. The beta-blocker thus prevents stimulation of the heart by these catecholamines, which would only further increase heart rate, contractile force, and myocardial oxygen demand. In addition, cardioselective beta1-blockers such as atenolol block the ß$_1$-adrenergic receptors on the surface of the heart. This reduces myocardial stimulation, which in turn reduces heart rate, slows conduction through the atrio-ventricular node, prolongs sinoatrial-node recovery, and decreases myocardial oxygen demand by decreasing myocardial contractile force (contractility).

3. Table 20-4 lists beta-blocker–induced adverse effects. Patient teaching should include instructions to monitor the apical pulse for 1 full minute and monitor blood pressure (because of the cardiac depression that can occur) and to notify the health care provider if systolic blood pressure decreases to lower than 100 mm Hg or pulse decreases to less than 60 beats per minute. Patients should also report any weight gain, especially a gain of 1 kg or more in a 24-hour period or 2 kg or more in a week, as well as any weakness, shortness of breath, and edema. The patient should also be taught about orthostatic changes and cautioned to rise slowly when getting up, to avoid syncope.

4. Make sure that patients are weaned off these medications slowly, if this is indicated, because of the possible rebound hypertension or chest pain that rapid withdrawal can precipitate. Beta-blockers may cause impotence, which may be the reason Bruce wants to stop the medication, but the nurse needs to ask him about his reason for wanting to stop atenolol.

CHAPTER 21
Cholinergic Drugs

Chapter Review

1. h
2. g
3. f
4. b
5. j
6. e
7. i
8. a
9. c
10. b
11. b
12. d
13. c
14. b, c, d, f
15. a
16. 17 gtts/min (16.7 gtts rounded to 17 gtts)
17. 26.7 mg

Critical Thinking and Application

18. *S*alivation, *L*acrimation, *U*rinary incontinence, *D*iarrhea, *G*astro-intestinal cramps, *E*mesis
19. a. Bethanechol is the drug of choice.
    b. None; bethanechol is contraindicated in patients with a genitourinary obstruction. The drug should be discontinued immediately.

20. a. Cholinergic crisis
    b. Ensure that atropine, the antidote, is readily available.
21. a. She should experience less eyelid drooping (ptosis), less double vision (diplopia), less difficulty swallowing and chewing, and less weakness.
    b. She needs to report any increased muscle weakness, abdominal cramps, diarrhea, or difficulty breathing.

Case Study

1. There are no "cures" for Alzheimer's disease, but there are several drugs available for the management of symptoms. Their use can sometimes yield enough improvement in a patient's mental status to make a noticeable improvement in the quality of life for patients as well as their caregivers and family members. However, individual response to these medications does vary from patient to patient. Available drugs include donepezil (Aricept), galantamine (Reminyl), rivastigmine (Exelon), and memantine (Ebixa).
2. Rivastigmine is also approved for treating dementia that is associated with Parkinson's disease.
3. Direct-acting cholinergic agonists bind to cholinergic receptors and activate them. Indirect-acting cholinergic agonists act by making more acetylcholine (ACh) available at the receptor site. As a result, ACh binds to and stimulates the receptors; it does this by inhibiting the action of cholinesterase, the enzyme responsible for breaking down ACh.
4. Adverse effects of rivastigmine include dizziness, headache, nausea and vomiting, diarrhea, and anorexia (loss of appetite). Administering this drug with meals helps decrease the gastro-intestinal adverse effects, although absorption may also be decreased. Patients who become dizzy with the therapy must be assisted with ambulation. Doses are titrated carefully to help minimize adverse effects.
5. Rivastigmine is also available in rapid orally disintegrating tablets, which may be easier for the patient to take.

CHAPTER 22
Cholinergic-Blocking Drugs

Chapter Review

1. a, c, f
2. a, c, d
3. b
4. c
5. b
6. d
7. 0.6 mL
8. a. 40 mcg
   b. 0.2 mL

Critical Thinking and Application

9. Atropine sulphate is used preoperatively to reduce salivation and excessive secretions in the respiratory and gastro-intestinal tracts. Glycopyrrolate is also used for this purpose.
10. a. Initially, this patient should be treated with hospitalization and close, continuous monitoring (including continuous electrocardiographic monitoring). Consultation with a Poison Control Centre is recommended. Activated charcoal can be administered to remove drug that is already absorbed. Fluid therapy and other standard measures used to treat shock should be instituted as needed.
    b. In the case of hallucinations, physostigmine has proved helpful, although its use is somewhat controversial because of severe adverse effects with routine use. It is available in Canada only under the Special Access Programme.
11. Antihistamines can have additive effects with cholinergic blockers, resulting in increased effects.
12. a. In the treatment of symptomatic bradycardia, higher dosages of atropine result in an increase in heart rate because of the cholinergic-blocking effects on the heart's conduction system. Atropine blocks the inhibitory vagal (cholinergic) effects on the pacemaker cells of the sinoatrial and atrio-ventricular nodes, which can lead to an increased heart rate due to unopposed sympathetic stimulation.
    b. Atropine has a therapeutic effect in cases of exposure to organophosphate insecticides because of its anti-cholinesterase effects.

Case Study

1. Tolterodine should not be used in patients with narrow-angle glaucoma or urinary retention. If patients have a history of decreased liver function or are taking drugs that inhibit cytochrome P-450 enzyme 3A4, the tolterodine dose will be reduced. Sashima's "eye problems" need to be evaluated further to rule out glaucoma.
2. Tolterodine appears to be associated with a much lower incidence of dry mouth. This may be due to tolterodine's specificity for the bladder as opposed to the salivary glands.
3. When these cholinergic-blocking drugs are used to treat urinary incontinence, the inability to sweat or

perspire should be managed with an increase in fluids and an avoidance of extreme heat. Sashima needs to avoid overheating when working outside.

4. Although this drug may be associated with a lower incidence of dry mouth, it may still cause this unpleasant adverse effect because it is a cholinergic-blocking drug. Dry mouth may be managed best by drinking adequate fluids, chewing gum, performing frequent mouth care, sucking on sugar-free hard candy, and using saliva-substitute products.

CHAPTER 23
Antihypertensive Drugs

Chapter Review

1. c
2. b, d, e
3. c
4. a
5. d
6. a, c
7. 2 tablets per dose
8. 4 mL

Critical Thinking and Application

9. Because nitroprusside has a very short half-life (10 minutes), the nurse will first discontinue the infusion. Treatment for the hypotension is supportive; pressor drugs can be given to raise the blood pressure quickly if necessary.

10. a. Captopril is probably best for Irene. In critically ill patients, a drug with a short half-life (such as captopril) is better, because if problems arise, they will be short-lived. Also, Irene has liver dysfunction, so captopril has an advantage because it is not a pro-drug. (A pro-drug is inactive in its initial form and must be biotransformed in the liver to its active form to be effective.)
    b. Because of his history of poor adherence, Kory would benefit from a drug with a long half-life and a long duration of action, a drug he would need to take only once a day. Therefore, one of the newer angiotensin-converting enzyme (ACE) inhibitors—benazepril, fosinopril, lisinopril, quinapril, or ramipril— would be best.

11. There is a first-dose effect with prazosin. This means that the patient will experience a considerable drop in blood pressure after taking the first dose; thus, Lance should take it if he will be lying down for a while or before bedtime and then should arise

slowly. This effect decreases with time or with a reduction in the dosage as ordered by the health care provider.

12. a. Beta-blockers and ACE inhibitors
    b. Calcium channel blockers and diuretics

Critical Thinking Crossword

Across
1. secondary
5. idiopathic
7. orthostatic
8. vasodilators

Down
2. essential
3. primary
4. diuretics
6. ACE

Case Study

1. Initial drug therapy would include thiazide-type diuretics. Other drugs that may also be started include ACE inhibitors, angiotensin II receptor blockers, beta-blockers, calcium channel blockers, or a combination of these. Because John is Black, calcium channel blockers and diuretics would most likely be chosen over beta-blockers and ACE inhibitors.
2. Teach him about the possibility of orthostatic hypotension, and instruct him to change positions slowly—especially after stooping or bending over or when rising from a supine or sitting position to a standing one.
3. Exercise is an important part of a healthy lifestyle. However, emphasize the importance of safety and the need to avoid excessive exercise, hot climates, saunas, hot tubs, and hot environments. Heat may precipitate vasodilation and lead to a worsening of hypotension, with the risk of fainting and injury to himself.

CHAPTER 24
Antianginal Drugs

Chapter Review

1. c
2. c
3. a, c, e (Note: d is also an available form; however, dysphagia is contraindicated for this form.)
4. d
5. a
6. b

7. a
8. 2 capsules

Critical Thinking and Application

9. The nurse MUST NOT cut the patch in half! The nurse needs to call the pharmacy to obtain the correct dosage of the transdermal patch, one that delivers 0.2 mg/hr.

10. The nurse will call 911 and assist the patient until the ambulance arrives and will check the "ABCs" and administer cardiopulmonary resuscitation (CPR) if it becomes necessary. At this time, the nurse does not know the man's condition and certainly cannot administer someone else's medication to him. Iso-sorbide dinitrate (Isordil) is available in a sublingual form, but the nurse cannot administer one person's medication to another person, especially to someone with an undetermined condition.

11. Victoria might be taking a beta-blocker. Fatigue and lethargy are the most common patient complaints with the use of beta-blockers, and mental depression can be exacerbated, particularly in older adults. Also, one of the central nervous system adverse effects of beta-blockers is the occurrence of unusual dreams.

12. Taylor has a good start, but she also needs to include in her journal a description of the activity she was performing at the time her angina occurred and the number of tablets she had to take before the pain subsided. Also, she must keep the tablets in an airtight, dark glass bottle away from sunlight, because the active ingredient in nitroglycerin is easily destroyed. The fact that she had no adverse effects such as headache may indicate that the drug is no longer active and needs to be replaced.

Case Study

1. Chronic stable angina, also known as classic or effort angina, can be triggered by either exertion or stress (cold temperatures or emotions).

2. When experiencing an acute anginal attack, Gideon should take one sublingual tablet as soon as possible after the pain begins, lie down immediately, remain calm, and rest. He can take up to three sublingual tablets every 5 minutes if relief is not experienced after the first tablet.

3. If Gideon experiences no relief after 15 minutes (three sublingual tablets), his handball partner should call 911 and have the emergency response team take him to the hospital. The emergency response team will be better equipped to help him should further complications occur.

4. The beta-blockers are most effective in the treatment of typical exertional angina.

CHAPTER 25
Heart Failure Drugs

Chapter Review

1. b
2. c
3. d
4. a
5. b
6. a, c, d, e, f
7. c, e, f
8. 2 mL
9.

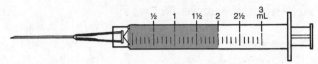

10. 250 mcg

Critical Thinking and Application

11. Vomiting, headache, fatigue, and dysrhythmia are adverse effects of cardiac glycosides. The presence of a serum potassium level of more than 5 mmol/L along with these symptoms means that administration of digoxin immune Fab is indicated for the treatment of severe digoxin toxicity.

12. Increased urinary output and decreased dyspnea and fatigue are therapeutic effects of digoxin. The constipation needs to be assessed. Fredrick should not consume large amounts of bran or other foods high in fibre because the bran will bind to the digitalis and make less of the drug available for absorption.

13. a. Milrinone increases the force of contraction (positive inotropic effect) and relaxes the blood vessels (vasodilation), causing a reduction in afterload, or the force against which the heart must pump to eject its volume.
    b. Phosphodiesterase inhibitors have a wider therapeutic window than digoxin does.
    c. Ventricular cardiac dysrhythmias

Case Study

1. a. Positive inotropic effect: increase in myocardial contractility
   b. Negative chronotropic effect: decrease in heart rate
   c. Negative dromotropic effect: Slowing of the conduction of electrical impulses in the heart
2. a. Stroke volume: increased
   b. Venous blood pressure and vein engorgement: decreased

c. Coronary circulation: increased

d. Diuresis: increased due to improved circulation

3. First, complete your assessment by checking the patient's apical pulse, heart and lung sounds, and blood pressure. In addition, check her potassium level, because low levels of potassium may lead to digoxin toxicity. If you have not yet given the digoxin dose, hold it and call the health care provider immediately. Monitor the patient for signs of digoxin toxicity, especially dangerous dysrhythmias. The digoxin level of 3.5 ng/mL is above the therapeutic range.

CHAPTER 26
Antidysrhythmic Drugs

Chapter Review

1. d
2. c, d, e
3. a
4. d
5. a
6. b
7. a, (3); b, (1); c, (2)
8. b, c, e
9. 150 mg
10. 2 mL

Critical Thinking and Application

11. a. Class II antidysrhythmics, or beta-blockers, are indicated because they have been shown to significantly reduce the incidence of sudden cardiac death after myocardial infarction.

    b. If Raj has had asthma, use of most of the class II drugs would be contraindicated. Noncardioselective beta-blockers block not only the ß₁-adrenergic receptors in the heart but also the ß₂-adrenergic receptors in the lungs. As a result, pre-existing asthma could be worsened.

12. Amiodarone is considered a drug of last resort. Although it is effective, amiodarone can penetrate and concentrate in the adipose tissue of any organ in the body, where it may cause unwanted effects. It may cause either hypothyroidism or hyperthyroidism, corneal microdeposits, pulmonary toxicity, and even dysrhythmias. Amiodarone has a long half-life, and the adverse effects may take months to subside.

13. a. Lidocaine must be injected intramuscularly or intravenously; when lidocaine is taken orally, the liver converts most of it to inactive metabolites.

    b. Lidocaine is extensively metabolized in the liver. For patients in liver failure or with a history of

cirrhosis, as with Warrick, a dosage reduction of 50% is recommended.

Case Study

1. As their name implies, calcium channel blockers work by inhibiting the slow-channel pathways, or the calcium-dependent channels. As a result, they depress phase 4 depolarization and slow sinoatrial and atrio-ventricular nodal conduction rates, thus reducing the incidence of paroxysmal supraventricular rhythms (i.e., paroxysmal supraventricular tachycardia [PSVT]).

2. Prevention or reduction of supraventricular rhythms

3. Taking phenytoin, an anticonvulsant, along with diltiazem may result in reduced effectiveness of the calcium channel blocker.

4. The health care provider may prescribe adenosine, which is useful for the treatment of PSVT that has failed to respond to verapamil.

CHAPTER 27
Coagulation Modifier Drugs

Chapter Review

1. a, c, d
2. b
3. a
4. c
5. b, c, d, e
6. d
7. b
8. 0.8 mL
9. 7.5 mg (patient weighs 75 kg)
10. k
11. n
12. j
13. l
14. m
15. b
16. a
17. c
18. i
19. h
20. e
21. g

Critical Thinking and Application

22. The injection site should not be massaged or rubbed before or after the injection because this may cause hematoma formation.

23. a. The anticoagulant effects of heparin can be reversed with protamine sulphate.

b. In general, 1 mg of protamine can reverse the effects of 100 units of heparin.

c. The activated partial thromboplastin time is the test most commonly used.

24. The health care provider will probably prescribe one of the antifibrinolytic drugs that are used to stop excessive oozing from surgical sites such as chest tubes.

25. Desmopressin (DDAVP) is used for patients with type I von Willebrand's disease. It increases the levels of clotting factor VIII.

26. a. No; alteplase is present in the body in a natural state, so it does not induce an antigen–antibody reaction.

b. Alteplase (Activase) can be re-administered because it has a short half-life of 5 minutes. Because of the short half-life, it is given with heparin to prevent reocclusion of the infarcted blood vessel.

27. a. Ursula's symptoms are possible indications of bleeding problems related to the anticoagulation therapy.

b. Ursula might also be exhibiting a change in pulse rate or rhythm, blood pressure, or level of consciousness.

c. Notify the health care provider immediately. Do not administer any other anticoagulants. If Ursula is receiving a continuous infusion, stop the infusion. Prepare to administer the appropriate antidote.

28. Heparin is commonly used for deep vein thrombosis prophylaxis in a dose of 5000 units two or three times a day given subcutaneously. It does not need to be monitored when used for prophylaxis.

Case Study

1. Use of acetylsalicylic acid (Aspirin) is contraindicated in the presence of peptic ulcer disease. Doug has been started on clopidogrel therapy to reduce the risk of having a stroke.

2. Doug should be taught to watch for signs of abnormal bleeding and should immediately report any of the following signs and symptoms to the health care provider: respiratory difficulty, back pain, skin rash, evidence of gastro-intestinal bleeding, any other bleeding abnormality, diarrhea, acute severe headache, and change in vision (blurred vision or loss of vision).

3. Doug needs to take measures to prevent bleeding, such as using a soft toothbrush and an electric razor, and he should take care when trimming his nails, gardening, and participating in rough sports. Doug needs to take precautions to protect himself from injury and subsequent bleeding or bruising, which can be extremely dangerous while he is taking antiplatelet drugs.

4. Natural health products that contain garlic, ginger, ginseng, and ginkgo should be avoided because they have anticoagulant properties.

CHAPTER 28
Antilipemic Drugs

Chapter Review

1. d
2. a, c, d, e
3. a
4. b
5. d
6. c
7. a, c, d, e
8. 1.5 tablets
9. 750 mg per dose; 3 tablets per dose

Critical Thinking and Application

10. Unless José has additional risk factors, his high level of low-density lipoprotein (LDL) cholesterol alone does not warrant drug therapy at this time. All reasonable nonpharmaceutical means of controlling José's LDL level need to be tried and found to fail before he is given drug therapy. José needs to find time in his busy schedule to exercise and eat more wisely.

11. Katherine is experiencing constipation and belching associated with cholestyramine (Novo-Cholamine) use. (She may also be experiencing heartburn, nausea, and bloating.) Katherine requires extra patient teaching and support to help her maintain adherence to the drug therapy. She should be assured that these adverse effects will probably diminish over time.

12. No. Jim is not a candidate for niacin (Niaspan) therapy for two reasons: (1) niacin is not recommended with lovastatin because it can lead to the development of rhabdomyolysis, and (2) niacin (Niaspan) is contraindicated in patients with peptic ulcer.

13. Nila must take her antihypertensive and cholestyramine (Olestyr) at different times of the day because the bile acid sequestrant may interfere significantly with the absorption of other drugs taken at the same time. All other drugs should be taken at least 1 hour before or 4 to 6 hours after the administration of antilipemics. Cholestyramine should be taken just before or with meals. Also, the powder form of cholestyramine should be allowed to dissolve slowly in at least 60 mL of fluid, without stirring, for at least 1 minute, because stirring causes the powder to clump. The powder may not mix totally in the glass, and more fluid may need to be added. The powder

may also be mixed thoroughly with food, such as crushed pineapple.

Case Study

1. No, Matt is not right. Dietary measures are a part of antilipemic therapy. Nonpharmacological measures include consumption of a low-fat, low-cholesterol diet; supervised, moderate exercise; weight loss; cessation of smoking or drinking; and relaxation therapy.
2. Atorvastatin (Lipitor) is used primarily to lower the total and LDL cholesterol levels as well as triglyceride levels. It has been shown to raise the high-density lipoprotein (HDL) level as well.
3. Elevations in liver enzyme levels may also occur, and the patient should be monitored for excessive elevations, which may indicate the need for alternative drug therapy. In addition, total cholesterol level, LDL and HDL cholesterol levels, and triglyceride levels need to be monitored to evaluate therapeutic effect.
4. Myopathy (muscle pain) is an uncommon but clinically important adverse effect that may occur in some patients taking statins. It may progress to a serious condition known as rhabdomyolysis, in which the breakdown of muscle protein occurs, leading to myoglobinuria and possible kidney damage. Patients receiving statin therapy should be taught to report unexplained muscle pain to their health care provider immediately.

CHAPTER 29
Diuretic Drugs

Chapter Review

1. a, c, d, e
2. c
3. a
4. d
5. b
6. b, e
7. 15 mL
8. 150 mL (Hint: 20% indicates 20 g per 100 mL.)
   20 g = 30 g
   100 mL   x mL
   (20 g)(x mL) = (100 mL)(30 g); 20x = 3000;
   x = 150 mL
9. c
10. f
11. e
12. i
13. g
14. j
15. h
16. a
17. d
18. b

Critical Thinking and Application

19. a. Madison was probably prescribed a carbonic anhydrase inhibitor (CAI).
    b. An undesirable effect of the CAIs is that they elevate the blood glucose level, causing glycosuria in diabetic patients. They may also interact with some oral anti-hyperglycemic drugs.
20. a. In order for mannitol to be effective in treating acute renal failure, enough kidney blood flow and glomerular filtration must exist to enable the drug to reach the tubules.
    b. Mannitol is always administered intravenously through a filter because it can crystallize when exposed to low temperatures (which is more likely to occur when concentrations exceed 15%).
    c. The patient's headache and chills are most likely adverse effects of the mannitol therapy. At this time, the therapy should be continued, but the patient should be monitored for the development of more serious adverse effects.
21. a. Jeff will be prescribed spironolactone (Aldactone) in high doses; this drug is used often for the treatment of ascites associated with cirrhosis of the liver.
    b. His serum potassium level will need to be monitored frequently because his kidney function is impaired.
22. a. Impotence and reduced libido are among the adverse effects of thiazide; Byron is possibly experiencing these effects.
    b. Byron should stop eating licorice because its consumption can lead to an additive hypokalemia in patients taking thiazide. Byron's fatigue may be the result of drug toxicity and should be evaluated.
23. It is likely that Barbara's neighbour was prescribed one of the potassium-sparing diuretics and thus was not instructed to eat additional potassium-rich foods. Barbara should follow the dietary recommendations provided for her, not for her neighbour.
24. Loop diuretics have a distinct advantage over thiazide diuretics in that their diuretic action continues even when creatinine clearance decreases below 25 mL per minute. This means that even when kidney function diminishes, loop diuretics can still work. As renal function decreases, the efficacy of thiazides diminishes, because delivery of the drug to the site of activity is impaired. Thiazides are not to be used if creatinine clearance is less than 30 to 50 mL per minute. Normal

creatinine clearance is 125 mL per minute, depending on the patient's age. However, metolazone remains effective to a creatinine clearance of 10 mL per minute and thus can be used in cases of renal failure.

Case Study

1. These symptoms suggest hypokalemia. Furosemide (Lasix) is a kaliuretic diuretic, which means that potassium is excreted along with sodium and water.
2. Foods high in potassium; these include bananas, oranges, dates, raisins, plums, fresh vegetables, potatoes (white and sweet), meat, fish, apricots, whole-grain cereals, and legumes.
3. Spironolactone (Aldactone) is a potassium-sparing diuretic. It causes sodium and water to be excreted, but potassium is retained.
4. The combined use of angiotensin-converting enzyme (ACE) inhibitors or potassium supplements in combination with potassium-sparing diuretics can result in hyperkalemia. When taken together, lithium and potassium-sparing diuretics can result in lithium toxicity. The use of nonsteroidal anti-inflammatory drugs with potassium-sparing diuretics can reduce the effectiveness of the diuretics.

CHAPTER 30
Fluids and Electrolytes

Chapter Review

1. a, b, d, e
2. c
3. d
4. c
5. b
6. b
7. 42 mL per hour
8. 100 mL per hour (50 mL : 0.5 hr = x mL : 1 hr; x = 100 mL/hr)

Critical Thinking and Application

9. **Advantages**: Crystalloids are (1) less expensive than colloids and blood products for replacing fluids and (2) better for emergency short-term plasma volume expansion. They also promote urinary flow. They do not carry the risk of transmission of viral diseases or anaphylaxis and do not promote bleeding.
Disadvantages: The fluids can leak out of the plasma into the tissues and cells, which results in edema, such as peripheral edema or pulmonary edema. They may dilute plasma proteins, result-ing in lower colloid oncotic pressure (COP), and

dilute erythrocyte concentration, resulting in decreased oxygen tension. Large volumes are needed to be effective, but prolonged infusions and administration of large volumes may worsen acidosis or alkalosis. Last, their effects are relatively short-lived compared with those of colloids.

10. a. Blood products
b. They are the only fluids that contain hemoglobin.
c. They are natural products that require human donors, which means that they can be incompati-ble with a recipient's immune system; these products can also transmit pathogens from the donor to the recipient.
11. a. The patient is exhibiting early symptoms of hypokalemia.
b. The patient should eat foods high in potassium, such as bananas, orange juice, and apricots. She may be placed on oral potassium supplements for a short time.
12. a. Hyponatremia
b. Vomiting is a possible adverse effect of oral administration of sodium chloride. If vomiting occurs, Samuel needs to be careful about monitoring for further fluid and electrolyte loss.
13. a. Signs of transfusion reaction include apprehen-sion, restlessness, flushed skin, increased pulse and respiration rates, dyspnea, rash, joint or lower back pain, swelling, fever and chills, nausea, weakness, and jaundice.
b. Although it is possible for pathogens such as that causing human immunodeficiency virus (HIV) infection to be transmitted via blood products, Vanessa's husband should be reassured that techniques that have drastically reduced the incidence of such problems are now being used.
c. Vanessa's restlessness and increased pulse are signs of a reaction to the blood product. The nurse will stop the transfusion immediately and change the infusion to normal saline. The nurse will stay with the patient and assess her vital signs and have another nurse notify the health care provider immediately; the facility's protocol for transfusion reactions will be followed.

Case Study

1. The normal total protein level should be 74 g/L. If this level drops below 53 g/L, the colloid oncotic pressure becomes less than the hydrostatic pressure, and fluid shifts into the tissues, which results in edema.
2. Colloids increase COP and move fluid from outside the blood vessels to inside the blood vessels, thus reducing the edema.

3. Colloids are the choice for this patient. Crystalloids can leak out of the plasma into the tissues and cells, which results in edema anywhere in the body. Crystalloids also dilute the proteins that are in the plasma, further reducing COP. Finally, crystalloids are more likely to cause edema because of the larger volumes needed to achieve the desired clinical effect. Colloids reduce edema and expand plasma volume by pulling fluid from the extravascular space into the blood vessels.

4. Colloids can alter the coagulation system, which results in impaired coagulation and possible bleeding. They have no oxygen-carrying ability and contain no clotting factors. They may also dilute the plasma protein concentration, which may impair the function of platelets.

CHAPTER 31
Pituitary Drugs

Chapter Review

1. d
2. d
3. b
4. a, d
5. c
6. a
7. a. Total dose per week for this child (44 lb = 20 kg) is 6 mg.
   b. Dose per injection (6 daily injections) = 1 mg per dose per day for 6 days
8. 0.5 mL

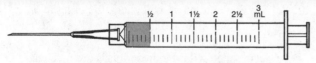

9. a. Glucocorticoids, mineralocorticoids, androgens
   b. cosyntropin
   c. Regulates anabolic processes related to growth and adaptation to stressors; promotes skeletal and muscle growth; increases protein synthesis; increases liver glycogenolysis; and increases fat mobilization.
   d. somatropin (Humatrope) and octreotide (Sandostatin)
   e. antidiuretic hormone
   f. vasopressin and desmopressin
   g. Promotes uterine contractions.
   h. oxytocin

Critical Thinking and Application

10. In addition to information about proper subcutaneous injection techniques, the teaching plan should include reminders of the dosage form and amount and of the importance of adherence to therapy. The parents should be shown how to keep a journal of growth measurements.

11. Cosyntropin (Cortrosyn) is used for the diagnosis of adrenocortical insufficiency, not for treatment. Once a diagnosis is made, the actual drug treatment generally involves replacement hormonal therapy using drug forms of the deficient corticosteroid hormones.

Case Study

1. Vasopressin or desmopressin.
2. Vasopressin should be given cautiously in patients with migraine headaches, seizures, cardiovascular disease, renal disease, or asthma.
3. Treatment will be injections, either intramuscular or subcutaneous, two to four times a day. This drug therapy will increase water resorption in the distal tubules and collecting ducts of the nephron, performing all the physiological functions of an antidiuretic hormone. As a result, water excretion is diminished.
4. Therapy should eliminate his severe thirst and decrease his urinary output.

CHAPTER 32
Thyroid and Antithyroid Drugs

Chapter Review

1. c
2. d
3. a
4. a, c, d
5. c
6. b
7. 0.088 mg
8. 1.5 mL
9. This patient's condition may result in the formation of a goitre, an enlargement of the thyroid gland resulting from its overstimulation by elevated levels of thyroid-stimulating hormone. She may benefit from one of the thyroid agents, including thyroid, thyroglobulin, levothyroxine (Eltroxin), or liothyronine. Levothyroxine is generally preferred because as a chemically pure formulation of 100% thyroxine, its hormonal content is standardized; therefore, its effect is predictable.
10. Surgery to remove all or part of the thyroid gland is an effective way to treat hyperthyroidism, but as a result, lifelong hormone replacement is normally required.
11. The most damaging or serious adverse effects of propylthiouracil (PTU) medications are liver and bone

marrow toxicity. Therefore, it is important to conduct liver function studies as well as a complete blood count (white blood cells, red blood cells, and platelets). In addition, PTU is rated as a pregnancy category D drug; a pregnancy test will be needed.

Critical Thinking Crossword

Across

3. secondary
6. thyroxine
7. primary

Down

1. levothyroxine
2. hyperthyroidism
4. propylthiouracil
5. tertiary
6. thyrotropin

Case Study

1. The symptoms suggest hypothyroidism. A thyroid replacement hormone, such as levothyroxine, is indicated for this condition.
2. The thyroid preparations are given to replace what the thyroid gland cannot itself produce in order to achieve normal thyroid levels (known as a "euthyroid condition").
3. Thyroid preparations should be taken at the same time every day to maintain constant blood levels. Taking the medication in the morning will help reduce problems with insomnia, which may result when the medication is taken later in the day or in the evening.

CHAPTER 33
Antidiabetic Drugs

Chapter Review

1. b
2. d
3. a
4. c
5. c
6. b
7. b
8. 4.9 units of insulin (13.2 mmol − 8.3 mmol = 4.9)
9.

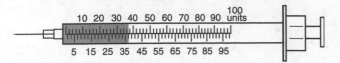

Critical Thinking and Application

10. a. Sitagliptin (Januvia) is indicated in combination with metformin in adult patients with type 2 diabetes mellitus to improve glycemic control when diet and exercise and use of metformin do not provide adequate control. Sitagliptin is a highly selective inhibitor of the dipeptidyl peptidase 4 (DPP-4) enzyme that enhances incretin hormones. The incretin hormones are released by the intestine throughout the day, and levels that have increased in response to a meal are part of an endogenous system involved in the physiological regulation of glucose homeostasis. Consequently, treatment with sitagliptin improves cell responsiveness to glucose and stimulates insulin release.
    b. Metformin works primarily by inhibiting hepatic glucose production and increasing the sensitivity of peripheral tissue to insulin, thus lowering blood glucose levels.

11. a. Alisa's diet should include a high intake of protein and a low intake of carbohydrates.
    b. The brain requires a constant supply of glucose to function. Thus, the central nervous system manifestations of hypoglycemia (such as irritability) are often the first to appear.
    c. For the conscious person, oral forms of glucose are used, such as rapidly dissolving buccal tablets or semisolid gel forms designed for rapid mucosal absorption. Alisa could also try corn syrup, honey, fruit juice, a nondiet soft drink, or a small snack such as crackers or half a sandwich.

12. a. The graduate nurse will check the order at least three times and then have another licensed nurse check the prepared injection to be sure it is in accordance with the prescriber's order. These second checks may vary with facilities.
    b. The co-worker is right. Humulin-R is regular insulin, and regular insulin is clear.
    c. If left at room temperature, the insulin in the vial must be discarded after 1 month.

13. a. The patient requires an intermediate-acting insulin.
    b. The patient's religious beliefs might prohibit him from using insulin made from pork. Because of the availability of human biosynthetic and analogue insulins, the patient should not need to use any insulins containing pork.

14. Francine needs to make some significant lifestyle changes. She must lose weight, stop smoking, and exercise regularly, which will help with both the high blood glucose level and the hypertension. The American Diabetes Association also recommends that (in addition to lifestyle changes) the oral

biguanide metformin (Glucophage) be started as initial therapy for lowering blood glucose levels.

15. a. 20 units of NPH (Novolin ge NPH) insulin plus 4 units regular insulin
    b. No coverage
    c. 6 units of regular insulin
16. If the patient receiving metformin is to undergo diagnostic studies with contrast dye, the prescriber will need to discontinue the drug on the day of the tests and restart it 48 hours after the tests. It may be necessary to re-evaluate the patient's renal status.
17. a. Hypoglycemia
    b. Hyperglycemia
    c. Hyperglycemia
    d. Hypoglycemia
    e. Hypoglycemia

Case Study

1. Glipizide works best if given 30 minutes before meals. This allows the timing of the insulin secretion induced by the glipizide to correspond with the elevation in blood glucose level induced by the meal in much the same way as endogenous insulin levels are raised in a person without diabetes. Its effect is much like the body's normal response to meals, and it will help to keep the blood glucose levels from becoming too high.
2. To provide a picture of the patient's adherence to the therapy regimen for the previous several months, hemoglobin A_{1c} is measured. This value reflects how well the patient has been doing with diet and drug therapy.
3. Deepak should contact his health care provider immediately. He may require a change in his diabetic treatment while he is sick, because vomiting and the inability to eat can cause a change in his blood glucose levels. If he is unable to eat and yet takes the glipizide, he is at risk for experiencing severe hypoglycemia.

CHAPTER 34
Adrenal Drugs

Chapter Review

1. a
2. c
3. a, b, c
4. c
5. d
6. c
7. One-half tablet
8. 3.2 mg per dose

Critical Thinking and Application

9. Inform Rachel that glucocorticoid can interact with acetylsalicylic acid (Aspirin) and other nonsteroidal anti-inflammatory drugs (NSAIDs), producing additive effects. Also, she should avoid persons with infections, because her own immune system is suppressed; for example, the children she visits in hospital may have infections. In addition, she should report any fever, increased weakness and lethargy, or sore throat.
10. a. The use of systemic glucocorticoids with antidiabetic agents may reduce the hypoglycemic effect of those drugs. A baseline blood glucose level should be determined, and Peter should be monitored for any problems.
    b. Oral systemic adrenal agents should be taken with milk, food, or nonsystemic antacids (such as aluminum-, calcium-, or magnesium-containing antacids), unless contraindicated, to minimize gastro-intestinal upset. Another option is for the health care provider to order a histamine-2 (H_2) receptor antagonist or proton pump inhibitors to prevent ulcer formation (glucocorticoids may cause gastric ulcers). Patients should be encouraged *not* to take the drug with alcohol, acetylsalicylic acid (Aspirin), or other NSAIDs to minimize gastric irritation and gastric bleeding.
11. The nurse should intervene. The student nurse should, while wearing gloves, apply the medication with a sterile tongue depressor or cotton-tipped applicator if the skin is intact. If the skin is not intact, a sterile technique should be used.
12. In addition to receiving routine teaching about inhaler administration technique, Lila should be instructed to rinse with lukewarm water after using the inhaler, to prevent the development of an oral fungal infection.

Case Study

1. Administration of prednisone causes the body to stop producing hormones; tapering the dose allows the body time to start making them again. Sudden discontinuation of this drug can precipitate an adrenal crisis caused by a sudden drop in the serum levels of cortisone. Also, a short term of therapy will reduce the effects that often occur with long-term therapy.
2. Short- or long-term therapy may cause steroid psychosis. In addition, long-term effects cause Cushings symptoms, including moon face, weight gain, muscle wasting, and increased deposition of fat in the trunk area, leading to truncal obesity.
3. A glucocorticoid. Biological functions of glucocorticoids include anti-inflammatory actions, maintenance

of normal blood pressure, carbohydrate and protein metabolism, fat metabolism, and stress effects. Biological functions of mineralocorticoids include sodium and water resorption, blood pressure control, and potassium levels and pH of blood.

4. The best time for the patient to take this drug is early in the morning (0600 to 0900) because this results in the least amount of adrenal suppression.

CHAPTER 35
Women's Health Drugs

Chapter Review

1. b, c, d, e, f
2. a
3. a
4. b
5. b
6. c, e, f
7. a, d
8. 1.3 mL (1.25 rounds to 1.3)

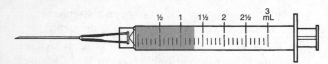

9. 10 mL

Critical Thinking and Application

10. a. The nurse should ask Osvalda if she is taking medication for depression. Estrogen therapy is indicated for the symptoms of menopause, but the use of estrogen with a tricyclic antidepressant may result in toxicity of the latter drug.
    b. The smallest dose of estrogen that alleviates the symptoms is used for the shortest possible time.
11. a. The health care provider will probably prescribe medroxyprogesterone, which is indicated for treatment of secondary amenorrhea.
    b. Brenda's dose of antidiabetic drug may need to be adjusted because of a possible decrease in glucose tolerance when progestins and antidiabetic drugs are taken together.
12. a. Perhaps the patient's prescription could be switched to a 28-day form of norethindrone/ethinyl estradiol, which is taken for all 28 days of the menstrual cycle rather than for 3 weeks with 1 week off.
    b. One of the benefits of oral contraceptive use is decreased blood loss during menstruation.
13. a. Choriogonadotropin alfa is often given in a carefully timed fashion after follicle-stimulating hormone–active therapy with a drug such as

mentropin or clomiphene, when patient monitoring indicates insufficient maturation of ovarian follicles. Once the ovaries have been sufficiently stimulated (with 9 to 12 days of therapy), then a single large dose of choriogonadotropin alfa is given the next day.
    b. This course of drugs may be repeated a second and third time if needed.
14. Ilsa needs to know that smoking can diminish the therapeutic effects of the estrogen she is taking and can add to the risk of thrombosis. Also, she should be cautioned to wear sunscreen while in Aruba, because estrogen makes the skin more susceptible to sunburn.
15. a. Vee is assuming that the medication is estrogen therapy. Alendronate (Fosamax) is indicated to prevent osteoporosis in postmenopausal women. The nurse will need to explain to her that alendronate is the first nonestrogen, nonhormonal medication used for prevention of bone loss in the early postmenopausal period; for women who experience early menopause, the dose of 5 mg daily is recommended.
    b. Besides the early menopause Vee experienced, other risk factors associated with the development of postmenopausal osteoporosis include thin body build, White or Asian race, a family history of osteoporosis, and moderately low bone mass. She would need to be assessed for these other risk factors.
16. Megestrol is used in the management of anorexia, cachexia, or unexplained substantial weight loss in patients with acquired immune deficiency syndrome (AIDS). In addition, it may be used to stimulate appetite and promote weight gain in patients (male or female) with cancer.

Case Study

1. The nonpharmacological treatment of premature labour includes bed rest, sedation, and hydration. Olivia should be placed in the left lateral recumbent position to minimize hypotension and increase blood flow to the kidneys and blood flow to the fetus.
2. In theory, tocolytic drugs are used to delay premature labour for up to 48 hours in order to gain time to allow steroids to hasten fetal lung development. One example of a tocolytic drug is ritodrine, a β_2-adrenergic agonist, which relaxes the uterus by stimulating the β_2-adrenergic receptors of the uterine muscle, resulting in a decrease in the intensity and frequency of uterine contractions. Ritodrine was removed from the Canadian market because of adverse effects of maternal pulmonary edema. Magnesium sulphate acts as competitive antagonist to calcium entry into the myocyte, resulting in

decreased myometrial contractility. However, the use of tocolytics has not reduced the risk of preterm births, the risk of low birth weights, or improved neonatal outcomes. In addition, tocolytics are associated with maternal adverse effects. Health Canada has not approved any drug for use as a tocolytic.

CHAPTER 36
Men's Health Drugs

Chapter Review

1. b
2. b, d, f
3. a
4. d
5. c
6. a
7. a, b, e
8. a. The 200 mg/mL strength is most appropriate. Using the 100 mg/mL strength would require 3 mL, which may require two separate injections.
   b. The nurse will administer 1.5 mL of the 200 mg/mL strength.

Critical Thinking and Application

9. a. Testosterone's poor performance in the oral dosage form is due to the fact that most of a dose is metabolized and destroyed by the liver before it can reach the circulation.
   b. Methyltestosterone (Android) and fluoxymesterone (Halotestin). These are both testosterone derivatives that are effective when given orally (or buccally in the case of methyltestosterone).
   c. With either of the above-mentioned drugs, contraindications that could apply to Manuel include significant cardiac, hepatic, or renal disease; male breast cancer; genital bleeding; and prostate cancer.
10. a. With actuated metered-dose pumps, each forced depression (actuation) of the pump will expel a specific (metered) dose of drug through a mouthpiece (the actuator). The label "60 actuation metered-dose" means the pump can be depressed 60 times, delivering 1.25 g of gel per actuation, for a total of 75 g of gel (the product usually has 88 g to take into account priming; see *b*, below). Ky should therefore be careful to note how many times he is pumping the canister in order to get the right dosage of testosterone, which would usually be 5 g of gel (equivalent to 50 mg of testosterone) per day.

b. The metered-dose AndroGel pump has to be primed prior to use; this usually takes about five depressions to remove the air, followed by gel discharge. The initial two gel discharges should be discarded so that an accurate gel dose is delivered. Ky should be especially careful when discarding the waste gel, to make sure other household members do not accidentally eat or touch it, especially since he is living with two small children.

11. With finasteride, education about the drug's therapeutic effects as well as adverse effects should be provided at the patient's education level. Female family members, significant others, and caregivers who are pregnant or of childbearing age should be educated about the need to avoid exposure while handling this drug, especially the need to avoid touching any broken or crushed tablets, which could result in exposure to the drug and the risk of teratogenic effects. Wearing gloves is recommended. Finasteride may be given orally without regard to meals. It should be protected from exposure to light and heat.

12. The Testoderm patch is applied only to the scrotal skin. The skin should be clean dry scrotal skin that has been shaved for optimal skin contact. These patches are replaced every day. Androderm patches should be applied to clean dry skin on the back, abdomen, upper arms, or thighs; the scrotum and bony areas (shoulder, hip) should be avoided. These patches are often ordered to be changed every 7 days. AndroGel is applied daily to the shoulders, arms, or abdominal skin.

Case Study

1. Sildenafil (Viagra) should be used cautiously in patients with renal disorders, hypertension, diabetes, and cardiovascular disease. It is contraindicated if Abu is taking nitrates, because of the danger for severe hypotensive effects.
2. He should be told that headache, dizziness, flushing, and dyspepsia are the most common reported adverse effects of sildenafil. In addition, sildenafil is highly protein bound and may interact with many drugs. Abu should check with the doctor before taking any other medication.
3. Older adults experience declining liver function, so drugs may not be metabolized as effectively as when these individuals were younger. In addition, there have been reports of vision loss in men who have been taking this class of drug.
4. He should take sildenafil 1 hour before intercourse.

CHAPTER 37
Antihistamines, Decongestants, Antitussives, and Expectorants

Chapter Review

1. a, b, c, e
2. a
3. b, e
4. c
5. b
6. d
7. a. 15 mL (See Overview of Dosage Calculations, Section II.)

   b.

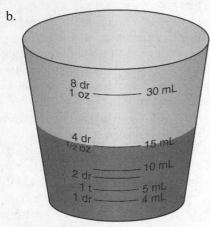

8. 2.5 mL

Critical Thinking and Application

9. No. Ling is likely experiencing rebound congestion caused by sustained use of oxymetazoline HCl (Afrin Sinus and Allergy) for several days.
10. Keith is exhibiting symptoms of the cardiovascular effects that can occur when a topically applied adrenergic nasal decongestant is somewhat absorbed into the bloodstream.
11. The mechanism of action of dextromethorphan (Benylin) is the same as that of the other drugs. It suppresses the cough reflex through direct action on the cough centre in the central nervous system (medulla). It also provides analgesia and has a drying effect on the mucosa of the respiratory tract, also increasing the viscosity of respiratory secretions. This helps to reduce such symptoms as runny nose and postnasal drip. However, because it is not an opioid, it does not have analgesic properties, nor does it cause addiction or central nervous system depression. Dextromethorphan may potentiate the serotonergic effects of monoamine oxydase inhibitors, and thus concurrent administration is contraindicated.
12. First, Lisa's brother received Robitussin AC, a narcotic antitussive containing codeine, for his cough; Lisa has been prescribed Robitussin, an expectorant, for her nonproductive cough associated with acute bronchitis. Second, even if the two children were prescribed the same drug, Lisa is only 5 years old and requires a smaller dosage than her brother requires.
13. The best answer is that antihistamines should generally be used with caution in lactating mothers. The decision is made by weighing the drug's potential effect on the baby against the need for Britney to take the medication.

Case Study

1. James's diabetes should not affect his treatment.
2. The topical diphenhydramine (Anti-Itch Cream) might come in combination with a drug such as calamine, camphor, or zinc oxide.
3. James should be informed that taking any of the sedating antihistamines may precipitate drowsiness; thus, he should be told to avoid driving or operating heavy machinery should these adverse effects occur or until he knows how he will respond to the medication.
4. Yes. James should be instructed not to consume alcohol or take other central nervous system depressants, because they may interact with the diphenhydramine to exacerbate drowsiness and sedation.

CHAPTER 38
Respiratory Drugs

Chapter Review

1. b, d, e, f
2. d
3. d
4. b
5. c
6. a
7. After 25 days (8 puffs per day, divided into 200 doses)
8. 1.8 mg

Critical Thinking and Application

9. Tom is exhibiting some adverse effects of theophylline therapy, and the level in his blood is probably too high. (The common therapeutic range for theophylline in the blood is 55 to 110 mcmol/L.) Tom may require a reduction in dosage.
10. The nurse first needs to know how much Willie weighs. The dosage of subcutaneous epinephrine is 0.01–0.03 mg/kg q5 min prn.

11. Sylvia is exhibiting dose-related adverse effects of the salbutamol (Ventolin), possibly because she used it too frequently. Sylvia needs to be reminded to use her medication exactly as prescribed.

12. a. Anticholinergics, corticosteroids, and ß-agonists
    b. Of concern is Roberta's glaucoma. The use of ipratropium bromide, an anticholinergic, is contraindicated in patients with glaucoma, and corticosteroids should be used with caution in patients with glaucoma.

13. a. A disadvantage to administering the corticosteroids orally is that they can then have systemic effects, such as adrenocortical insufficiency; increased susceptibility to infection; fluid and electrolyte disturbances; and endocrine, dermatological, and nervous system effects. Another disadvantage is that they can also interact with other systemically administered drugs. (The advantage to administering corticosteroids by inhalation is that their action is limited to the topical site of action: the lungs. In that way, they have no systemic effects and cannot interact with other systemically administered drugs.)
    b. Yes. The use of an inhaled corticosteroid frequently allows a reduction in the daily dose of the systemic corticosteroid. This reduction should be gradual.

14. a. Advair contains fluticasone propionate (a corticosteroid) and salmeterol xinaforte (a long-acting bronchodilator). Advair is used for the maintenance treatment of asthma.
    b. A rapid-onset short-duration inhaled bronchodilator (e.g., salbutamol) should be used to relieve Sam's acute asthmatic symptoms.

15. His problem could be that he ingests foods and beverages that contain caffeine (e.g., chocolate, coffee, cola, cocoa, and tea); their consumption can exacerbate central nervous system stimulation.

Case Study

1. These drugs are not direct bronchodilators; they work to reduce the inflammatory response in the lungs.
2. The nurse should tell Jennie that antiasthma medications are primarily used for oral prophylaxis and chronic treatment of asthma and are not recommended for treatment of acute asthma attacks.
3. There are no interactions between ibuprofen and montelukast; however, the nurse should advise Jennie to continue to check with her health care provider before taking other over-the-counter medications.
4. No. These agents should be taken every night on a continuous schedule even if symptoms improve.

CHAPTER 39
Acid-Controlling Drugs

Chapter Review

1. b
2. c
3. d
4. b, d, e
5. b
6. 2 mL
7. 200 mL/hr

Critical Thinking and Application

8. Omeprazole (Losec, Nexium) should be taken before meals, and the entire capsule should be taken whole—not crushed, opened, or chewed. Omeprazole may also be given with antacids, if ordered. As with omeprazole, most of the proton pump inhibitors are given on a short-term basis, and this should be emphasized to patients.
9. Patients (such as Kurt) who have hypertension or a history of heart failure should use antacids that are low in sodium. Kurt should also be told to take the antacid alone, not at the same time as other medications (unless specifically instructed to do so), because the antacid will interfere with the absorption of the other medications. Antacids should be taken 1 hour before or 1 to 2 hours after other medications. If symptoms continue or worsen, he should consult his health care provider.
10. The nurse should tell Vlad that antacids may promote premature dissolving of the enteric coating; if the coating is destroyed early in the stomach, gastrointestinal upset may occur. Vlad should take the acetylsalicylic acid (Aspirin) tablets with food, not with antacids.
11. Frank will likely be placed on a combination drug therapy that is referred to as "triple therapy," which involves the use of a proton pump inhibitor such as lansoprazole (Apo-Lansoprazole) in addition to two different antibiotics, such as amoxicillin and clarithromycin, for 7 to 14 days. Often the recommended drug combinations are packaged together for convenience.
12. Stress ulcer prophylaxis (or therapy to prevent severe gastro-intestinal damage) is undertaken in almost every critically ill patient in an Intensive Care Unit and for many patients in general medical surgical units.
13. e
14. i
15. a, b

16. f
17. d
18. b
19. g

Case Study

1. Although histamine-2 (H₂) antagonists are available over the counter, the dose of the over-the-counter preparation is generally half the strength of the usual prescription dose.
2. The drug effects of H₂ blockers are limited to specific blocking actions on the parietal cells of the gastric glands in the stomach. As a result, hydrogen ion production is decreased, which leads to an increase in the pH of the stomach (i.e., decreased stomach acid).
3. The use of H₂ receptor antagonists is contraindicated in patients who have a known drug allergy or who have impaired kidney function or liver disease. Cautious use is recommended in patients who are confused or disoriented or in older adults. Interactions may occur with drug that have a narrow therapeutic range. Caution should be used if Eda is taking theophylline (Theolair) for her asthma. Patients requiring these medications should avoid acetylsalicylic acid (Aspirin) and other nonsteroidal anti-inflammatory drugs, alcohol, and caffeine because of their ulcerogenic or gastro-intestinal tract–irritating effects.
4. Smoking has been shown to decrease the effectiveness of H₂ blockers because the absorption of H₂ antagonists may be impaired in individuals who smoke. Hopefully, if Eda is not smoking, this will not be a problem for her, but spending several hours in a smoke-filled room may have an effect. Also, the beer and possibly spicy pizza may aggravate the underlying condition.

CHAPTER 40
Antidiarrheal Drugs and Laxatives

Chapter Review

1. d
2. a
3. d
4. c
5. a, d
6. a. 1.5 mg per dose (6 mg per day)
   b. 3 mL per dose
7. 7.5 mL

Critical Thinking and Application

8. The nurse should inform Anna that darkening of the tongue or stool is a temporary and harmless adverse effect associated with bismuth subsalicylate (Pepto-Bismol).
9. The nurse can explain that the use of belladonna alkaloid preparations, also known as anticholinergics, is contraindicated for patients with narrow-angle glaucoma. In Canada, belladonna is available only in combination with opium, so Martina's choices are limited even if she had no contraindications for this drug.
10. Several factors may be causing Hillary's constipation: lack of proper exercise, poor diet (which might involve inadequate roughage and an excess of dairy products), use of aluminum-containing antacids, and stress.
11. a. The bulk-forming laxatives tend to produce normal stools, have few systemic effects, and are among the safest available.
    b. Ira should be instructed to mix the medication with at least 180 to 240 mL of fluid and to drink it immediately. It should be taken alone (i.e., not with food) and, as per the package insert instructions, usually in the morning and evening.
12. a. Because glycerin is mild. (Thus, it is often used in children.)
    b. Abdominal bloating and rectal irritation

Critical Thinking Crossword

Across
6. emollient
7. probiotic
8. saline
9. bulk forming

Down
1. adsorbent
2. opiates
3. hyperosmotic
4. stimulant
5. anticholinergic

Case Study

1. The probable cause of Charles's diarrhea is the antibiotic therapy, which destroys the balance of normal flora in the intestines, and diarrhea-causing bacteria proliferate.
2. *Lactobacillus acidophilus* is indicated for diarrhea caused by antibiotic treatment that has destroyed the normal intestinal flora.
3. By exogenously supplying these bacteria, which helps restore the balance of normal flora and suppress the growth of diarrhea-causing bacteria.

4. It is considered a dietary supplement; it is often used for uncomplicated diarrhea, even though this is an off-label (non–Health Canada–approved) use.

CHAPTER 41
Antiemetic and Antinausea Drugs

Chapter Review

1. a, b, d, e
2. c, e
3. d
4. c
5. b
6. 2 mL

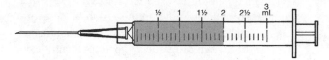

7. 30 mL

Critical Thinking and Application

8. a. The nurse should tell Petra that she should take the metoclopramide 30 minutes before meals and at bedtime.
   b. Petra should be cautioned about taking the medication with alcohol owing to the possible toxicity and central nervous system depression that can occur.
9. This drug is available in oral, intramuscular, intravenous, and rectal forms, but because Nellie is on "nil per os" (nothing-by-mouth) status and has no intravenous access, the intramuscular route was ordered. The nurses can call Nellie's health care provider for an alternative route, but the route cannot be changed without an order because the dosage may be different.
10. Dronabinol is a synthetic derivative of the major active substance in marijuana. The nurse should explain to Chuck that dronabinol is used to stimulate appetite and weight gain in patients with acquired immune deficiency syndrome.

Case Study

1. The only listed contraindication is drug allergy.
2. Antiemetics are often administered before a chemotherapy drug is given, frequently 30 minutes to 3 hours before treatment. Taking it only at the onset of nausea would have no useful effect.
3. Headache is caused by the ondansetron and can be relieved with acetaminophen.

CHAPTER 42
Nutritional Supplements

Chapter Review

1. a
2. c
3. a, c, d, e
4. c
5. a
6. d
7. 900 mL

Critical Thinking and Application

8. a. The advantages of the newer tubes are that they are thinner and more pliable for better patient tolerance. However, they also make checking for gastric aspiration more difficult.
   b. If Pauline is lactose intolerant, she would experience cramping, diarrhea, abdominal bloating, and flatulence with the ingestion of lactose. In this case, lactose-free solutions should be used.
   c. The residual amount should not be more than 2 hours' worth of feeding, which in this case is no more than 100 mL. The nurse should return the aspirate, withhold the feeding, elevate the head of the bed, and notify the health care provider.
9. Ronaldo shows signs of fluid overload. The first thing the nurse should do is slow his infusion rate, then remain with him and contact the health care provider immediately. The nurse should continually assess his vital signs. Next time, the nurse can prevent this by maintaining intravenous rates, assessing the intravenous infusion every hour, and monitoring the patient's fluid status.

Critical Thinking Crossword

Across
1. erythromycin
4. anabolism
5. gastrostomy
8. absorptive
10. fatty acid
11. essential
12. nitrogen

Down
2. catabolism
3. enteral
6. semiessential
7. metabolism
8. arginine
9. phlebitis

Case Study

1. If total parenteral nutrition is discontinued abruptly, rebound hypoglycemia may occur because the pancreas has not had time to adapt to the reduced blood glucose levels. Hypoglycemia is manifested by cold clammy skin, dizziness, tachycardia, and tingling of the extremities.
2. To prevent hypoglycemia, the nurse should hang a solution of 5% to 10% glucose to infuse until bag four is ready. The nurse should also call to make sure the pharmacy is preparing the infusion bag.
3. During this infusion, Genevieve's blood glucose levels should be monitored on a regular basis. The nurse should assess for signs of hyperglycemia as well as hypoglycemia, signs of infection, and signs of fluid overload.

CHAPTER 43
Antibiotics Part 1: Sulphonamides, Penicillins, Cephalosporins, Macrolides, and Tetracyclines

Chapter Review

1. b, d, e
2. a
3. b
4. c
5. d
6. d
7. 10 mL

Critical Thinking and Application

8. Cefoxitin is frequently used for patients undergoing abdominal or colorectal surgeries, because it can kill intestinal bacteria such as gram-positive, gram-negative, and anaerobic bacteria.
9. a. Sean should not take the doxycycline (Doxycin) with milk because doing so can result in a significant reduction in the oral absorption of the medication. Sean should also be aware that tetracyclines can cause photosensitity; he should avoid sunlight.
   b. The diarrhea is probably the result of an alteration of the intestinal flora, caused by the drug therapy.
10. Sandra is experiencing a superinfection because the antibiotics that she has been taking for the bronchitis have reduced the normal vaginal bacterial flora, and the yeast that is usually kept in balance by this normal flora has an opportunity to grow and cause an infection.

Critical Thinking Crossword

Across
3. prophylactic
6. tetracycline
7. penicillin
8. bactericidal
9. cephalosporin

Down
1. macrolide
2. sulphonamide
4. bacteriostatic
5. superinfection

Case Study

1. This patient should be assessed for severe hepatitis, glomerular nephritis, and uremia. Also, the use of sulphamethoxazole trimethoprim is contraindicated in cases of known drug allergy to sulphonamides or chemically related drugs such as sulphonylureas (used for diabetes), thiazide and loop diuretics, and carbonic anhydrase inhibitors.
2. Yes. If he is taking a sulphonylurea for the type 2 diabetes, close monitoring is needed because sulphonamides can potentiate the hypoglycemic effects of sulphonylureas in diabetes. In addition, even though he is currently receiving intravenous heparin and not warfarin, he may be placed on oral anticoagulants soon, so the nurse should keep in mind that sulphonamides can potentiate the anticoagulant effects of warfarin and lead to hemorrhage.
3. These antibiotics achieve high concentrations in the kidneys, through which they are eliminated. Therefore, they are primarily used in the treatment of urinary tract infections.
4. Sulphonamides do not actually destroy bacteria, but they inhibit bacterial growth. For this reason, they are considered bacteriostatic antibiotics; bactericidal antibiotics kill bacteria.

CHAPTER 44
Antibiotics Part 2: Aminoglycosides, Fluoroquinolones, and Other Drugs

Chapter Review

1. c
2. a
3. a, b, c, d, e
4. a
5. b, c, d
6. 40 mL
7. 187.5 mg

Critical Thinking and Application

8. The current practice is once-a-day aminoglycoside dosing. Thus, the nurse can explain to Angie that studies have shown that once-daily dosing provides a sufficient plasma drug concentration to kill bacteria and also has equal or lower risk of toxicity compared with multiple-daily dosing. Hopefully, this type of dosing will be safer and more effective for Angie.

9. A blood sample for measurement of "trough" level is drawn at least 18 hours after a dose is administered (24 hours if the patient has kidney impairment). The therapeutic goal is a trough level at or below 1 mcg/mL. If the trough level is above 2 mcg/mL, the patient is at greater risk for ototoxicity and nephrotoxicity. Trough levels should be monitored once every 3 days until the drug is stopped. In addition, kidney function is monitored by measuring serum creatinine levels. A rising serum creatinine suggests reduced creatinine clearance by the kidneys. Serum creatinine level should be measured at least twice weekly.

10. Yes. In patients who receive amiodarone therapy, dangerous cardiac dysrhythmias are more likely to occur when quinolones are taken. Another drug besides levofloxacin may show effectiveness against the bacteria that is causing the infection.

11. Nitrofurantoin (MacroBID) is used primarily to treat urinary tract infections because it is excreted via the kidneys and concentrates in the urine. It can cause significant kidney impairment but is usually well tolerated if the patient is kept well hydrated. The purpose of forcing fluids is to facilitate the elimination of the drug. Consequently, the drug will exert its desired effect, and the patient will not be at risk for kidney damage.

Case Study

1. Ototoxicity and nephrotoxicity. Symptoms of ototoxicity include dizziness, tinnitus, and hearing loss. Symptoms of nephrotoxicity include urinary casts, proteinuria, and increased blood urea nitrogen and serum creatinine levels. Keeping the drug blood levels (peak and trough) within a specific therapeutic range can help prevent those toxicities.

2. Aminoglycosides and penicillins are often used together because they have a synergistic effect; that is, the combined effect of the two drugs is greater than that of either drug alone.

3. There is certainly a concern. The desired trough level is 1 mcg/mL, so a level of 3 mcg/mL could mean that Virgil is receiving a dose that is too high. The increased serum creatinine level is also a concern because it could be an indication of impaired kidney

function. The health care provider should be notified immediately and doses of the aminoglycoside withheld until the health care provider responds.

CHAPTER 45
Antiviral Drugs

Chapter Review

1. d
2. d
3. a
4. c
5. a, b
6. b
7. 5 mL
8. 22 mg

Critical Thinking and Application

9. Yes. Zidovudine (Retrovir [AZT]), one of the few anti-HIV drugs known to prolong patient survival, can be used for maternal and fetal treatment. Between 14 and 34 weeks of pregnancy, Amy can receive oral zidovudine capsules. During labour, she can receive zidovudine intravenously. Oral drug therapy (syrup) for the infant can begin within 12 hours of delivery and continue for 6 weeks. However, transmission to infants may still occur in some cases despite the use of this regimen.

10. a. Acyclovir (Zovirax) is indicated for the varicella-zoster virus (shingles). The greatest benefit occurs when treatment is initiated within 48 hours of the onset of lesions.
    b. Bailey can be treated with acyclovir again; it is the drug of choice for treatment of both initial and recurrent episodes of shingles.

11. a. Ribavirin (Virazole) is used to treat infections caused by respiratory syncytial virus.
    b. Yes. Brenda's treatment will last at least 3 days but not more than 7 days. Treatment with ribavirin should be started as soon as possible within the first 3 days of an infection with respiratory syncytial virus.

12. No. The nurse's co-worker is doing fine. Acyclovir administered by intravenous infusion is first diluted in sterile water or in a solution recommended by the manufacturer and is administered slowly over at least 1 hour.

13. No. Therapy with oseltamivir (Tamiflu) should begin within 2 days of the onset of influenza. It is probably too late for this drug to be effective for Stacey.

Case Study

1. The nurse teaches Simon to wear a glove or finger cot when applying topical acyclovir (Zovirax) to the affected area, which should be kept clean and dry. Also, he should not use any other creams or ointments on the area.
2. The nurse should tell Simon that his herpes cannot be "cured," although the acyclovir will help manage the symptoms.
3. The nurse should stress the importance of treatment for Simon and his sexual partner and should discuss how to prevent transmission of the virus.
4. There are several viruses in the Herpesviridae family, including herpes simplex type 1 (HSV-1), which causes mucocutaneous herpes, usually manifest by blisters around the mouth; varicella-zoster virus (herpes simplex type 3 [HSV-3]), which causes both chicken pox and shingles; herpesvirus type 4 (also called Epstein-Barr virus [EBV]); and herpesvirus type 8, which is believed by some to cause Kaposi's sarcoma, a cancer associated with acquired immune deficiency syndrome.

CHAPTER 46
Antitubercular Drugs

Chapter Review

1. a
2. b
3. a, b, c
4. c
5. a
6. 3 tablets
7. 1800 mg; yes, maximum dose is 2 g (2000 mg)

Critical Thinking and Application

8. a. Liver function studies should be performed because isoniazid can cause liver impairment. A complete blood count, including hemoglobulin and hematocrit value, should be done because of the hematological disorders isoniazid can cause.
   b. Diane may be a slow acetylator. Acetylation, the process by which isoniazid is metabolized in the liver, requires certain enzymes to break down the isoniazid. In slow acetylators, who have a genetic deficiency of the enzymes, the isoniazid accumulates. The dosage of isoniazid may need to be adjusted downward in these patients.
9. a. Streptomycin is administered intramuscularly, deep in a large muscle mass, and the sites are rotated.

   b. Although it may not be a concern in terms of Ina's streptomycin therapy, oral contraceptives become ineffective when given with rifampin. If rifampin is part of her therapy, Ina should switch to another form of birth control.
10. A thorough eye examination may be called for before the institution of therapy because ethambutol can cause a decrease in visual acuity resulting from optic neuritis, which is also a contraindication to the use of ethambutol.
11. a. Fabian needs to know that his adherence to therapy is essential for achieving a cure. Although he is keeping his follow-up appointments, Fabian also needs to take his medication as ordered. He should be warned to not consume alcohol, and he should be encouraged to take care of himself with adequate nutrition, rest, and relaxation.
    b. The therapeutic response can be confirmed by results of laboratory studies (sputum culture and sensitivity tests) and chest radiographic findings.
12. a. Frannie, as with all patients taking antituberculosis drugs, needs to adhere to the therapy and keep her follow-up appointments. She should be reminded that she can spread the disease during the initial period of the illness; she should wash her hands frequently and cover her mouth when coughing or sneezing. Frannie also needs adequate nutrition and rest.
    b. The nurse thinks it is likely that Frannie is on rifampin therapy. She should be told that her urine, stool, saliva, sputum, sweat, or tears may become red-orange-brown and that this is an effect of rifampin therapy.

Case Study

1. George's gout is a consideration; pyrazinamide (Tebrazid) can cause hyperuricemia, so gout or flare-ups of gout can occur in susceptible patients. His diabetes is a concern as well; ethambutol (Etibi) should be used cautiously in patients with diabetes. A baseline hearing test should be performed if streptomycin is considered, because this drug may cause ototoxicity.
2. An individual with a genetic deficiency of the liver enzymes that metabolize medications can be classified as a "slow acetylator." When isoniazid is taken by slow acetylators, the drug accumulates because there is not enough of the enzymes to break down the isoniazid. As a result, the dosage of isoniazid may need to be reduced.
3. Results of liver function tests should be assessed carefully before therapy is initiated, because some drugs (isoniazid, pyrazinamide) are

heptatotoxic. Liver function test results should be monitored closely during therapy as well.

4. Patients should take pyridoxine (vitamin B_6) as prescribed by the health care provider to prevent some of the neurological adverse effects of isoniazid, such as peripheral neuritis.

CHAPTER 47
Antifungal Drugs

Chapter Review

1. c
2. b, c, e, g
3. d
4. b
5. a
6. 50 mL per hour
7. 660 mg for the 6 mg/kg dose; 440 mg for the 4 mg/kg dose

Critical Thinking and Application

8. a. Fluconazole (Diflucan), unlike itraconazole, can pass into the cerebrospinal fluid, making fluconazole effective in the treatment of cryptococcal meningitis. It is considered to be the most effective of the imidazoles for treating several infections.
   b. The nurse will explain that unfortunately, Yun will need to remain on a reduced dosage of the medication for 10 to 12 weeks after the negative results of the cerebrospinal fluid culture.

9. a. The amphotericin B (Fungizone) should be diluted according to the manufacturer's guidelines. Sterile water without a bacteriostatic agent (such as benzyl alcohol, which may cause precipitation of the antibiotic) is recommended for its reconstitution, and 5% dextrose in water may be used for infusion. Amphotericin B is administered by *slow* intravenous infusion over 2 to 6 hours.
   b. Fever, chills, hypotension, tachycardia, malaise, muscle and joint pain, anorexia, nausea and vomiting, and headache. These are the possible adverse effects the nurse should closely monitor for.
   c. No. Almost all patients experience these effects. To decrease the severity, the patient may be pretreated with an antipyretic (e.g., acetaminophen), an antihistamine, and an antiemetic.

10. Lewis should be made aware that he will be taking the medication for 2 to 6 weeks, until the infection clears. During that time, he should avoid alcohol because of the increased risk for hepatoxicity, and

he should take the medication with food to avoid gastro-intestinal upset. Ketoconazole also causes photophobia, so Lewis should avoid sunlight or use sunscreen and sunglasses with ultraviolet protection.

11. Nystatin oral troches or lozenges are to be dissolved slowly and completely in the mouth for the best effects and should not be chewed or swallowed. Chrissie needs a review of how to use this medication.

12. j
13. e
14. f
15. g
16. a
17. c
18. h
19. i
20. d
21. b

Case Study

1. Voriconazole (Vfend) is used for major fungal infections in patients who do not tolerate or respond to other antifungal agents.
2. Because of the risk of inducing serious cardiac dysrhythmias, the use of voriconazole is contraindicated in patients taking other drugs that are metabolized by the cytochrome P-450 enzyme 3A4 (e.g., quinidine).
3. Careful cardiac monitoring should be done if Sally is taking quinidine while taking voriconazole.

CHAPTER 48
Antimalarial, Antiprotozoal, and Anthelmintic Drugs

Chapter Review

1. a
2. b
3. c
4. b, c, d, e
5. b, e
6. d
7. a, c
8. The dose is 280 mg (4 mg/kg × 70 kg); the nurse will draw up 4.7 mL of the diluted solution for the infusion.
9. 5 tablets

Critical Thinking and Application

10. Malaria is caused by *Plasmodium* organisms. During the asexual stage of the *Plasmodium* life cycle,

which occurs in the human host, the parasite resides for a short time outside the erythrocyte. This is called the exoerythrocytic phase. The most effective agent for eradicating the parasite during this phase is primaquine.

11. Mefloquine (Lariam) is indicated for the treatment of chloroquine-resistant malaria.

12. a. Each of these three patients has a protozoal infection.

   b. The patient with the intestinal disorder has giardiasis; the patient with acquired immune deficiency syndrome has pneumocystosis; and the patient with the sexually transmitted infection has trichomoniasis.

   c. The most likely drug treatment for the patient with giardiasis is metronidazole. For the patient with acquired immune deficiency syndrome who has pneumocystosis, the most likely drugs for treatment include dapsone, atovaquone, primaquine, and clindamycin. For the patient with the sexually transmitted infection who has trichomoniasis, the most likely drug for treatment is metronidazole.

Case Study

1. Intestinal roundworms are diagnosed on the basis of symptoms and examination of stool specimens.

2. Contraindications to pyrantel (Combantin) include pregnancy and allergy to the medication. Even though Sandra is only 15 years of age, she should be assessed for possible pregnancy before this medication is given.

3. Based on Sandra's weight of 57 kg, the dose would be 627 mg (57 mg × 57 kg).

4. Pyrantel is generally well tolerated. The infrequent adverse effects are limited to vomiting and diarrhea. Headache, insomnia, irritability, drowsiness, dizziness, anorexia, abdominal cramps, nausea, and rash have also been reported.

CHAPTER 49
Anti-Inflammatory and Antigout Drugs

Chapter Review

1. b
2. b
3. a, b, d, e
4. c
5. a, c, d
6. c
7. No. The child weighs 15 kg, and the appropriate dose for that weight is 50 mg PO twice daily, not 100 mg.

8. 1.3 mL

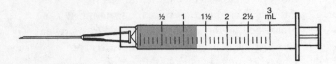

Critical Thinking and Application

9. Her symptoms and history suggest chronic salicylate intoxication, which occurs as a result of either high dosages of Aspirin or prolonged therapy with high dosages of Aspirin.

10. Sergio has an acute overdose of a nonsalicylate nonsteroidal anti-inflammatory drug (NAID). If the condition progresses, symptoms can include intense headache, dizziness, cerebral edema, cardiac arrest, and even death in extreme cases.

11. Sammy needs to know that compliance with the entire medical regimen is important for the success of his treatment for gout. Allopurinol needs to be taken with meals to help prevent the occurrence of gastro-intestinal symptoms such as nausea, vomiting, and anorexia. Increase fluids to 3 L per day, and hazardous activities must be avoided if dizziness or drowsiness occurs with the drug. Also, alcohol and caffeine need to be avoided because these drugs will increase uric acid levels and decrease the levels of allopurinol.

12. a. The nurse will tell Eileen that ketorolac (Toradol) is indicated for the short-term management (up to 5 days) of moderate to severe acute pain that requires analgesia at the opioid level. It is not indicated for treatment of minor or persistent painful conditions.

   b. The main adverse effects of ketorolac (Toradol) include renal impairment, gastro-intestinal pain, dyspepsia, and nausea. These problems limit the length of time that the medication can be used.

Case Study

1. The specific cyclooxygenase-2 (COX-2) selectivity of these drugs allows them to control the inflammation and pain while not producing some of the toxicity associated with therapy with nonsteroidal anti-inflammatory drugs.

2. The most common adverse effects include fatigue, dizziness, lower-extremity edema, hypertension, dyspepsia, nausea, heartburn, and epigastric discomfort. The nurse should report to the health care provider immediately any stomach pain, unusual bleeding, or blood in vomit or stool. Chest pain, palpitations, and any gastro-intestinal problems should be reported as well.

3. The nurse will tell Sadie that she should avoid alcohol and acetylsalicytic acid (Aspirin) while taking this medication and should check with her health care provider before taking any over-the-counter medications.

CHAPTER 50
Immunosuppressant Drugs

Chapter Review

1. b
2. c
3. c
4. a
5. a, c, d, e
6. a, d
7. a, c, f
8. 4 capsules
9. a. 750 mg for this dose
   b. 15 mL (See Overview of Dosage Calculations, Section II.)

Critical Thinking and Application

10. The patient should be encouraged to take cyclosporine (Neoral) with meals or mixed with milk, to prevent stomach upset.
11. Glatiramer acetate (Copaxone) is the only immunosuppressant drug that is currently indicated for the treatment of relapsing remitting multiple sclerosis. Glatiramer is used to reduce the frequency of relapses.

Case Study

1. Yes, immunosuppressant therapy will be lifelong.
2. White patches on the tongue, mucous membranes, and oral pharynx would be indicative of candidiasis.
3. She should tell Kellum that he needs to be seen by a health care provider immediately; these symptoms could indicate that he has a severe infection.
4. Patients taking immunosuppressant drugs need to avoid live vaccines. There may be a risk of an infection developing due to the administration of a live vaccine to a person with lowered immunity.

CHAPTER 51
Immunizing Drugs and Pandemic Preparedness

Chapter Review

1. b
2. d

3. a
4. a
5. c
6. a, c
7. 0.005 mg

Critical Thinking and Application

8. She will most likely receive the diphtheria, tetanus, and acellular pertussis (DTaP) vaccine (Adacel). With the recent increase in cases of pertussis, the DTaP vaccine is recommended for adults in place of the tetannus and diphtheria (Td) vaccine, which lacks the pertussis component.
9. The nurse will tell Jim that occasionally, after vaccination, the levels of antibodies against a particular pathogen decline over time, and a second dose of the vaccine is given to restore the antibody titres to a level that can protect the person against the infection. This second dose is referred to as a "booster shot."
10. The nurse explains to her that each year, a new influenza vaccine is developed, one that contains the three influenza virus strains that represent the strains that are likely to circulate in North America in the upcoming winter. The vaccination from the previous year may not be effective for the influenza virus strains in the current year.
11. Paul is experiencing more than the expected adverse effects of his vaccinations. He is probably experiencing "serum sickness," which may occur after repeated injections of equine immunizing drugs. Because his symptoms may indicate respiratory impairment, he needs to be taken to the hospital for evaluation and monitoring. He may receive analgesics, antihistamines, epinephrine, or corticosteroids to treat this reaction.
12. a. Varicella vaccine
    b. Active
    c. Active
    d. *Haemophilus influenzae* type b prophylaxis
    e. Hepatitis B virus vaccine inactivated
    f. $Rh_0(D)$ immunoglobulin
    g. Passive
    h. Active
    i. Tuberculosis prophylaxis
    j. Active
    k. Diphtheria, tetanus, acellular, and pertussis prophylaxis (pediatric)
    l. Passive
    m. Postexposure passive tetanus prophylaxis
    n. Active
    o. Diphtheria, tetanus, and acellular pertussis prophylaxis (adolescents)

Case Study

1. Rabies is a potent virus.
2. Those at high risk for rabies exposure, such as veterinarians, will receive the rabies virus vaccine (Imovax, Rabavert) as pre-exposure prophylaxis, followed by booster shots based on blood titres. This is a type of active immunization.
3. As a volunteer, the nurse will receive drugs that give both active and passive immunization. Postexposure prophylaxis is given with injections of the rabies virus vaccine (see Answer 2) and also with rabies immunoglobulin. Because rabies can progress rapidly, the body has insufficient time to mount an adequate immune defence, and death occurs before it can do so. Even though it does not stimulate an antibody response, the passive immunization confers a temporary protection that is usually sufficient to keep the invading organism from causing death. The active immunization will stimulate an antibody response.

CHAPTER 52
Antineoplastic Drugs Part 1: Cancer Overview and Cell Cycle–Specific Drugs

Chapter Review

1. a, b, c, e, f
2. d
3. a
4. b
5. c
6. d
7. a, e
8. 25,000 units; yes
9. a. 8.2 mg
   b. 8.2 mL

Critical Thinking Crossword

Across

3. spread
4. folic
7. extravasation
8. nadir
9. limiting
10. leukemia

Down

1. malignant
2. leucovorin
5. nonspecific
6. benign
7. emetic

Case Study

1. Methotrexate is an antimetabolite—specifically, a folic acid antagonist. It inhibits the action of an enzyme that is responsible for converting folic acid to a substance used by the cell to synthesize deoxyribonucleic acid for cell reproduction. As a result, the cell dies.
2. Laboratory results of white blood cell and red blood cell counts, hemoglobin level and hematocrit, platelet counts, and renal and liver function studies should be checked.
3. The concurrent administration of nonsteroidal anti-inflammatory drugs (NSAIDs) and methotrexate may lead to severe bleeding tendencies. Allen should be instructed to avoid all NSAIDs (including acetylsalicylic acid [Aspirin]) while taking methotrexate.
4. Antiemetic therapy and antacids are often needed to decrease nausea, vomiting, and gastro-intestinal upset. Because methotrexate may cause hyperuricemia (i.e., increased uric acid levels) associated with tumour lysis syndrome, allopurinol (Zyloprim) may be given. Leucovorin may be used to protect the patient from potentially fatal bone marrow suppression, a toxic effect of methotrexate.

CHAPTER 53
Antineoplastic Drugs Part 2: Cell Cycle–Nonspecific and Miscellaneous Drugs

Chapter Review

1. c
2. a
3. b
4. a, c, e, f
5. b
6. d
7. b, c, d
8. 83 mL per hour
9. 50 mL per hour

Critical Thinking and Application

10. Selena should be assessed and monitored carefully for the development of pulmonary fibrosis and pneumonitis, which can occur during treatment with bleomycin.
11. The nurse should not prepare the drug for infusion. In most facilities, institutional guidelines direct that the pharmacy department prepare these drugs. Special requirements must be met for the safety of those working with these drugs,

including the use of a laminar airflow hood and appropriate personal protection equipment (e.g., gown, mask, and gloves). It would not be safe for the nurse or for those around the nurse to mix the chemotherapy drug on the nursing unit.

12. Cytoprotective drugs help to reduce the toxicity of various antineoplastics. As a result, the adverse effects may be reduced so that increased dosages of the antineoplastic medication may be tolerated, which allows greater killing of cancer cells. Examples include the following:
    - Amifostine, used during therapy with cisplatin to reduce renal toxicity
    - Dexrazoxane, used during therapy with doxorubicin to reduce cardiac toxicity

Case Study

1. Cisplatin is associated with nephrotoxicity, peripheral neuropathy, and ototoxicity.
2. Baseline renal studies need to be performed because this drug is highly nephrotoxic. If Gabby is receiving any other therapy that is potentially nephrotoxic (such as aminoglycoside therapy), dosage changes will need to be considered. If she has gout, concurrent use of cisplatin may result in hyperuricemia or worsening of the gout. Baseline auditory studies are needed, as well as baseline liver function studies and measurements of white blood cell count, hemoglobin level, hematocrit, and platelet level, because of the anticipated bone marrow suppression.
3. Because peripheral neuropathies may occur, numbness, tingling, or pain in the extremities should be reported to the health care provider immediately to prevent complications and enhance comfort.
4. Yes. This is a concern because dehydration while the patient is taking cisplatin may lead to kidney damage. Gabby should be reminded of the importance of hydration and should be told to contact the health care provider if she experiences dry mucous membranes, has dark amber urine or little or no urinary output, or vomits large amounts over a period of 8 hours or less. It may be a challenge, but Gabby needs to try to take in 3000 mL of fluid per day to prevent dehydration.

CHAPTER 54
Biological Response–Modifying Drugs and Antirheumatic Drugs

Chapter Review

1. b
2. a, b, c, d, e

3. c
4. a, b, d, e
5. 1.3 mL (See Overview of Dosage Calculations, Section III.)

Critical Thinking and Application

6. The major dose-limiting adverse effect of interferon is fatigue. Patients taking high dosages become so exhausted that they are often confined to bed. Pedro needs to know this before he starts the therapy in order to make an informed decision.
7. Colony-stimulating factors (CSFs) such as filgrastim (Neupogen) and pegfilgrastim (Neulasta) can be given for chemotherapy-induced leukopenia. These drugs should be administered 24 hours after the chemotherapy drugs have been administered, because the myelosuppressive effects of the chemotherapy drugs tend to cancel out the therapeutic benefits of the CSFs.
8. Methotrexate is given weekly, not daily! The nurse needs to clarify and correct this mistranscribed order. It is very important to note that the drug is given once per week, not once per day. Serious drug errors, including deaths, have occurred when the drug is given daily instead of once a week.
9. e
10. a
11. g
12. b
13. h
14. d
15. c

Case Study

1. Epoetin alpha (Epogen) is a synthetic derivative of the human hormone erythropoietin, which is produced primarily by the kidneys. It promotes the synthesis of erythrocytes (red blood cells) by stimulating the production of red blood cell precursors.
2. The hemoglobin level and hematocrit should be monitored carefully. If therapy is not halted when the target hemoglobulin of 120 g/L is reached or if the hemoglobin level and hematocrit rise too quickly, hypertension and seizures can result.
3. The nurse can tell Connie that epoetin is synthetically manufactured in mass quantities by means of recombinant deoxyribonucleic acid (DNA) technology. This technology allows the medication to be essentially identical to its endogenously produced counterpart in the body.
4. Epoetin can be given either intravenously or subcutaneously. For administration at home, Connie will need to be taught subcutaneous administration.

5. Darbepoetin alpha can be administered weekly, so the number of injections will obviously be less.

CHAPTER 55
Anemia Drugs

Chapter Review

1. d
2. b, c, f
3. c
4. b, c
5. b, c, d, e
6. d
7. a
8. 26 mg (rounded up from 25.9)

Critical Thinking and Application

9. Jack, who is about to receive his first dose of iron dextran, is at risk for fatal anaphylaxis. Because of this, a test dose of 25 mg of iron dextran should be administered by the chosen route and appropriate method of administration. An anaphylactic reaction should occur within a few moments, although waiting at least 1 hour before giving the rest of the initial dose is recommended. Iron should be administered deep in a large muscle mass via a Z-track method and a 23-gauge 4-cm needle.
10. The orange juice contains ascorbic acid (vitamin C), which enhances the absorption of iron.
11. Treatment should include suction and maintenance of the airway, correction of acidosis, and control of shock and dehydration with intravenous fluids or blood, oxygen, and a vasopressor. Abdominal radiographs can allow visualization of the tablets. A serum concentration greater than 54 mmol/L will place the child at serious risk for toxicity. Consultation with a Poison Control Centre is recommended. The child's stomach should be emptied immediately. Because many of the iron products are extended-release formulations that release their contents in the intestines rather than in the stomach, whole-gut irrigation with a polyethylene glycol solution is generally believed to be superior and more effective for decontaminating the bowel, followed by possible surgical removal of intake iron tablets. A child with severe symptoms of iron intoxication will exhibit coma, shock, or seizures. Chelation therapy with deferoxamine should be initiated.

Case Study

1. Oral forms can be given with juice (but not antacids or milk) between meals for maximal absorption.

Should gastro-intestinal distress occur, however, the iron can be taken with meals.
2. Maureen should be reminded that the use of any iron product will cause the stools to turn tarry and black.
3. Maureen should be told that one iron product cannot be substituted for another, because each product contains different forms of the iron salt in different amounts.
4. Liquid oral forms of iron should be diluted per the manufacturer instructions and taken through a plastic straw to avoid discolouration of tooth enamel.

CHAPTER 56
Dermatological Drugs

Chapter Review

1. a
2. b
3. a
4. b
5. a, b, d
6. d
7. a
8. a, b, d, e
9. 100 mL per hour
10. 167 mL per hour

Critical Thinking and Application

11. The nurse would first ask Lester about any allergies to other forms of drugs. If he has an allergy to a particular antibacterial drug, that drug should not be used topically either. If culture and sensitivity testing is to be carried out, the specimen should be collected before the first application of the antibacterial drug. In this case, the nurse can apply a thin film of clindamycin and monitor for signs of allergy to clindamycin and other antibiotics.
12. Gloves are used not only to prevent contamination from secretions but also to prevent absorption of the medication through the skin of the person applying the medication.

Case Study

1. The nurse should assess any allergies Judy may have, especially any allergies to sulphonamide drugs. Silver sulphadiazine cream should be applied only to areas that have been cleansed and debrided. The wound bed may need to be debrided before the cream can be applied.

2. The dressing helps keep the medication at the intended site and provides protection to the wound. In addition, it keeps the cream from soiling the patient's clothing.
3. The use of gloves prevents contamination of the medication and avoids exposure to Judy's wound secretions. The health care provider should apply the cream with a sterile, gloved hand.
4. The adverse effects of silver sulphadiazine are similar to those of other topical drugs and include pain, burning, and itching.

CHAPTER 57
Ophthalmic Drugs

Chapter Review

1. c
2. b
3. b
4. d
5. b, c, d, e
6. c
7. 19 drops per minute

Critical Thinking and Application

8. The effect is less pronounced in individuals with dark eyes (brown or hazel) because pigment absorbs the drugs and dark eyes have more pigment than light eyes (blue).
9. a. Dipivefrin (Propine), a pro-drug of epinephrine, has better lipophilicity than epinephrine and can penetrate into the anterior chamber of the eye. It is 4 to 11 times more potent than epinephrine in reducing intraocular pressure.
   b. Jin should report any stinging, burning, itching, lacrimation, or puffiness of the eye.
   c. No. Systemic effects are rare. They include cardiovascular effects and possibly headaches and faintness.
10. Ned may have had an allergic reaction to a preservative, such as benzalkonium chloride, in the first drug that was tried. Timolol is available in a preservative-free product.
11. The nonsteroidal anti-inflammatory drugs are considered less toxic, and they are preferred over the corticosteroids as initial topical therapy.
12. The nurse would explain that stinging is normal after instillation of the drops and that Luna should not wear her contact lenses while taking this medication.
13. The eye drops need to be administered first, then the pilocarpine gel, at least 5 minutes after the drops are administered.
14. c

15. h
16. j
17. k
18. a
19. d
20. b
21. f
22. g
23. e

Case Study

1. The ointment should be applied to the conjunctival sac, not directly onto the cornea or eyeball, moving from the inner canthus to the outer edge of the eye. Excess medication can be removed with a tissue, but Wey should not rub his eyes.
2. You tell Wey that ointments may cause a temporary blurriness to the vision because of the film that bathes the eye. This film will decrease once absorbed, and vision should become clearer. He will need to be careful and prevent himself from falling if his vision is blurry. In addition, he should not touch the tip of the drugs container to his eye or to his fingers, in order to prevent contamination of the medication.
3. You will tell Wey that burning and stinging are common but transient effects of ophthalmic antimicrobial drugs and they should subside shortly.
4. Tell Wey that he should not take this medication! It is most likely contaminated, and it is not ordered for his current problem. In addition, if the drops are a corticosteroid, there could be immunosuppressive effects, which may interfere with the antimicrobial's action.

CHAPTER 58
Otic Drugs

Chapter Review

1. a, b, d, e
2. d
3. b
4. a
5. c
6. a. 375 mg
   b. Low range (20 mg/kg): 220 mg; high range (40 mg/kg): 440 mg
   c. Yes, 375 mg is in the range of 220 mg and 440 mg.

Critical Thinking and Application

7. The nurse tells the patient he needs medical care immediately because his symptoms may be indicative of head trauma.

8. Anti-infective otic drugs are frequently combined with steroids to take advantage of the steroidal anti-inflammatory, antipruritic, and antiallergic drug effects.

9. a. Clean the ear, remove all cerumen by irrigation, and clean the dropper with alcohol. The drops also need to be at room temperature.

   b. André might become dizzy, so he should be supine when the drops are instilled.

10. a. The hydrocortisone will help to reduce the inflammation and itching associated with the infection.

    b. A drug hypersensitivity or a perforated eardrum

11. Many otic combination products contain local anaesthetic drugs because many ear disorders involve pain and inflammation. The anaesthetic effect of the local anaesthetic drugs makes them beneficial in treating these conditions.

12. a. The instructions are different for each boy. The pinna should be held up and back during the instillation of eardrops in children older than 3 years, like Drew. For children 3 years of age and younger, like Ben, the pinna should be gently pulled down and back.

    b. Reduced pain, redness, and swelling are therapeutic effects of the drug.

13. a. No. Esther's husband should warm up the eardrops to body temperature by holding the bottle under warm running water, not soaking it in hot water, particularly because he should be careful not to let water get into the bottle or damage the label.

    b. The nurse will tell Esther that she should not sit up right away. She should lie down on the side opposite the side of the affected ear for about 5 minutes after the drug is instilled. As an alternative, Esther can gently insert a small cotton ball into the ear canal to keep the drug in place, but the cotton ball should not be forced into the ear canal.

Case Study

1. Mark probably has an impaction of earwax in his ear canal. Such a buildup can cause pain and temporary deafness.

2. He should be taught that he should not insert anything into his ear canal. He will need to know how to clean his ears properly and how to use cerumen-removal drugs. The nurse may need to irrigate his ear canals before drug therapy is started.

3. This drug is given as otic drops (eardrops). Mark will need to follow the manufacturer's recommendations for administration. He should lie on the side opposite the side of the affected ear for about 5 minutes after instillation of the drug. A small cotton ball may be inserted gently into the ear canal to keep the medication there, but it should not be forced into the ear or jammed down into the ear canal. When administering the drops, Mark should pull the pinna of his ear up and back.

OVERVIEW OF DOSAGE CALCULATIONS

Introduction

Interpreting Medication Labels

1. Generic name: rifampin
   Trade name: Rifadin
   Unit dose: 150 mg capsule
   Total in container: 100 capsules
   Route: oral

2. Generic name: medroxyprogesterone acetate
   Trade name: Depo-Provera
   Unit dose: 50 mg per mL
   Total in container: 5 mL
   Route: intramuscular use only

Section I

Basic Conversions Using Ratio and Proportion

1. 600,000 mcg
2. 1,500,000 mcg
3. 5 mg
4. 5000 mg
5. 2500 mg
6. 0.9 g (Do not forget the leading zero.)
7. 8000 g
8. 0.75 L (Do not forget the leading zero.)
9. 975,000 mL
10. 0.5 L (Do not forget the leading zero.)
11. 1.5 g
12. 20 mL
13. 12 tsp
14. 6 tbsp
15. 198 lb
16. 68.2 kg (rounded to tenths)
17. 24.2 lb

Section II

Calculating Oral Doses

1. 1 tablet
   0.5 g = 500 mg. Each tablet is 500 mg; therefore, 1 tablet is needed.

2. 2 tablets
   0.5 mg = 500 mcg
   250 mcg : 1 tablet :: 500 mcg : x tablet
   Proof: 250 × 2 = 500; 1 × 500 = 500

3. 0.5 tablet
   0.25 g = 250 mg
   500 mg : 1 tablet :: 250 mg : x tablet
   Proof: 500 × 0.5 = 250; 1 × 250 = 250

4. 20 mL
   12.5 mg : 5 mL :: 50 mg : x mL
   Proof: 12.5 × 20 = 250; 5 × 50 = 250

5. 4 mL
   0.1 g = 100 mg
   125 mg : 5 mL :: 100 mg : x mL
   Proof: 125 × 4 = 500; 5 × 100 = 500

6. 3 tablets
   0.3 g = 300 mg
   100 mg : 1 tablet :: 300 mg : x tablet
   Proof: 100 × 3 = 300; 1 × 300 = 300

7. 22.5 mL
   20 mmol : 15 mL :: 30 mmol : x mL
   Proof: 20 × 22.5 = 450; 15 × 30 = 450

8. 3 capsules
   0.15 g = 150 mg
   50 mg : 1 capsule :: 150 mg : x capsule
   Proof: 50 × 3 = 150; 1 × 150 = 150

9. 4 tablets
   2 g = 2000 mg
   500 mg : 1 tablet :: 2000 mg : x tablet
   Proof: 500 × 4 = 2000; 1 × 2000 = 2000

Section III

Reconstituting Medications

1. 2 mL
   100 mg : 1 mL :: 200 mg : x mL
   Proof: 100 × 2 = 200; 1 × 200 = 200

2. 1.5 mL
   40 mg : 1 mL :: 60 mg : x mL
   Proof: 40 × 1.5 = 60; 1 × 60 = 60

3. 0.8 mL
   10,000 units : 1 mL :: 8000 units : x mL
   Proof: 10,000 × 0.8 = 8000; 1 × 8000 = 8000

4. 1.5 mL
   500 mg : 1 mL :: 750 mg : x mL
   Proof: 500 × 1.5 = 750; 1 × 750 = 750

5. 20 mL
   125 mg : 5 mL :: 500 mg : x mL
   Proof: 125 × 20 = 2500; 5 × 500 = 2500

6. Choose the concentration using the 4.6 mL diluent.
   Using the 9.6 mL diluent would necessitate giving
   3 mL intramuscularly versus the 1.5 mL using the
   4.6 mL diluent.
   1.5 mL
   200,000 units : 1 mL :: 300,000 units : x mL

Proof: 200,000 × 1.5 = 300,000; 1 × 300,000 = 300,000

7. 0.75 mL
   First: Convert micrograms to milligrams : 750 mcg
   = 0.75 mg
   1:1000 indicates 1 g in 1000 mL, or 1000 mg in
   1000 mL, or 1 mg/mL.
   1 mg : 1 mL :: 0.75 mg : x mL
   Proof: 1 × 0.75 = 0.75; 1 × 0.75 = 0.75

8. 1 mL
   NOTE: 1:5000 indicates 1 g in 5000 mL, or 1000
   mg in 5000 mL, or 0.2 mg/mL.
   0.2 mg : 1 mL :: 0.2 mg : x mL
   Proof: 0.2 × 1 = 0.2; 1 × 0.2 = 0.2

9. 9 mL
   NOTE: 10% indicates 10 g per 100 mL, or 0.1 g/mL.
   Need to ensure that units are alike: 900 mg = 0.9 g
   0.1 g : 1 mL :: 0.9 g : x mL
   Proof: 0.1 × 9 = 0.9; 1 × 0.9 = 0.9

10. 8 mL
    NOTE: 50% indicates 50 g per 100 mL, or 0.5 g/mL.
    0.5 g × 1 mL :: 4 g : x mL
    Proof: 0.5 × 8 = 4; 1 × 4 = 4

Section IV

Child Calculations

1. a. 0.46 to 47.3 mg/hr
   40 lb = 18.2 kg
   Low dose: 0.025 mg/kg/hr × 18.2 kg = 0.455,
   rounded to 0.46 mg/hr
   High dose: 2.6 mg/kg/hr × 18.2 kg = 47.32,
   rounded to 47.3 mg/hr
   b. Yes, the ordered dose of 1 mg/hr falls within the
   safe range for this child.

2. a. 75 to 150 mg/dose
   33 lb = 15 kg
   Low dose: 5 mg/kg/dose × 15 kg = 75 mg/dose
   High dose: 10 mg/kg/dose × 15 kg = 150 mg/dose
   b. 600 mg (40 mg × 15 kg = 600 mg/kg per
   24 hours)
   c. Yes, the ordered dose of 120 mg falls within the
   safe and therapeutic range for this child.

3. a. 3180–4770 mg per 24 hours
   70 lb = 31.8 kg
   Low dose: 100 mg/kg per 24 hours × 31.8 kg =
   3180 mg per 24 hours
   High dose: 150 mg/kg/24 hr × 31.8 kg = 4770 mg
   per 24 hours
   b. 1060–1590 mg per dose
   Three doses in 24 hours; 3180 ÷ 3 = 1060 mg per
   dose; 4770 ÷ 3 = 1590 mg per dose
   c. No. 1.7 g 5 1700 mg, which exceeds the safe dosage range for this drug for this child. (Did you
   remember to convert grams to milligrams?)

4. a. 0.14–0.36 mg/d

   15 lb = 6.8 kg

   Low dose: 0.02 mg/kg/d × 6.8 kg = 0.136, rounded to 0.14 mg/d

   High dose: 0.05 mg/kg/d × 6.8 kg = 0.34 mg/d

   b. 0.07–0.18 mg/dose

   "bid" doses are given twice in 24 hours. 0.14 ÷ 2 = 0.07 mg per dose; 0.36 ÷ 2 = 0.18 mg per dose

   c. Yes, 150 mcg = 0.15 mg, which falls within the safe and therapeutic dose range for this child. (Did you remember to convert micrograms [mcg] to milligrams [mg]?)

5. a. 15.5 to 34.1 mg/kg per dose

   34 lb = 15.5 kg

   Low dose: 1 mg/kg per dose × 15.5 kg = 15.5 mg per dose

   High dose: 2.2 mg/kg per dose × 15.5 kg = 34.1 mg per dose

   b. Yes, the ordered dose of 30 mg is within the safe and therapeutic dose range for this child.

6. a. 60.8–76 mcg/kg/d

   50 lb = 22.7 kg

   Low dose: 4 mcg/kg/d × 17.2 kg = 68.8 mcg/d

   High dose: 5 mcg/kg/d × 17.2 kg = 86 mcg/d

   b. No. The ordered dose (0.2 mg = 200 mcg) exceeds the safe and therapeutic dose range for this child. (Did you remember to convert micrograms to millilitres?)

Section V

Basic Intravenous Calculations

1. Start at STEP 1. You need to calculate the hourly rate.

   a. 167 mL/hr

   1000 mL : 6 h :: x : 1 hr

   $(1000 \times 1) = (6 \times x)$; 1000 = 6 x;

   x = 1000/6 = 166.66 (Round to nearest whole number.)

   Proof: 1000 × 1 = 1000; 6 × 167 = 1002 (slight difference due to previous rounding)

   (Alternative method: 1000 mL ÷ 6 hr = 166.67 or 167 mL/hr)

   b. 42 gtt/min (Round to nearest whole number.)

   STEP 2:

   drop factor

   _____× hourly rate = 15/60 × 167 =

   time (minutes)

   1/4 × 200 = 41.75, rounded to nearest whole number

2. Start at STEP 1. You need to calculate the hourly rate.

   a. 200 mL/hr

   600 mL : 3 hr :: c : 1 hr

   $(600 \times 1) = (3 \times x)$; 600 = 3 x;

   x = 600/3 = 200

Proof: 600 × 1 = 600; 3 × 200 = 600

(Alternative method: 600 mL ÷ 3 hr = 200 mL/hr)

   b. 33 gtt/min (Round to nearest whole number.)

   STEP 2:

   drop factor

   _____× hourly rate = 10/60 × 200 =

   time (minutes)

   1/6 × 200 = 33.33, rounded to nearest whole number

3. Start at STEP 1. You need to calculate the hourly rate.

   a. 83 mL/hr

   1000 mL : 12 hr :: x : 1 hr

   $(1000 \times 1) = (12 \times x)$; 1000 = 12 x; x = 1000/12 = 83.33 (Round to nearest whole number.)

   Proof: 1000 × 1 = 1000; 12 × 83 = 996 (slight difference due to previous rounding)

   (Alternative method: 1000 mL ÷ 12 hr = 83.33 or 83 mL/hr)

   b. 21 gtt/min (Round to nearest whole number.)

   STEP 2:

   drop factor

   _____× hourly rate = 15/60 × 83 =

   time (min)

   1/4 × 83 = 20.75, rounded to nearest whole number

4. Start at STEP 1. You need to calculate the hourly rate.

   a. 100 mL/hr

   200 mL : 2 hr :: x : 1 hr

   $(200 \times 1) = (2 \times x)$; 200 = 2 x;

   x = 200/2 = 100

   Proof: 200 × 1 = 200; 2 × 100 = 200

   (Alternative method: 200 mL ÷ 2 hr = 100 mL/hr)

   b. 100 gtt/min

   STEP 2:

   drop factor

   _____× hourly rate = 60/60 × 100 = time

   (minutes)

   1 × 100 = 100

   c. The drop factor for microdrip tubing is 60 gtt/mL.

5. Start at STEP 2. The hourly rate has been provided (75 mL/hr).

   13 gtt/min (Round to nearest whole number.)

   STEP 2:

   drop factor

   _____× hourly rate = 10/60 × 75 =

   time (min)

   1/4 × 75 = 12.75, rounded to nearest whole number

6. Start at STEP 2. The hourly rate has been provided (75 mL/hr).

   19 gtt/min (Round to nearest whole number.)

   STEP 2:

   drop factor

   _____× hourly rate = 15/60 × 75 =

   time (minutes)

   1/4 × 75 = 18.75

7. Start at STEP 2. The hourly rate has been provided (75 mL/hr).
   19 gtt/min
   STEP 2:
   $$\frac{\text{drop factor}}{\text{time (minutes)}} \times \text{hourly rate} = 20/60 \times 75 =$$
   $1/3 \times 75 = 25$

8. As the drop factor increases, the drops per minute (gtt/min) also increase.

9. a. 100 mL/hr
   b. and c. Since the infusion pump delivers in millilitres per hour, it is unnecessary to calculate drops per minute.
   Start at STEP 1. You need to calculate the hourly rate. Remember, 30 min = 0.5 hr.
   50 mL : 0.5 hr :: x mL : 1 hr
   $(50 \times 1) = (0.5 \times x)$; $50 = 0.5 x$;
   $x = 50/0.5 = 100$
   Proof: $50 \times 1 = 50$; $0.5 \times 100 = 50$
   (Alternative method: 50 mL ÷ 0.5 hr = 100 mL/hr)

10. Start at STEP 1. You need to calculate the hourly rate.
    a. 125 mL/hr
    500 mL : 4 hr :: x : 1 hr
    $(500 \times 1) = (4 \times x)$; $500 = 4 x$;
    $x = 500/4 = 125$
    Proof: $500 \times 1 = 500$; $4 \times 125 = 500$
    (Alternative method: 500 mL ÷ 4 hr = 125 mL/hr)
    b. 125 gtt/min
    STEP 2:
    $$\frac{\text{drop factor}}{\text{time (minutes)}} \times \text{hourly rate} = 60/60 \times 125 =$$
    $1 \times 125 = 125$

Practice Quiz

1. 0.75 mg
   1000 mcg : 1 mg :: 750 mcg : x mg
   Proof: $1000 \times 0.75 = 750$; $1 \times 750 = 750$

2. 8000 mg
   1 g : 1000 mg :: 8 g : x mg
   Proof: $1 \times 8000 = 8000$; $1000 \times 8 = 8000$

3. 113.6 kg
   1 kg : 2.2 lb :: x kg : 250 lb
   Proof: $1 \times 250 = 250$; $2.2 \times 113.6 = 249.92$
   (rounds to 250)

4. 165 lb
   1 kg : 2.2 lb :: 75 kg : x lb
   Proof: $1 \times 165 = 165$; $2.2 \times 75 = 165$

5. 15 mL
   1 tsp : 5 mL :: 3 tsp : x mL
   Proof: $1 \times 15 = 15$; $5 \times 3 = 15$

6. 10 mL
   25 mg : 5 mL :: 50 mg : x mL
   Proof: $25 \times 10 = 250$; $5 \times 50 = 250$

7. 1 tablet
   STEP 1: Convert grams to milligrams: 0.5 g = 500 mg
   500 mg : 1 tablet :: 500 mg : x tablet
   Proof: $500 \times 1 = 500$; $1 \times 500 = 500$

8. 2 mL
   50 mg : 1 mL :: 100 mg : x mL
   Proof: $50 \times 2 = 100$; $1 \times 100 = 100$

9. 5 mL
   1% indicates 1 g in 100 mL, which equals 1000 mg/100 mL, or 10 mg/1 mL.
   10 mg : 1 mL :: 50 mg : x mL
   Proof: $10 \times 5 = 50$; $1 \times 50 = 50$

10. 0.25 mL
    1:1000 indicates 1 g in 1000 mL, which equals 1000 mg/1000 mL, or 1 mg/mL.
    1 mg : 1 mL :: 0.25 mg : x mL
    Proof: $1 \times 0.25 = 0.25$; $1 \times 0.25 = 0.25$

11. 1.5 mL
    10,000 units : 1 mL :: 15,000 units : x mL
    Proof: $10,000 \times 1.5 = 15,000$; $1 \times 15,000 = 15,000$

12. a. 0.2 mg per dose
    b. Yes, the dose of 1 mg does not exceed the safe and therapeutic dosage range for this child.
    22 lb = 10 kg
    Acceptable range: 0.2 mg/kg/dose × 10 kg = 2 mg/dose

13. a. 63 mL/hr
    500 mL ÷ 8 hr = 62.5, rounded to 63 mL/hr
    b. 16 gtt/min
    $$\frac{\text{drop factor}}{\text{time (minutes)}} \times \text{hourly rate} = 15/60 \times 63 =$$
    $1/4 \times 63 = 15.75$, rounded to nearest whole number

14. a. Infusion pumps deliver mL/hr.
    b. 50 mL/hr (as stated in the question)

15. a. 42 mL/hr
    1000 mL ÷ 24 hr = 41.67, rounded to 42 mL/hr
    b. 42 gtt/min (Remember, if the drop factor is 60, the rate is the same as the drops per minute [gtt/min]).
    $$\frac{\text{drop factor}}{\text{time (min)}} \times \text{hourly rate} = 60/60 \times 42 =$$
    1×42 gtt/min

16. a. 750 mg
    b. 5.6 mL
    90 mg : 1 mL :: 750 mg : x mL
    Proof: $90 \times 5.6 = 500$; $1 \times 500 = 500$

17. a. 200,000 units/mL
    b. 23 mL
    c. 1 mL (concentration is 200,000 units per 1 mL)
    d. Label the multidose vial with the date, time, amount of diluent used, and user's initials.

18. a. 6 mL
    100 mg : 1 mL :: 600 mg : x mL

Proof: $100 \times 6 = 600$; $1 \times 600 = 600$

b. Up to 1410 mg per 24 hours

31 lb = 14.1 kg; 14.1 kg $\times$ 100 mg/kg/d = 1410 mg per 24 hours (safe dose)

c. 705 mg/dose

There are two doses per day: 1410 mg ÷ 2 = 705 mg/dose

d. Yes

The ordered dose of 600 mg does not exceed the 705 mg maximum dose.

19. 2.5 mL

125 mcg = 0.125 mg

0.05 mg : 1 mL :: 0.125 mg : x mL

Proof: $0.05 \times 2.5 = 0.12502$ $1 \times 0.125 = 0.125$

20. 15 mL

1000 units : 1 mL :: 15,000 units : x mL

Proof: $1000 \times 15 = 15,000$; $15,000 \times 1 = 15,000$

21. 3 mL

50 mg : 2 mL :: 75 mg : x mL

Proof: (75 x 2) = (50 x x); 150 / 75 = 50 x; 3 = x

Notes